MICROBIOLOGY
Practical Applications and Infection Prevention

MICROBIOLOGY
Practical Applications and Infection Prevention

Bruce J. Colbert
MS, RRT

Luis S. Gonzalez III
Pharm.D., BCPS

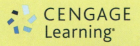

CENGAGE
Learning

Australia • Brazil • Mexico • Singapore • United Kingdom • United States

Microbiology
Practical Applications and Infection Prevention
Bruce J. Colbert, M.S., R.R.T
Luis S. Gonzalez III, Pharm.D.

SVP, GM Skills & Global Product Management:
Dawn Gerrain

Product Director: **Matthew Seeley**

Product Manager: **Laura Stewart**

Senior Director, Development: **Marah Bellegarde**

Product Development Manager: **Juliet Steiner**

Senior Content Developer: **Elisabeth F. Williams**

Product Assistant: **Deborah Handy**

Vice President, Marketing Services:
Jennifer Ann Baker

Marketing Manager: **Jonathan Sheehan**

Senior Production Director: **Wendy Troeger**

Production Director: **Andrew Crouth**

Senior Content Project Manager: **Kara A. DiCaterino**

Managing Art Director: **Jack Pendleton**

Cover and Interior Design Images:
©Eraxion/iStock.com,
©CLIPAREA/Shutterstock.com

For product information and technology assistance, contact us at
Professional & Career Group Customer Support, 1-800-648-7450

For permission to use material from this text or product, submit all requests
online at **www.cengage.com/permissions**
Further permissions questions can be e-mailed to
permissionrequest@cengage.com

Library of Congress Control Number: 2014949641

ISBN: 978-1-133-69364-2

Cengage Learning
20 Channel Center Street
Boston, MA 02210 USA

Cengage Learning is a leading provider of customized learning solutions with office locations around the globe, including Singapore, the United Kingdom, Australia, Mexico, Brazil, and Japan. Locate your local office at: www.cengage.com/global

Cengage Learning products are represented in Canada by Nelson Education, Ltd.

To learn more about Cengage Learning, visit www.cengage.com

Purchase any of our products at your local college store or at our preferred online store
www.cengagebrain.com

Notice to the Reader

Publisher does not warrant or guarantee any of the products described herein or perform any independent analysis in connection with any of the product information contained herein. Publisher does not assume, and expressly disclaims, any obligation to obtain and include information other than that provided to it by the manufacturer. The reader is expressly warned to consider and adopt all safety precautions that might be indicated by the activities described herein and to avoid all potential hazards. By following the instructions contained herein, the reader willingly assumes all risks in connection with such instructions. The publisher makes no representations or warranties of any kind, including but not limited to, the warranties of fitness for particular purpose or merchantability, nor are any such representations implied with respect to the material set forth herein, and the publisher takes no responsibility with respect to such material. The publisher shall not be liable for any special, consequential, or exemplary damages resulting, in whole or part, from the readers' use of, or reliance upon, this material.

Printed in the United States of America
Print Number: 01   Print Year: 2015

DEDICATION

To the memory of my parents, Robert and Josephine Colbert, who instilled the importance of education within me. In addition, to Patty, my loving wife of 33 years, and to my two wonderful sons, Joshua and Jeremy. Finally, to Ali who is a great daughter-in-law.

—*Bruce*

To the memory of my father, who taught me the value of hard work and learning from my failures. A special thanks to my wife, three sons, daughter-in-law, and grandson for your love and support. Finally, to my mother, who unselfishly cared for my father during his battle with cancer and made the end of his life worth living.

—*Luis*

CONTENTS

Preface — xiii

About the Authors — xix

Acknowledgments — xxi

Reviewers — xxiii

How to Use This Book — xxv

SECTION I

The Background and Science of Microbiology — 3

Chapter One: The Background of Microbiology — 5

Introduction 6

Classification of Microorganisms 8

Cellular Anatomy and Physiology 9

    Prokaryotes and Eukaryotes 9

Normal Flora versus Pathogens 15

Immunity and Infection 17

    Immune System 17

    Infection 24

Chapter Two: Medical Microbiology — 31

Introduction 32

History of Microbiology 32

    Evolution of the "Science" of Microbiology 35

Medical Microbiology..39
    Other Fields and Applications of Microbiology 40

Bacteriology 41
    Naming Bacteria 43
    Bacterial Structure and Morphology 43

Specimen Collection 46
    Bacterial Staining 47
    Growing and Testing Bacteria...50
    Bacterial Disease 55

General Principles of Antibiotic Therapy..56
    Antibiotic Classification 56

Chapter Three: More Medical Microbiology Specialties   63

Introduction 64

Virology..64
    Viral Identification..67
    Antiviral Agents 69

Parasitology 72
    Protozoa...73
    Helminths..75
    Ectoparasites 78

Mycology 79
    Yeasts 81
    Molds 84

Prions...86

SECTION II

Microbiology in Practice   91

Chapter Four: Infection Prevention   93

Introduction 94

Basic Definitions...95

Issues to Consider When Killing an Organism..98

Methods Used to Disinfect and Sterilize 98
    Heat 98
    Pasteurization 99
    Boiling Water 99
    Steam and Pressure 99
    Various Liquids and Compounds 100
    Gas Sterilization 103
    Radiation 104

Chapter Five: Protecting Patients and Ourselves   **111**

Introduction 112
Portals of Entry 112
Routes of Transmission 115
    Contact 115
    Common Vehicle 115
    Airborne 116
    Vector 116
Hand Hygiene 118
Fundamental Principles of Infection Prevention and Control 121
    Standard Precautions 122
    Cough Etiquette and Respiratory Hygiene 124
    Safe Injection Practices 127
    Safe Handling of Potentially Contaminated Surfaces or Equipment 127
    Transmission-Based Precautions 128
Occupational Safety and Health Administration (OSHA) Regulations 132

Chapter Six: Microbiology-Related Procedures   **139**

Introduction 140
Infectious Waste Disposal 140
Applying and Removing Nonsterile Disposable Gloves 141
Applying and Removing Sterile Gloves 142
Asepsis 147
    Hand Hygiene for Surgical Asepsis 148
Sterile Principles 149

Specimen Collection 150

    General Principles 151

    Blood Cultures 152

    Cerebrospinal Fluid (CSF) Cultures 153

    Sputum Cultures 153

    Wound Cultures 154

    Urine Specimens 155

    Stool Specimens 155

    Throat Culture 157

    Nasal Specimens 157

SECTION III

The Infectious Diseases: A Systems Approach   163

Chapter Seven: Immunizations and Antimicrobials   165

Introduction 166

General Disease Terminology 167

    Signs and Symptoms of Disease 167

Immunizations 168

Monitoring Antimicrobial Therapy 170

Microbial Resistance Mechanisms 171

Antibacterial Drug Classification 174

    Bacteriostatic versus Bactericidal 174

    Spectrum of Activity: Broad versus Narrow 175

    Based on Mechanism of Action 175

Antibacterial Agents 176

    Beta-Lactams 176

    Penicillins 176

    Cephalosporins 177

    Monobactams 179

    Carbapenems 179

    Quinolones 180

    Aminoglycosides 181

    Glycopeptides 182

    Macrolides 182

Tetracyclines 183

Folate Inhibitors 184

Oxazolidinones 184

Quinupristin-Dalfopristin 185

Daptomycin 185

Clindamycin 186

Metronidazole 186

Antituberculosis Agents 186

Antivirals 188

Antivirals to Treat Herpes Virus Infections 190

Antivirals to Treat Influenza Virus 190

Antivirals to Treat Respiratory Syncytial Virus 191

Antivirals to Treat Hepatitis C Virus 192

Antivirals to Treat Human Immunodeficiency Virus
(HIV) Infection 194

Antifungal Agents 194

Chapter Eight: Microbiological Diseases: Nonrespiratory Infectious Diseases   201

Introduction 202

Infectious Diseases of the Head and Neck 202

Meningitis 203

Encephalitis 204

Otitis Media 205

Parotitis 208

Infections of the Eye 209

Conjunctivitis 209

Keratitis 210

Cardiovascular Infections 210

Endocarditis 210

Catheter-Related Bloodstream Infections (CRBSIs) 211

Infectious Diseases of the Skin and Soft Tissues 213

Cellulitis and Erysipelas 213

Necrotizing Skin and Soft Tissue Infections 215

Intra-Abdominal Infections 216

Appendicitis 216

Acute Cholecystitis 217

Diverticulitis 218

Clostridium difficile Colitis 219

Infectious Diarrhea 221

Genitourinary Tract Infections 223

Sexually Transmitted Diseases 223

Urinary Tract Infections 227

Bone and Joint Infections 228

Osteomyelitis 228

Septic Arthritis 228

Chapter Nine: Respiratory-Related Microbiological Diseases **233**

Introduction 234

Upper Respiratory Airway Infections 235

Sinusitis 235

Pharyngitis 235

Epiglottitis 237

Croup 237

Infectious Diseases of the Lower Respiratory System 238

Acute Bronchitis and Bronchiolitis 239

Pneumonia 241

Tuberculosis 252

Bioterrorism 253

Avian Influenza 253

Appendix A: Answers to Chapter Stop and Review Questions **259**

Appendix B: Clinical Laboratory–Related Abbreviations and Acronyms **267**

Appendix C: Select Viral, Bacterial, Fungal, and Protozoa Conditions and Their Causative Agents **275**

Appendix D: Patient Education on Preventing Health Care–Associated Infections (HAIs) **279**

Glossary **281**

Index **295**

PREFACE

The goal of *Microbiology: Practical Applications and Infection Prevention* is to provide health profession students with a basic understanding of medical microbiology, with an emphasis on the practical application to health care. In essence, this book is envisioned to be a relevant and practical guide that serves as the core knowledge for readers who need to understand medical microbiology and how it relates to medical practice. The text offers foundational knowledge, then builds to practical application, so readers can learn simple to more complex topics in a progression. This learning path is reinforced in the ancillary materials that round out this robust learning system.

As the authors of this book, we hold that our mission is to provide students and educators with material that will be useful not only for their academic experience, but will also serve as a valuable future on-the-job reference. Great care has been taken to include the most up-to-date and relevant information for students as they transition into practitioners. For example, the term *infection control* has been ingrained in the medical literature for years and still is commonly found in printed material. However, the most recent and current thinking concerning infections is to prevent them from occurring in the first place. For years the CDC was known as the Centers for Disease Control until finally changing its name to the Centers for Disease Control and Prevention, emphasizing *prevention* of infection rather than controlling an infection once it occurs. In health care the focus should be on preventing infections. We hope that students and instructors alike will appreciate how this practical book and ancillary materials prepare the student for actual clinical practice.

Organization

The presentation and organization of *Microbiology: Practical Applications and Infection Prevention* offer educators optimal flexibility in their curriculum design. The book is organized and written in three sections based on the principle of building from knowledge to practice. Section One covers the background and science of microbiology to lay the conceptual foundation for the clinical application that follows. Topics covered include microorganisms, immunity and infection, medical microbiology, virology, parasitology, mycology, and prions. This section is written in a conversational tone to introduce students to some of these new areas and also to develop a comfort level with the material.

Next, readers will put this knowledge into action. Section Two focuses on the techniques and procedures related to medical microbiology. Core content areas include infection prevention, transmission routes and precautions, infectious waste disposal, sterile principles, and safe specimen and culture procedures. This section maintains a mix of conversational tone with more technical writing because of the focus on testing and procedures.

All of the content is pulled together in the final section, which focuses on the specific infectious diseases students are likely to encounter in practice. In Section Three, infectious diseases are related to each affected body system through a review of microbiological disease etiology, diagnosis, treatment, and prevention practices. Topics include signs and symptoms of disease, immunizations, antibacterial and antiviral agents, and respiratory and nonrespiratory diseases. Now readers are immersed in true medical writing similar to what they would see in a medical journal, where they should now feel comfortable given the building process of the textbook.

Material is also organized following a building block approach, with reinforcement activities in the text and online supplements to solidify understanding of concepts. For example, after reading various sections in the book, students will be directed to the companion website to view videos on infection control and prevention and also to watch procedures such as specimen collection, donning personal protective equipment, and so forth. At each step, readers will find multimedia assets to support the concepts they are learning in the core text.

Features

Special features in the text will facilitate understanding of microbiology by challenging readers to think critically and ask themselves what was learned.

- **Objectives** outline the targeted learning goals for each chapter to guide reading and study.

- **Key terms** are bolded in color and defined within each chapter. An extensive end-of-book glossary lists and defines all key terms used throughout the text.

- **Phonetic pronunciations** facilitate learning new terminology with the correct pronunciation.

- **Learning Hint** boxes include tips about the material, such as word origins, spelling hints, applying concepts in real life, and so on.

- **Clinical Application** boxes support students in putting new skills and knowledge to work in the clinical setting.

- **Stop and Review** boxes appear periodically throughout the chapters and offer students the chance to pause in reading to confirm that material was understood. Answers to Stop and Review exercises are included in Appendix A.

- **Food for Thought** boxes challenge readers to approach a situation with an open mind and consider a new perspective or solution.

- **Chapter Summaries** bring together the main points of each chapter and serve as a quick reference for study.

- **Chapter Review Questions** include matching, multiple choice, short answer, and other formats, to test understanding of the material.

- **Case Studies** close out each chapter and are designed to stimulate critical thinking through the presentation of reality-based situations relating to microbiology.

- **Additional Activities** offer ideas to engage readers in critical thinking.

- **Media Connection** boxes direct students to additional learning opportunities such as videos, interactive exercises, and practice questions, available on the **Online Resources** at http://www.CengageBrain.com.

- **MindTap** is a fully online, interactive learning platform which combines readings, multimedia, activities, and assessments into a singular learning path, elevating learning by providing real-world application to better engage students. MindTap includes an interactive eBook with highlighting and note-taking capability, self-quizzes, and learning exercises such as matching activities, multiple choice questions, flash cards, and more. MindTap can be accessed at http://www.CengageBrain.com.

Learning Package for the Student

MindTap

MindTap is the first of its kind in an entirely new category: the Personal Learning Experience (PLE). This personalized program of digital products and services uses interactivity and customization to engage students, while offering a range of choice in content, platforms, devices, and learning tools. MindTap is device agnostic, meaning that it will work with any platform or learning management system and will be accessible anytime, anywhere: on desktops, laptops, tablets, mobile phones, and other Internet-enabled devices. *Microbiology: Practical Applications and Infection Prevention on MindTap* includes:

- An interactive eBook with highlighting, note-taking, and more

- Drag-and-drop microbiology exercises

- Flashcards for mastering chapter terms

- Computer-graded activities and exercises

Online Resources

Additional resources can be found online at http://www.CengageBrain.com. Search by author name, ISBN, or title to gain access to videos, animations, and other valuable learning tools.

Teaching Package for the Instructor

Instructor Resources

The *Instructor Companion Website to Accompany Microbiology: Practical Applications and Infection Prevention* contains a variety of tools to help instructors successfully prepare lectures and teach within this subject area. This comprehensive package provides something for all instructors, from those teaching medical microbiology for the first time to seasoned instructors who want something new. The following components on the website are free to adopters of the text:

- A downloadable and customizable Instructor's Manual containing lecture notes, teaching strategies, class activities, and more.

- A Computerized Test Bank with several hundred questions and answers, for use in instructor-created quizzes and tests.

- Chapter slides created in PowerPoint® to use for in-class lecture material and as handouts for students.

MindTap

In the new *Microbiology: Practical Applications and Infection Prevention on MindTap* platform, instructors customize the learning path by selecting Cengage Learning resources and adding their own content via apps that integrate into the MindTap framework seamlessly with many learning management systems. The guided learning path demonstrates the relevance of basic principles in microbiology through engagement activities, interactive exercises, and animations, elevating the study by challenging students to apply concepts to practice. To learn more, visit www.cengage.com/mindtap.

To the Student Studying Microbiology

Welcome to the wonderful world of medical microbiology! You are about to embark on an exciting and challenging journey. With *Microbiology: Practical Applications and Infection Prevention*, authors Colbert and Gonzalez have collaborated to interweave their unique skill sets, creating an accurate, timely, and academically rewarding experience for you, the learner. The material in this book and its accompanying learning package has been carefully developed by author Colbert, an active educator and expert in the field, who is passionate about delivering educational material in an engaging and student-friendly manner. The relevance of the material is enhanced through author Gonzalez, who has a very active clinical practice dealing with infection prevention, health care–associated infections, and antimicrobial resistance on a daily basis. The sum of this collective work provides you with the classroom fundamentals of microbiology and then quickly shows you how this material is relevant to current clinical practice. So come with an open mind, be prepared to learn, and enjoy the journey!

ABOUT THE AUTHORS

Bruce Colbert is Clinical Associate Professor and Director of the Allied Health Department of the University of Pittsburgh at Johnstown. He has authored nine books, developed an interactive work text and DVD program on student success, and given over 300 invited lectures and workshops at both the regional and national level. Many of his workshops are with educational programs on improving teaching effectiveness by utilizing active teaching and learning techniques to make the medical sciences relevant to today's students. Bruce is most proud of his volunteer work with wounded veterans in helping them to successfully transition into the workplace.

Dr. Luis S. Gonzalez III is an Associate Program Director in the Department of Internal Medicine Residency Program at Conemaugh Memorial Medical Center, where he also serves as the Clinical Coordinator for Pharmacy Services and directs a Pharmacy Residency Program. He is the Chair of Conemaugh Health System's Institutional Review Board and is an active member of the Epidemiology and Infection Prevention Committee. His main area of clinical practice is Critical Care, where he has been a long-standing member of the Critical Care Team. He is a Clinical Associate Professor for the Schools of Pharmacy at the University of Pittsburgh, Duquesne University, and Ohio Northern University. He teaches nursing pharmacology as an Adjunct Professor in the department of nursing at the University of Pittsburgh at Johnstown. He has authored numerous peer-reviewed publications and has presented at regional and national conferences. Dr. Gonzalez is one of the original founders of the Johnstown Free Medical Clinic.

ACKNOWLEDGMENTS

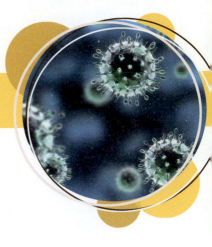

First and foremost, our gratitude goes to all the wonderful people at Cengage who helped to put this project together. While we cannot name them all personally, a few deserve special mention. Matt Seeley deserves a major thank you for his enthusiasm and support and for believing in this project and the authors. Our gratitude also goes to Deb Myette-Flis who does a phenomenal job of keeping track of everything and keeping everything together, including the two authors. Finally, we thank Beth Williams, who was brought in late on the project but added much to the production of not only the textbook but the newly developed interactive electronic assets that surround the textbook.

REVIEWERS

Anthony Avenido, MD
Allied Health Department Chair
Brown Mackie College
Cincinnati, Ohio

Cheryl H. Bordwine, BHA, MBA, RMA
Director/Associate Professor
Medical Assistant Program
College of the Mainland
League City, Texas

Marianne Bovee, CCMA, CHI, CET
Department Head
Medical Assistant/Phlebotomy Technician
Duluth Business University
Duluth, Minnesota

Liza Dee Cano, RMA, NRCMA
Allied Health Instructor
Texas City, Texas

Jill D. Henning, PhD
Assistant Professor of Biology
University of Pittsburgh at Johnstown
Johnstown, Pennsylvania

Brandon W. Montoya, MS
Program Coordinator Biological Sciences
iPad Champion
Allied Health Department
Brown Mackie College–Cincinnati
Cincinnati, Ohio

Eva Oltman, MEd, CMA, CPC
Professor and Division Chair
Allied Health
Jefferson Community and Technical College
Louisville, Kentucky

Jean Ann Rearick, RN, BSN, MPH, CIC, CPHQ
Executive Director of Performance Excellence and Quality
Conemaugh Memorial Medical Center
Johnstown, Pennsylvania

Darhon Rees-Rohrbacher, DMus, RN, MSN
Instructor
Bryant & Stratton College
Albany, New York

Karan Serowik, BS, RMA
Program Director of Healthcare
Heald College
Portland, Oregon

Gazelle Lynn Sexton, MSHSA, BS, CST
Surgical Technology Instructor
American Career College, Ontario Campus
Riverside, California

Jackie Uselton, RHD, CPhT, MEd
Health Science Instructor
Westlake High School
Austin, Texas

Alan M. Warren, DPM, Board Certified
American Board Podiatric Orthopedics and Primary Podiatric Medicine
    and
Faculty Department of Natural Sciences
Eastwick College
Ramsey, New Jersey
    and
Private Practice
Podiatric Medicine and Surgery
Parsippany, New Jersey

HOW TO USE THIS BOOK

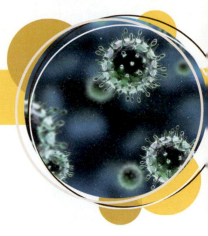

Microbiology: Practical Applications and Infection Prevention helps you learn microbiology in a concise format. The following features are integrated throughout the book to assist you in learning and mastering the core concepts and terms.

- **Objectives** Read this list of targeted objectives before you begin reading each chapter, so you have a grasp of the scope and depth of the content to be presented. Note any questions you may have about unfamiliar topics, then refer back to these questions as you study to test how well you have met these objectives.

- **Key Terms** Pretest your knowledge of the subject matter by reviewing the list of key terms at the beginning of each chapter, make a list of terms you need to learn, and watch for them as you read the material. Once you complete the chapter, revisit the list to gauge how your mastery of the terms has changed; then use the list of terms as you prepare to take your exams.

- **Phonetic pronunciations** Sound out new words as you read the Key Terms list. Having a correct pronunciation in your head will help you learn and retain new terminology. If you are unsure how to say a new word after reading the suggested pronunciation, check with your instructor.

Learning Hint
Why Do We Call It Flora?

The word *flora* actually means "flowers" from the ancient Greek language. However, in the eighteenth century it became used to describe all general plants found in a certain area. So although microorganisms such as bacteria are not small plants, the term *flora* has stuck and still is widely used today to describe normal microbial inhabitants of the human body. So when you hear that probiotics are used to replace the normal flora in the intestinal tract, you can think of this as the "general population of good microorganisms in that region."

- **Learning Hint** Skim through these boxes before you start your chapter reading to stimulate your thinking and to get a taste of what you will be learning.

Clinical Application
Infectious Proteins

Prions are infectious particles that do not fit into any of these cellular categories. They do not contain a nucleus and are basically infectious proteins that can cause severe diseases of the central nervous system in humans and mammals, which will be covered in the infectious disease section. They are the only known infectious pathogen that is lacking in nucleic acid.

- **Clinical Application** Learn how to use the knowledge you have gained in a real-world situation. Read through these boxes to get a framework for how microbiology is linked to our everyday life.

1-1
Stop and Review

1. Microorganisms that normally exist in our body are referred to as normal _____.
2. _____ is the term used for an organism that can produce an infection.
3. Cellular energy is stored in the _____.
4. Eukaryotic cells are different from prokaryotic cells because they contain a(n) _____.

- **Stop and Review** Sprinkled throughout the text at key spots, these boxes encourage you to stop and ask yourself how well you have processed the material presented. Are you able to answer the questions or respond to the challenges? If you feel uneasy or unsure, reread the content until you can confidently respond. Suggested answers can be found in Appendix A.

Food for Thought
Friendly Bacteria

Probiotics are live microorganisms that are similar to beneficial microorganisms found in the human intestine. They are also called "friendly, or good, bacteria." If you take an antibiotic, you may kill "good" as well as "bad," or pathogenic, bacteria. Probiotics are available to consumers in the form of foods (yogurt) and dietary supplements. They can be used to replace or restore the "good bacteria" that were present in our intestines before antibiotic use. The jury is still out on the use of probiotics. In people with suppressed immune systems, these products may even be dangerous because the organisms they contain may cause illness.

- **Food for Thought** Have you considered different aspects of a situation or different perspectives? Have you thought about how you might resolve a certain dilemma? These boxes will challenge you to do just that.

- **Chapter Summary** Use this listing of the main content points covered in the chapter as you study and prepare to take exams. Identify areas where your knowledge is not as strong as you would like it to be and reread those sections of the chapter.

Chapter Summary

- This chapter laid the foundation for you to understand how microorganisms are classified. We discussed the differences between prokaryotic and eukaryotic cells. The inner workings of a eukaryotic cell were described along with the structure and function of each component. Remember that eukaryotic cells are the more complex of the two and contain a true nucleus.

- The distinction was made between bacteria that can be considered as normal flora in our bodies and bacteria that do not normally reside in our bodies unless they are causing us to be ill (pathogens). Normal flora help keep our body free of pathogenic microbes because they, in a sense, do not allow any room at the inn. Our bodies are the inn, and our normal flora are the inhabitants of the inn.

- **Chapter Review** When you complete the chapter, answer these questions to determine how well you have mastered the content. Answers are included in the Instructor's Manual.

Chapter Review

Match the cellular component with its function

1. _____ nucleus
2. _____ lysosome
3. _____ Golgi apparatus
4. _____ cell membrane

a. contains structures of the cell
b. forms a barrier and contains components of cell
c. brain of cell
d. powerhouse of cell

- **Case Study** These real-world scenarios give you a chance to apply your knowledge to a patient situation. Challenge yourself to identify additional areas of patient care or interaction that you might encounter in each case.

Case Study

A 69-year-old male patient presents to the department of emergency medicine at a local hospital with a fever, cough, and low blood pressure. He had a dual kidney and liver transplant 3 months ago and was taking a medicine called tacrolimus, which suppresses cellular immunity (prevents T-cell activation) to prevent organ rejection. He was found to have cytomegalovirus (CMV) pneumonia. The donor of these organs tested positive for this virus but according to his family was not ill prior to his untimely death in an automobile accident. Why did the transplant recipient get sick from the virus but the organ donor was not ill? What broad category of immunity was suppressed in this transplant patient?

- **Additional Activities** Once you complete the reading, look over these activities, which invite you to think critically and engage in activities beyond the classroom. Meet with fellow students to brainstorm how you might approach these activities and try something new.

Additional Activities

1. Currently there is a "perfect storm" brewing in public health. Microbes are becoming more resistant to anti-infective agents (e.g., antivirals, antifungals, and antibiotics), and at the same time very few new anti-infective agents are being approved by the U.S. Food and Drug Administration to treat these resistant "bugs." At times, existing drugs end up in short supply because of drug manufacturers shifting production to more profitable medications. Although we will be discussing this in future chapters, research some of the reasons why drug resistance occurs and the dangers it poses.

2. Research the mandatory reporting of infections within your state. How do they relate to your surrounding states? Why are there differences?

3. Invite a medical technologist who works in a hospital microbiology lab to discuss bacterial resistance in your area.

- **Media Connection** This is your lifeline to online resources that support your learning. Be sure to visit our MindTap learning platform at www.CengageBrain.com as you work through each chapter, to engage in multimedia presentations, view videos, and take quizzes.

Media Connection

Go to the accompanying online resources and have fun learning as you play games, view animations and videos, and take practice tests to help reinforce key concepts you learned in this chapter.

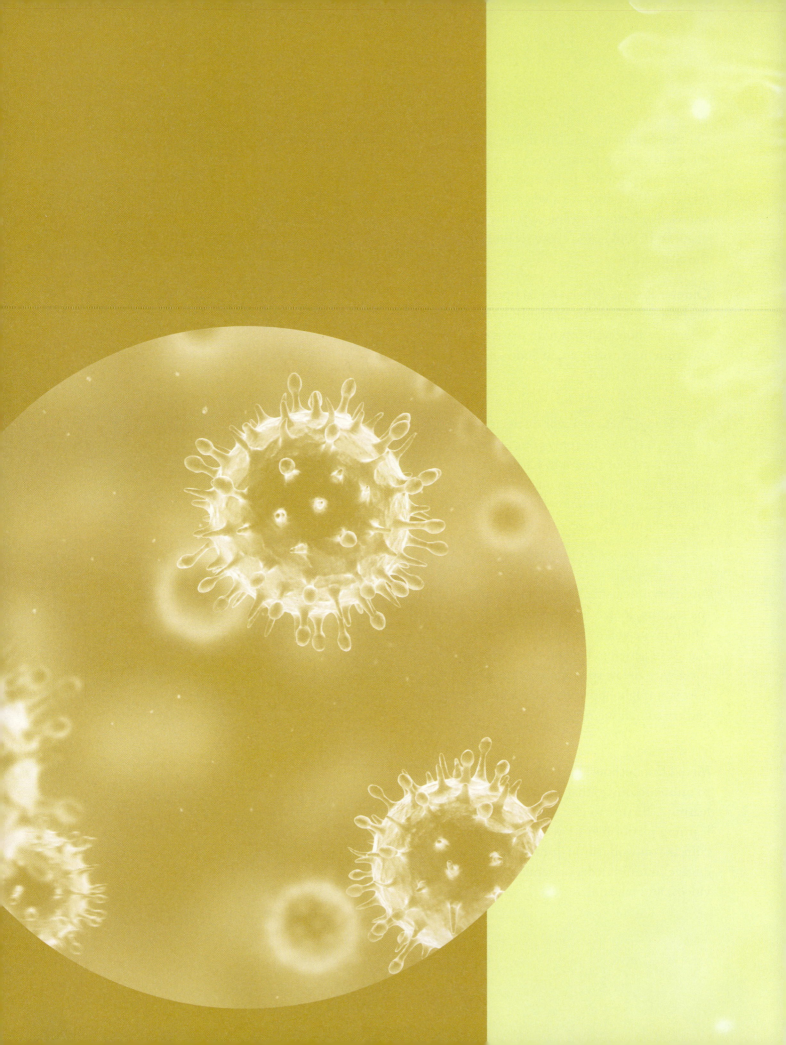

The Background and Science of Microbiology

In between studying for exams, you have probably seen movies with killer viruses that threaten to wipe out humankind. Even though you may chuckle and think this does not happen in real life, think again. Outbreaks of disease occur all the time and can be deadly to large numbers of people. You have probably read or maybe even experienced firsthand becoming ill from eating contaminated food caused by "bugs" with difficult to pronounce names like *Escherichia coli* or *Salmonella*. This section (Chapters 1–3) presents the background and foundation for you to understand the various clinical applications and procedures related to medical microbiology and its relevancy to you as a health care practitioner.

In Section Two (Chapters 4–6), we focus on the clinical procedures related to medical microbiology and infection prevention, and we conclude in Section Three (Chapters 7–9) with microbiological diseases organized by each body system.

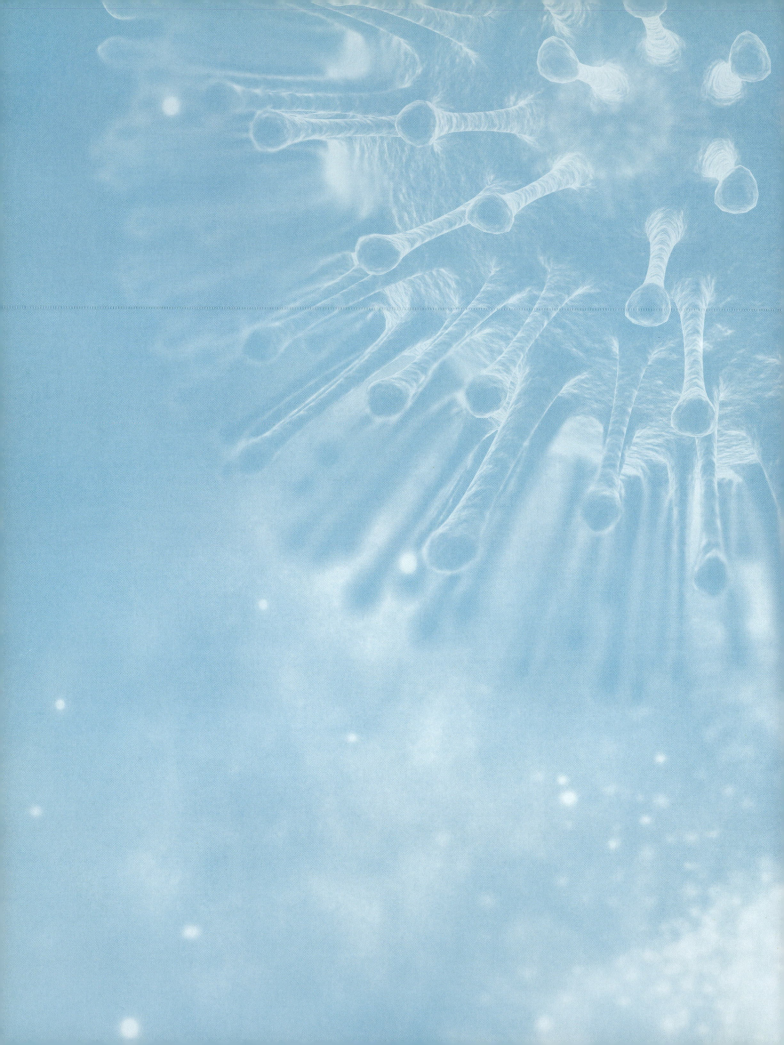

The Background of Microbiology

OBJECTIVES

After studying this chapter, the learner will be able to:

- List the classification of microorganisms.

- Describe the function of each structure of a eukaryotic cell.

- Differentiate between normal flora and pathogens.

- Describe the immune system, listing the various components and how they work to eliminate microbes.

- Contrast modes of disease transmission.

- Discuss how infections develop in humans.

KEY TERMS

adaptive immune response

airborne transmission

antibodies

antigen-presenting cells (APCs)

B cells

biological vector

capsule

cell membrane

chromosomes

cilia [SILL ee ah]

common vehicle transmission

contact transmission

cytoplasm [SIGH toh plazm]

endoplasmic reticulum (ER)

endotoxins

eukaryotes [you CARE ee oats]

exotoxins

flagella [fla JEL ah]

fomite [FO might]

Golgi apparatus [GOAL jee app ah RA tuss]

humoral immune response [hu MORE al]

infection

innate immune response

inoculum

lysosomes [LIE soh soamz]

macrophage [MACK roh fayj]

mechanical vector

microbiology

mitochondria [MITE oh KAHN dree ah]

mitosis

monocytes

mononuclear phagocyte system (MPS)

(Continues)

KEY TERMS *(Continued)*

mucous membranes

neutrophils [NEW troh fills]

normal flora

nucleolus [new clee OL us]

nucleus [NEW clee us]

pathogen [PATH oh jen]

pathogenic
　[PATH oh JEN ick]

phagocyte [FAG oh sight]

pinocytic vesicles
　[PIN oh sit ik]

prokaryotes
　[pro CARE ee oats]

protists [PRO tists]

spores

T cells

vector borne

vectors

virulence [VEAR you lence]

Introduction

microbiology: the scientific study of microorganisms, that is, of bacteria, fungi, intracellular parasites, protozoans, viruses, and some worms

normal flora: mixture of bacteria normally found at specific body sites

pathogenic [PATH oh JEN ick]: productive of disease

virulence [VEAR you lence]: the relative power and degree of pathogenicity possessed by organisms

Microbiology is the study of microscopic or small organisms that can be seen only with the aid of a microscope. There are a variety of microscopes that can give various levels of resolution and are used in different clinical settings. Figure 1-1 shows three different types of microscopes and representative samples of the images they produce.

Microorganisms can exist in the body, and it is important to keep in mind that the majority of microorganisms are beneficial to the body and are known as **normal flora**. However, a small percentage can cause disease or be classified as **pathogenic**. **Virulence** is the term used to describe the increased ability for an organism to produce an infection.

Learning Hint
Why Do We Call It Flora?

The word *flora* actually means "flowers" from the ancient Greek language. However, in the eighteenth century it became used to describe all general plants found in a certain area. So although microorganisms such as bacteria are not small plants, the term *flora* has stuck and still is widely used today to describe normal microbial inhabitants of the human body. So when you hear that probiotics are used to replace the normal flora in the intestinal tract, you can think of this as the "general population of good microorganisms in that region."

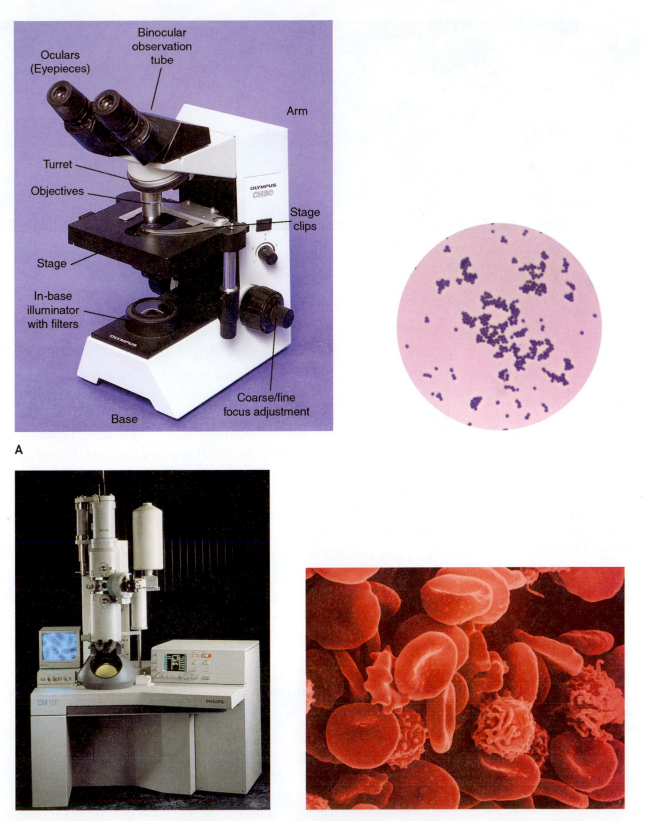

FIGURE 1-1 A. Basic compound microscope with an image of cocci bacteria. © Cengage Learning®. **B.** A scanning electron microscope with an image of red blood cells. Courtesy of Philips Electronic Instruments Company   (*Continues*)

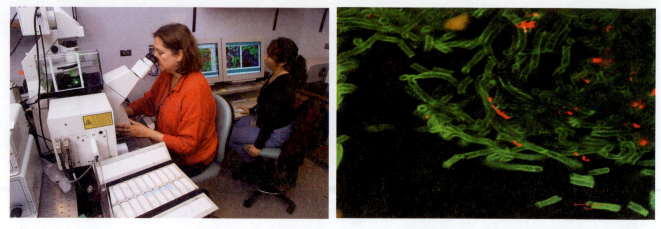

C

FIGURE 1-1 *(Continued)* **C.** Confocal laser microscope with three-dimensional colorized image of *Bacillus anthracis*. Source: CDC/James Gathany (Left), CDC/Dr. Sherif Zaki, Dr. Kathi Tatti, Elizabeth White (Right)

Classification of Microorganisms

Microorganisms are classified according to their cell type, and some of the classification systems do vary. Historically, living organisms were broadly divided into two "kingdoms" called plants and animals. With the invention of the microscope, a whole new kingdom was discovered that was neither plant nor animal. This new kingdom was classified as *protista*, and the one-celled organisms of this kingdom were known as *protists*. Two groups of **protists** are important in health care. The first group of protists are called **prokaryotes** and consist of bacteria, blue-green algae, rickettsiae, and mycoplasmas. The second group of protists is classified as **eukaryotes** and includes animals, plants, algae (other than blue-green), protozoa, fungi, and slime molds. Another separate category of microorganisms was also discovered called *viruses*, and this category has huge implications in the field of medicine. See Table 1-1 for a simplified classification of microorganisms.

protists [PRO tists]: any member of the kingdom *Protista*; organisms that include the protozoa, unicellular and multicellular algae, and the slime molds

prokaryote [pro CARE ee oat]: in taxonomy, the kingdom of organisms with prokaryotic cell structure; that is, they lack membrane-bound cell organelles and a nuclear membrane around the chromosome

eukaryote [you CARE ee oat]: organisms in which the cell nucleus is surrounded by a membrane

 Clinical Application

Infectious Proteins

Prions are infectious particles that do not fit into any of these cellular categories. They do not contain a nucleus and are basically infectious proteins that can cause severe diseases of the central nervous system in humans and mammals, which will be covered in the infectious disease section. They are the only known infectious pathogen that is lacking in nucleic acid.

TABLE 1-1 Simplified Classification of Microorganisms

Classification	Microorganism	Definitions
Plant	Algae	Simple plants that are important in the maintenance of freshwater and marine ecosystems. Most species are not harmful to humans. Blue-green and red algae may produce toxins that, if consumed by animals or humans, can cause disease.
	Bacteria	Microscopic, one-celled organisms that have both beneficial and harmful kinds.
	Fungi	Large group of simple plants that have some disease-producing forms; some examples include mushrooms, molds, and yeast.
Animal	Protozoa	One-celled animals much larger than bacteria; found in bodies of water; an amoeba is an example.
Unclassified	Viruses	Organisms that are so small they can be viewed only through a special electron microscope. They contain either DNA or RNA that is surrounded by a protective protein coat. Because they are incapable of reproducing on their own, they take up residence within a healthy host cell, take over the cellular machinery, and reproduce using the host cell's reproductive machinery. Some examples include measles, HIV, and the common cold.
	Rickettsiae	Similar to bacteria but smaller; cannot exist outside living host and are therefore parasitic; can cause scrub typhus and Rocky Mountain spotted fever.

© 2016 Cengage Learning®.

Cellular Anatomy and Physiology

When you look at a human, animal, or plant, it is hard to visualize that all of these living things are made up of millions of cells. The following sections take a more in-depth look at the structure and function of a cell.

Prokaryotes and Eukaryotes

Prokaryotes and eukaryotes are the two major categories of cells. Eukaryotes (means "true nucleus") are the more complex of the two and consist of cells from humans, animals, plants, protozoa, fungi, and most algae. Prokaryotes (means "before nucleus") are less complex and consist, for our purposes, primarily of bacteria. Figure 1-2 contrasts a eukaryotic human cell with the

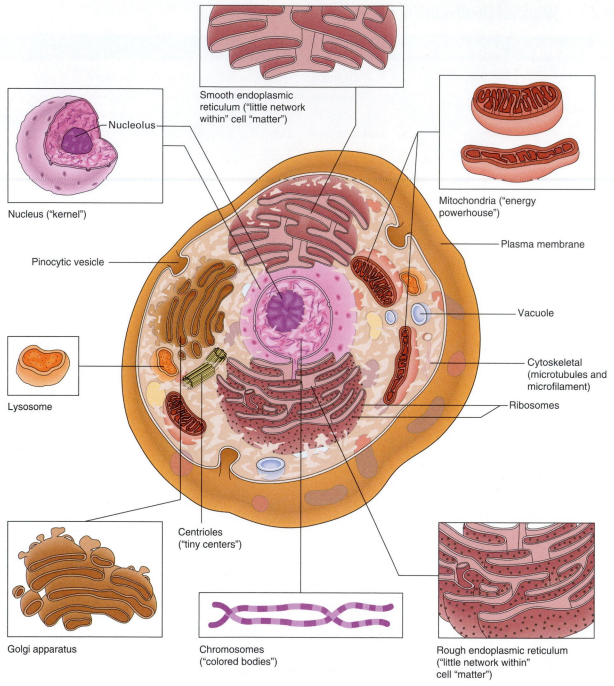

Smooth endoplasmic reticulum ("little network within" cell "matter")

Nucleolus

Nucleus ("kernel")

Pinocytic vesicle

Lysosome

Golgi apparatus

Centrioles ("tiny centers")

Chromosomes ("colored bodies")

Mitochondria ("energy powerhouse")

Plasma membrane

Vacuole

Cytoskeletal (microtubules and microfilament)

Ribosomes

Rough endoplasmic reticulum ("little network within" cell "matter")

A

FIGURE 1-2 A. Eukaryotic human cell with organelles (tiny cellular organs). © 2016 Cengage Learning®. (*Continues*)

prokaryotic bacterial cell. Notice how the human cell is more complex, with a nucleus (control center), multiple chromosomes, and many organelles with specific cellular functions. The bacterial cell contains no nucleus or organelles. Now we explore the structure and function of each cell type in a little more depth.

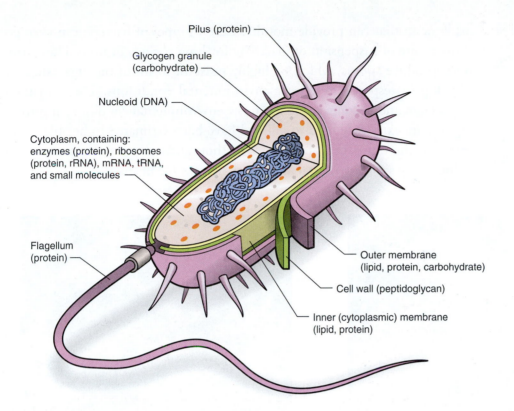

Pilus (protein)

Glycogen granule
(carbohydrate)

Nucleoid (DNA)

Cytoplasm, containing:
enzymes (protein), ribosomes
(protein, rRNA), mRNA, tRNA,
and small molecules

Flagellum
(protein)

Outer membrane
(lipid, protein, carbohydrate)

Cell wall (peptidoglycan)

Inner (cytoplasmic) membrane
(lipid, protein)

B

FIGURE 1-2 *(Continued)* **B.** Prokaryotic bacterial cell. © 2016 Cengage Learning®.

Learning Hint
Make the Material Come Alive

As you try to learn material, make use of analogies, comparisons, and even stories to make learning the material more familiar and more understandable. We will be using these throughout the textbook, but feel free to come up with your own. In addition, having a medical dictionary close by would be helpful.

Prokaryotes

As can be seen in Figure 1-2B, a bacterial cell (prokaryotic cell) contains a cell membrane, a cell wall, and no nucleus. However, it does contain a nucleus-like (nucleoid) region where the DNA is stored. Some bacteria can form a protective covering around the cell wall known as a **capsule**, or **slime layer**, that can increase their resistance to antibacterial agents. Although many bacteria have no independent forms of locomotion or movement, others do possess short fine filaments called **cilia** or longer filaments known

capsule or **slime layer:** a sheath or continuous enclosure around an organ or structure

cilia [SILL ee ah]: threadlike projections from the free surface of certain epithelial cells used to propel or sweep materials across a surface

flagella [fla JEL ah]: threadlike structures that provide motility for certain bacteria, protozoa, and spermatozoa

spores: cells produced by fungi for reproduction; a resistant cell produced by bacteria to withstand extreme heat or cold or dehydration

as **flagella** that can provide motility. Certain types of bacteria can even go into a state of suspension or inactivity for long periods of time. These bacteria produce **spores**, which are highly resistant forms of the organism that develop in response to adverse environmental conditions. They can then regenerate and become active when the environmental conditions improve. Spores are extremely hard to kill and have been estimated to be able to remain in the dormant state for tens of thousands of years. See Figure 1-3, which shows some bacterial forms and an example of spores.

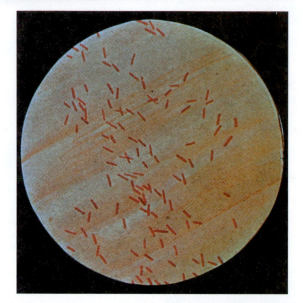

A

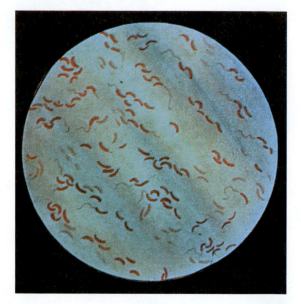

B

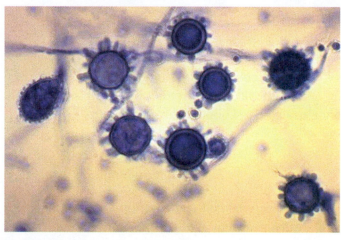

C

FIGURE 1-3 A. *Escherichia coli.* **B.** Bordetella pertussis. **C.** Notice the tough outer wall of spores, which make these bacteria harder to kill and allow them to remain dormant for long periods of time. Source: CDC/Atlanta, GA

Eukaryotes

To get a better understanding of how cells work, we can compare the structure and function of eukaryotic cellular components to a human being. For example, cells have an outer layer, or "skin," which is called a **cell membrane**. It protects the integrity of the cell just as our skin protects us. Just like us, inside the cell membrane there are structures that help the cell with its day-to-day functions. Extending our analogy, these structures are actually called organelles, which means "tiny organs."

Eukaryotic cells contain a **nucleus** that could be compared with a central processing unit of a computer (CPU) (see Figure 1-2A). It is the command center for the cell and contains the cell's DNA (deoxyribonucleic acid). As the cell grows, it reaches a size that stimulates the cell to divide. The cell divides into two equal parts by a process called **mitosis**. Each new cell contains the same amount of nuclear material in structures called **chromosomes**, which are the basic units of heredity.

The outer covering, or cell membrane, protects the cell from other cells and the environment. It allows the passage of nutrients and waste into and out of the cell, respectively. It also serves as a semipermeable barrier to *selectively* allow needed substances to enter and prevent unwanted intruders or substances from entering the cell.

If you pinch your skin, it returns to its original shape because of fluid contained in your tissues. The **cytoplasm** is the cell's fluid, and it not only maintains the shape of the cell but has important substances in it such as proteins, fats, carbohydrates, minerals, salts, and water. The structures of the cell are contained within the cytoplasm.

The nucleoli (plural) or **nucleolus** (singular) of the cell takes part in protein synthesis by manufacturing ribosomes, which contain cellular ribonucleic acid (RNA). The ribosomes assist with protein synthesis. Each protein produced by a cell has an important function. For example, a specialized protein called an enzyme controls the speed of chemical reactions within the cell.

The powerhouses of the cell are called **mitochondria** (singular: mitochondrion). Cells can contain one or many of these tiny powerhouses depending on the type and purpose of the cell. See if you can guess whether heart cells would contain more mitochondria than skin cells. Energy within the mitochondria is stored in the form of adenosine triphosphate (ATP). Glucose (simple sugar) and oxygen are needed for cellular respiration to take place and form ATP. By the way, if you guessed heart cells contain more mitochondria than skin, you are correct because the workload of the heart requires constant energy to pump blood throughout the body.

cell membrane: a semipermeable phospholipid bilayer that separates the interior of cells from the outside environment and controls movement into and out of the cell

nucleus [NEW clee us]: the structure within a cell that contains the chromosomes and is responsible for the cell's metabolism, growth, and reproduction

mitosis: type of cell division of somatic cells in which each daughter cell contains the same number of chromosomes as the parent cell

chromosome: a linear strand made of DNA that carries genetic information (genes)

cytoplasm [SIGH toh plazm]: a gel-like matrix contained within the cell membrane that holds all of the cell's internal substructures

nucleolus [new clee OL us]: a spherical structure in the nucleus of a cell made of DNA, RNA, and protein; the site of synthesis of rRNA

mitochondria (MITE oh KAHN dree ah): cell organelles of rod or oval shape that contain the enzymes for the aerobic stages of cell respiration and are the site of most ATP synthesis

Golgi apparatus [GOAL jee app ah RA tuss]: stacks of membrane-bound structures that package proteins inside the cell before they are sent to their destination; important in the processing of proteins for secretion

lysosomes [LIE soh soamz]: cell organelles containing hydrolytic enzyme capsules used to break down proteins and carbohydrates to aid in intracellular digestion

endoplasmic reticulum (ER): organelle that consists of a network of channels that transport materials within the cell

pinocytic vesicles [PIN o sit ik VES ih kuls]: compartments made when cells ingest extracellular material and its contents by invaginating the cell membrane and pinching off

Carbohydrates are combined with proteins by a cellular structure named the **Golgi apparatus** (also called Golgi bodies) named after Camillo Golgi, an Italian scientist who discovered them in 1898. These manufactured molecules are stored until needed, when they are secreted from the cell. Carbohydrates are nutrients used by our bodies as a source of energy. Cells of the pancreas, stomach, and salivary glands contain numerous Golgi bodies because they store enzymes that aid in digestion of food.

Lysosomes are manufactured in a cellular structure called the **endoplasmic reticulum (ER)**, which has both rough and smooth components. Rough ER has ribosomes surrounding the outer membrane, while smooth ER does not. Once the lysosomes are manufactured, they are matured by the Golgi apparatus. Once matured, they are stored within the cytoplasm of the cell. Lysosomes contain enzymes that can digest foreign material, bacteria, or old worn-out cells. Enzymes must be safely contained within lysosomes, otherwise the cell would auto-digest itself. You can think of them as the waste disposal unit. If the contents of a lysosome are released prematurely, they can cause the cell to die by digesting itself.

Fortunately, if we want to get a steak or our favorite food into our body, we have to eat it (just imagine the joy you would miss if you could just absorb it through your skin). However, nutrients and materials needed by the cell do not pass as easily through the cell membrane. The cell membrane prevents passage of substances such as fats (lipids) and proteins. These substances enter cells via **pinocytic vesicles**. Pinocytic vesicles are like bubbles and are formed when the cell membrane surrounds the protein or fat. Once the substance is fully surrounded, it is taken up into the cell by the vesicle "pinching" itself away from the cell membrane and entering the cytoplasm. See Table 1-2, which describes human eukaryotic cellular structure and function.

1-1
Stop and Review

1. Microorganisms that normally exist in our body are referred to as normal _____.

2. _____ is the term used for an organism that can produce an infection.

3. Cellular energy is stored in the _____.

4. Eukaryotic cells are different from prokaryotic cells because they contain a(n) _____.

TABLE 1-2 Cellular Function and Structure

Cellular Function	Cellular Structure	Organelle Tasks
Structure	Plasma or cell membrane	Protective covering; allows for semipermeability
Control	Nucleus	Controls most cellular activity and reproduction
Reproduction	Chromatin	Found in nucleus and contains DNA; condenses to form chromosomes, which contain genes
	Centrosomes	Contain centrioles, which play a major role in cell division
Build and repair	Nucleolus	Contains ribosomes made of RNA; synthesizes and produces protein
Energy	Mitochondria	Energy powerhouse found throughout cytoplasm
Environmental control	Golgi apparatus	Stores and packages secretions for removal
	Lysosomes	Digest old cells and foreign material
Intracellular communication	Endoplasmic reticulum	Network of tubes that facilitates transport of materials in and out of nucleus; synthesizes and stores protein

© 2016 Cengage Learning®.

Normal Flora versus Pathogens

It is sometimes difficult to understand that microorganisms can be beneficial, harmful, or both depending on the state of their human host and where they reside. A microorganism that can produce disease is considered to be a **pathogen**. In general, only a small number of microorganisms are capable of producing disease in humans, and these will be discussed in more detail later.

pathogen [PATH oh jen]: a microorganism capable of producing a disease

There is a very large number of microorganisms that do not cause disease in healthy individuals, and they are called normal flora. They can exist either on, in, or around us in very large numbers. In fact, the human body is made up of about one trillion eukaryotic cells but has about ten trillion prokaryotic cells living within it that make up our normal flora.

Most normal flora are found in the eyes, nose, mouth, throat, urethra, small and large bowel (intestines), and the skin. This has implications later on when we discuss specimen collection. It is important to collect specimens properly to prevent contamination of the specimen with normal flora. See Table 1-3, which provides a few examples of body sites and microorganisms that would potentially be considered pathogens or normal flora if found when cultured. Notice that some body sites such as the blood and cerebrospinal fluid (CSF) do not contain any normal flora. These sites and body fluids normally are sterile.

Pathogens are microorganisms that are capable of producing disease in humans. Not to confuse you, but under certain conditions, normal flora can even cause disease in humans and be pathogenic. This occurs if, for example, an organism such as *Escherichia coli* (better known as *E. coli*), which is normal flora in the bowel, gets into the bloodstream or the kidney, where it can cause serious disease.

TABLE 1-3 Body Sites and Representative Pathogenic and Normal Flora

Body Site	Pathogens	Normal Flora
Throat	*Streptococcus pyogenes*	*Streptococcus viridans*
	Haemophilus influenzae	Diphtheroids
Stool	*Salmonella typhi*	*Enterobacter* species
	Giardia lamblia	*Escherichia coli*
	Clostridium difficile	*Klebsiella* species
Blood	Any microorganism*	none
Cerebrospinal fluid (CSF)	*Neisseria meningitides*	none
	Streptococcus pneumoniae	
	Haemophilus influenzae	
Sputum	*Streptococcus pneumoniae*	Diphtheroids
	Legionella pneumophila	*Staphylococcus epidermidis*
	Mycobacterium tuberculosis	*Streptococcus viridans*
	Staphylococcus aureus	
	Haemophilus influenzae	
	Klebsiella pneumoniae	

*Blood and CSF should be sterile, meaning we do not have any microorganisms living in our bloodstream or central nervous system that are normal flora.

Food for Thought
Friendly Bacteria

Probiotics are live microorganisms that are similar to beneficial microorganisms found in the human intestine. They are also called "friendly, or good, bacteria." If you take an antibiotic, you may kill "good" as well as "bad," or pathogenic, bacteria. Probiotics are available to consumers in the form of foods (yogurt) and dietary supplements. They can be used to replace or restore the "good bacteria" that were present in our intestines before antibiotic use. The jury is still out on the use of probiotics. In people with suppressed immune systems, these products may even be dangerous because the organisms they contain may cause illness.

1-2
Stop and Review

1. What normal flora exist in the blood and CSF?

2. _____ are bacteria that inhabit our bodies but do not cause disease. _____ are bacteria that cause disease when they infect humans.

3. Name a microorganism that would be considered a pathogen if found in the stool.

Immunity and Infection

Did you ever wonder how your body prevents an infection? First we explore the various components of our immune system and how they work to prevent infection. Then we discuss what happens if a microorganism evades our immune defense and causes disease.

Immune System

Before we discuss how microorganisms cause disease, it would be a good idea to review how our bodies may prevent or fight off disease. In general, there are three lines of defense against pathogens:

1. protective barriers such as **mucous membranes**, skin, body secretions, and excretions;

2. circulatory or bloodstream response; and

mucous membranes: linings of mostly *endodermal* origin, covered in *epithelium,* which are involved in *absorption* and *secretion*

3. specific types of immune system responses called innate (those you were born with) and adaptive, which can be divided into cellular and antibody (humoral).

Protective Barriers

Unless the skin is damaged, it normally provides the first line of defense and an effective barrier to keep out intruders. The barrier is not just the intact skin itself but the secretions found on the skin from sweat and sebaceous glands. These fatty acid secretions cause our skin to be acidic, which creates an inhospitable environment for many microbes.

Other protective barriers also exist within the body systems. In the respiratory tract, tiny hairlike projections called cilia are found from the nose down to the lungs. The mucus within the respiratory tract traps inhaled foreign particles that can then be propelled upward by the cilia. These particles can then be expelled by sneezing or coughing or can be destroyed by enzymes in the fluid lining the respiratory tract.

The digestive system provides several protective barrier first lines of defense activities. The saliva washes microbes from the teeth, gums, and mouth and contains lysozyme, an antibacterial enzyme. The acidic pH of the stomach supports a hostile environment for most microorganisms. Moving on to the intestines, the acidic environment now turns alkaline, which is just as hostile to most bacteria. As we move down the small intestine, normal flora such as *Escherichia coli* and *anaerobes* (bacteria that can grow and thrive without oxygen) provide a barrier to invasion by organisms because pathogens have difficulty competing for nutrients and room to grow. Mucus secreted by the intestines helps to trap invaders until they can either be expelled by muscular contractions or in stool. Of course, activities such as defecation and vomiting can expel microorganisms from the body.

The genitourinary tract is protected from foreign microorganisms by the frequent flushing of urine, and in females, vaginal secretions. Males are

Learning Hint

MUCUS VS. MUCOUS

The terms *mucus* and *mucous* are often confused because they sound exactly the same. The difference is that mucus is the noun representing the actual secretion, and mucous is the adjective that would describe, for example, the membrane that secretes the substance. Therefore, the mucous membrane secretes mucus.

less likely than females to get infections in this area because of anatomy. The length of the male urethra provides a mechanical barrier against bacterial invasion. Normal flora that are found in the digestive tract can sometimes enter the urethra of females, especially during sexual intercourse. This may cause a bladder or kidney infection in the female.

Circulatory and Bloodstream Response

If a pathogen manages to enter our bodies, it faces formidable foes in our circulatory system, or bloodstream. Specific types of cells found in our bloodstream called phagocytes love to feast on these intruders. **Phagocyte** means "to eat," and *neutrophils, monocytes, macrophages,* and *dendritic cells* make up the body's phagocytic cells. **Neutrophils** and **monocytes** are formed in the bone marrow and circulate in the bloodstream. When monocytes leave the bloodstream, they migrate into tissues and the spleen, forming either dendritic cells or **macrophages**. These cells use a process called phagocytosis to ingest microorganisms. This process is like wrapping your arms around someone but then ingesting them. The body is constantly purging itself of all types of dead and foreign material, much of which is dead or worn-out cells. Once bacteria are ingested, they can then be destroyed by lysosomes, which contain digestive enzymes.

Phagocytes are found in fixed locations within the body such as the reticular connective tissue, spleen, liver, bone marrow, and lymph nodes. The **mononuclear phagocyte system (MPS)** (this used to be called the **reticuloendothelial system [RES]**) contains phagocytic cells located in the reticular connective tissue. The phagocytes may also roam the body, rushing to the site once a foreign substance is discovered. Certain white blood cells (WBCs) such as neutrophils, eosinophils, basophils, and monocytes are types of mobile phagocytes that can rush to an area of invasion, engulf the bacteria or foreign material, ingest it by phagocytosis, and then kill it by combining the phagocytized intruder with a lysosome. Eventually this is a suicide mission for the WBC, which continues to ingest until it ages and then is eaten by a macrophage who basically is the cleanup crew. See Figure 1-4.

phagocyte [FAG oh sight]: white blood cells that can ingest and destroy microorganisms, cell debris, and other particles in the blood or tissues

neutrophils [NEW troh fills]: granular white blood cells responsible for much of the body's protection against infection. They play a primary role in inflammation and are readily attracted to foreign antigens, destroying them by phagocytosis

monocyte: a mononuclear phagocytic white blood cell derived from myeloid stem cells that circulate in the bloodstream and act as the first line of defense in the inflammatory process

macrophage [MACK roh fayj]: a monocyte that has left the circulation and settled and matured in a tissue such as the spleen, lymph nodes, alveoli, and tonsils

mononuclear phagocyte system (MPS) or **reticuloendothelial system (RES):** the system of fixed macrophages and circulating monocytes that serve as phagocytes, engulfing foreign substances in a wide variety of immune responses

Learning Hint

Use Your Medical Terminology

"Phago" is the medical term related to swallowing and "cyte" is the medical term for cell. Therefore, a phagocyte is literally a cell that eats.

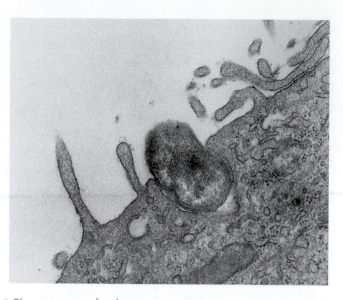

FIGURE 1-4 Phagocytosis of rickettsia. Source: CDC/Dr. Edwin P. Ewing, Jr.

Immune System Responses: Innate and Adaptive Immune Responses

If a pathogen has broken through our previous lines of defense, it first encounters our **innate** (born with) **immune response**. No previous exposure to the intruder is required to summon this immune response. Its primary functions are to kill invading microbes and to alert the adaptive immune response of the invasion. Some of the cells we talked about earlier are important components of this response. The neutrophils' job is to kill microbes. Macrophages and dendritic cells kill microbes but also *present* the intruding microorganisms to helper T cells and thus are called **antigen-presenting cells (APCs)**. An antigen is any marker that our body's immune system recognizes as foreign. Phagocytosis by the APCs engulfs the invading pathogen, breaks it into fragments, and then *presents* these fragments of the invading antigen on its surface. This is like raising a flag to let everyone know there is an invasion and exactly who the invader is. This process serves to alert and activate our **adaptive immune response**. See Figure 1-5.

The other important component of innate immunity, along with the physical barriers previously discussed, is the inflammatory response generated by proteins produced by the macrophages (e.g., interleukins 1 and 6 and tumor necrosis factor). This response produces the redness, swelling, and pain of the infected tissue that causes the body to recognize that something is wrong. The swelling helps to wall-off the inflamed area so the attack can be focused to that site.

Next they may encounter either our cell-mediated or humoral (antibodies circulating in the bloodstream) immune response. Collectively these

innate immune response: the ability to protect one's self from pathogens, the immunity you have when you are born

antigen-presenting cells (APCs): a group of immunocompetent cells that mediate cellular immune response by engulfing, processing, and presenting antigens to the T-cell receptor. Traditional antigen-presenting cells include macrophages, dendritic cells, Langerhans cells, and B lymphocytes.

adaptive immune response: immune mechanisms that "learn" to deal with specific invaders

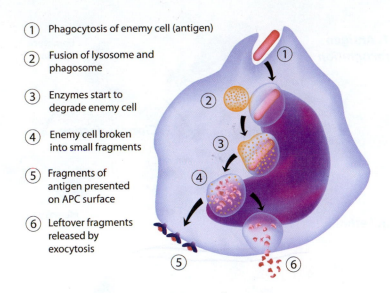

① Phagocytosis of enemy cell (antigen)

② Fusion of lysosome and phagosome

③ Enzymes start to degrade enemy cell

④ Enemy cell broken into small fragments

⑤ Fragments of antigen presented on APC surface

⑥ Leftover fragments released by exocytosis

FIGURE 1-5 Role of an antigen-presenting cell. © Alila Medical Media/Shutterstock.com.

responses are termed our adaptive immune response. The cellular immune response can be thought of like a bouncer at a bar. The unruly patron has broken through several lines of defense at the bar that keep out unsavory customers but now has become rowdy and needs to be dealt with in a different manner. The bouncer's response generally occurs in four phases. First, we must recognize the pathogen or intruder. Macrophages and dendritic cells present the intruder to helper T cells, the bouncers, which recognize the pathogen as foreign. Second, the bouncer calls for reinforcements, which in the case of our cellular immune response are additional **T cells**. Again, the T cells are presented to the intruder by the macrophages or dendritic cells, they become activated, and then they either enter peripheral tissues or interact with other cells (**B cells**) in lymphoid tissue. These activated T cells secrete cytokines that are specific to the cell and certain types of invading microorganisms. When T cells are activated, some become memory cells that can last a long time (in case the pathogen comes back later), while others are short-lived effector cells and deal with the situation at hand. See Figure 1-6, which shows cytotoxic (cell-killing) T-cell activation and actions on a cancer cell.

Not to be outdone, our **humoral** (B-cell mediated) **immune response** comes to the bouncer's rescue. If the person fighting the infection has not encountered the microbe before, there is a lag time before antibodies will be produced by B cells. However, if the individual has either encountered the intruder before or has been immunized against the intruder, antibodies

T cell: a type of white blood cell that matures in the thymus, contains a T-cell receptor, and plays a central role in cell-mediated immunity

B cell: a type of lymphocyte, developed in bone marrow, that circulates in the blood and lymph and, upon encountering a particular foreign antigen, differentiates into a clone of plasma cells that secrete a specific antibody and a clone of memory cells that make the antibody on subsequent encounters

humoral immune response [hu MORE al]: immunity associated with circulating antibodies

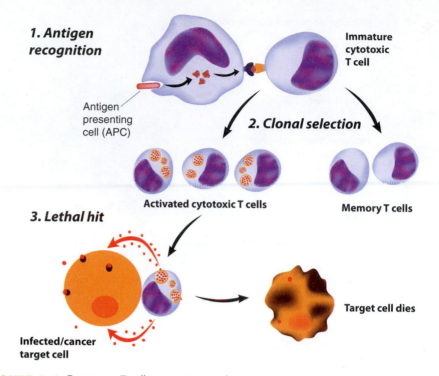

1. Antigen recognition

Antigen presenting cell (APC)

Immature cytotoxic T cell

2. Clonal selection

Activated cytotoxic T cells

Memory T cells

3. Lethal hit

Infected/cancer target cell

Target cell dies

FIGURE 1-6 Cytotoxic T-cell activation and actions on a cancer cell. © Alila Medical Media/Shutterstock.com.

antibody: a substance produced by a B lymphocyte in response to a unique antigen, which it can then combine with to destroy or control it

specific for the microbe will be quickly produced from the plasma cells (B cells) previously formed. The antibodies recognize the intruder by antigens located on the pathogen's cell wall. The **antibodies**, also called immunoglobulins, latch onto the antigen causing the invader to be either destroyed or engulfed. If by now the bouncer, with assistance from our cell-mediated and humoral immune responses, has destroyed the pathogen or at least controlled him, it is time to clear out the bar. T and B cells go home; antibodies, however, are still there after last call, hanging around in case the pathogen shows up again in the future. To put this all together for you, see Table 1-4, which compares the body's humoral and cell-mediated lines of defense, in addition to Figure 1-7, which illustrates the integrated immune response.

TABLE 1-4 Comparison of Humoral and Cell-Mediated Immunity

Type of Immunity	Cells	Mediated by	Provides Protection from
Humoral (circulating in blood)	B cells (plasma cells)	Antibodies	Bacteria, toxins
Cell-mediated	T cells	Cells, cytokines, and chemokines	Viruses, fungi

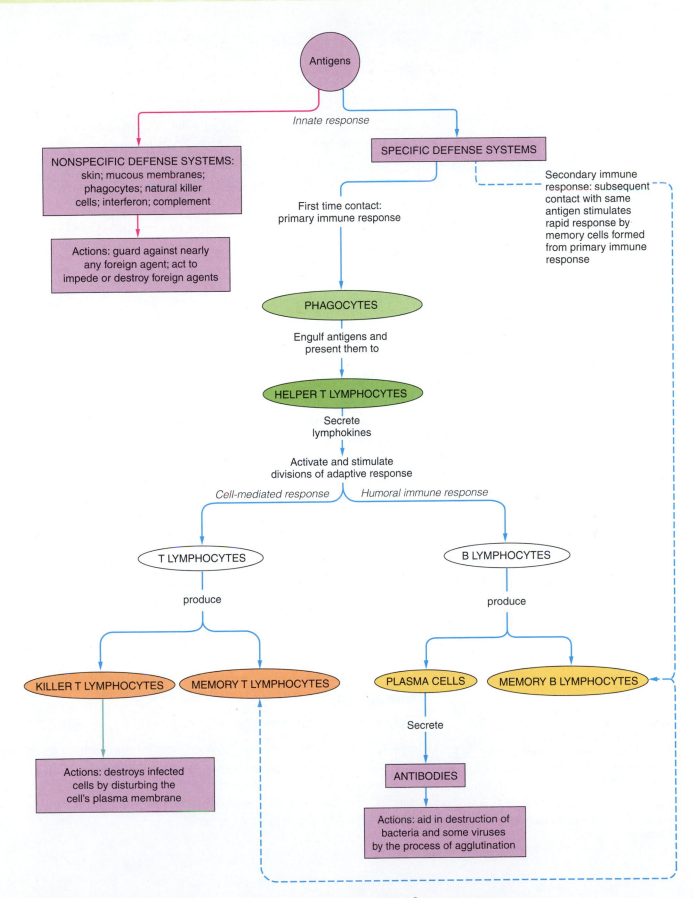

FIGURE 1-7 The integrated immune response. © 2016 Cengage Learning®.

Infection

infection: a disease caused by microorganisms, especially those that release toxins or invade body tissues

If a microbe is able to gain entrance into our bodies, it may cause an **infection**. The infection could be localized to a specific area of the body such as an infected cut on your skin, or it could spread into a generalized infection affecting our entire body, possibly resulting in death. The ability of a microorganism to cause disease in a human is termed pathogenicity, while the severity of the disease caused defines the *virulence* of the pathogen. The virulence of a microbe is determined by certain cell structures and the ability of the microbe to produce endo- or exotoxins.

Hopefully, you recall our previous discussion concerning normal flora and pathogens. It is important to understand that even organisms with potentially low virulence can cause disease in a compromised human host (weakened or absent immune response). Likewise, organisms that are normal flora in our bodies can become pathogenic if they invade tissues where

endotoxin: a lipopolysaccharide that is part of the cell wall of gram-negative bacteria released after the cell's death

exotoxin: a poisonous substance produced by certain bacteria

💡 **Learning Hint**
Applying Medical Terminology

The word *toxins* of course means "poisons," and **endotoxins** are literally poisons contained within (*endo*) the microorganism as, for example, within the cell wall of certain gram-negative bacteria. *Exo* means "outside," and therefore **exotoxins** are produced by bacteria and secreted outside the bacterial cell.

they don't belong. In general, for a microbe to cause infection, it must enter our bodies, resist our immune system, multiply or enter in sufficient numbers to overwhelm our bouncers (immune system), and either be highly virulent or enter a human host who has been weakened by diseases or aging. You may have seen newspaper or magazine covers warning of flesh-eating bacteria. This highly virulent species of *Streptococci* can cause disease and possibly death even in young healthy persons.

Bacteria, viruses, fungi, and parasites are the most commonly encountered types of microorganisms causing disease in humans. We discuss each of these classes in detail in upcoming chapters.

Direct and Indirect Disease Transmission

For microbes to cause an infection, they somehow must be transmitted to a human host by contact. **Contact transmission** can occur either by *direct contact* with a person who is infected or *indirect contact* by coming in contact with something contaminated by an infectious person. Examples of direct contact would be traveling on a crowded subway with people sneezing and coughing (especially when they forget to cover their noses and mouths). The other way infection may occur is by indirect contact such as handling tissues that someone else sneezed into (okay, yucky example) or touching secretions on a doorknob someone else used. Stethoscopes have also been known to be possible conduits for the indirect transmission of microorganisms. The stethoscope in this case is called a **fomite**. Fomites are inanimate (not living) objects that are capable of transmitting disease.

A medical example of *direct contact* is when a patient has a bowel movement in bed and the feces come into contact with an open wound on the patient's buttocks. Direct contact can also occur when a health care provider doesn't wash his or her hands or "glove up" before tending to an open wound. A clinical example of *indirect contact* is when medical equipment is not properly sterilized before it is used on the next patient, and pathogens from the previous patient are transferred to the next. An example at home would be touching a doorknob that had been previously handled by someone with the flu.

In addition to contact transmission, other main routes of transmission include **vectors**, common vehicle, and airborne spread. Although rarely occurring in hospitals, the vector route of transmission is quite common in the community. A **vector borne** transmission is one in which the organism is carried by an insect, other animal, or human. This can occur in one of two ways. The insect may have the pathogen living inside it, and when it bites you, it infects your blood with that organism. This is known as a **biological vector**.

contact transmission: occurs when microorganisms are transferred from one infected person to another

fomite [FO might]: object that may harbor microorganisms and is capable of transmitting them

vectors: carriers of disease

vector borne: transmitting a pathogenic microorganism from an infected individual to another individual by an arthropod or other agent, sometimes with other animals serving as intermediary hosts

biological vector: A vector that is essential in the life cycle of a pathogenic organism

mechanical vector: a vector that simply conveys pathogens to a susceptible individual and is not essential to the development of the organism

common vehicle transmission: the mode of transmission of infectious pathogens from a source that is common to all the cases of a specific disease, by means of a vehicle such as water, food, air, or the blood supply

airborne transmission: a transmission mechanism in which the infectious agent is spread as an aerosol and usually enters a person through the respiratory tract

inoculum: a substance or microorganism introduced by inoculation

An example of a biological vector is the spread of malaria through the bite of an infected female *Anopheles* mosquito. Alternatively, the insect may have that organism *on* its body and spread it to you by landing on an open wound. This is known as a **mechanical vector**. If a fly walks over cow feces, and then lands on an open bowl of potato salad sitting in the warm sun at your picnic, that would be considered disease spreading via a mechanical vector.

Common vehicle transmission is one you may hear about in the news. This occurs when consumable goods (such as blood or blood products; IV fluids; food such as ground meat, vegetables, or seafood) become contaminated. This sets up the potential for a major epidemic and is readily recognizable by the sudden occurrence of many infections caused by the same pathogen.

Airborne transmission is a result of the spread of droplets that contain the pathogen. Examples include the spread of tuberculosis by sneezing or even laughing or pathogens growing in an air conditioner and being spread when the air conditioner is turned on, as happened in the case of the outbreak of Legionnaires' disease in 1977 in Philadelphia. See Figure 1-8, which clearly demonstrates the need to cover your mouth when you sneeze to prevent airborne or droplet transmission.

Once the organism comes into contact with a human host, the ability to cause infection is determined by organism virulence, number of organisms (also called **inoculum**), host immune system status, and portal of entry, which will be expanded on in the infection control chapter.

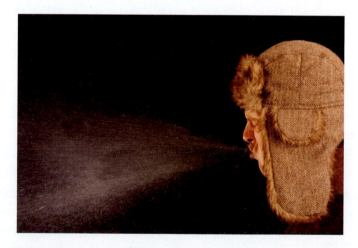

FIGURE 1-8 The aerosol produced by a sneeze. Source: Courtesy of Lester V. Bergman/Corbis

Fever and the Inflammatory Response

When an infection occurs, it is usually accompanied by fever and the previously discussed inflammatory response. Fever is a biologically important defense mechanism mounted by the body to assist in clearing infections. Inflammation is part of the innate immune response and is caused by the dilation of blood vessels, which allows the passage of fluid, antibodies, and WBCs into the infected body area. This generally results in pain, swelling, redness, and warmth that can be seen and felt. The antibodies and WBCs cause the death of microbes and result in the formation of a thick, creamy-appearing liquid known as pus. These responses aid in containing and hopefully eliminating the pathogen from its human host. We will be learning other disease and infection prevention terminology and concepts as we journey through the chapters.

Chapter Summary

- This chapter laid the foundation for you to understand how microorganisms are classified. We discussed the differences between prokaryotic and eukaryotic cells. The inner workings of a eukaryotic cell were described along with the structure and function of each component. Remember that eukaryotic cells are the more complex of the two and contain a true nucleus.

- The distinction was made between bacteria that can be considered as normal flora in our bodies and bacteria that do not normally reside in our bodies unless they are causing us to be ill (pathogens). Normal flora help keep our body free of pathogenic microbes because they, in a sense, do not allow any room at the inn. Our bodies are the inn, and our normal flora are the inhabitants of the inn.

- We discussed how our immune systems keep microbes at bay and what happens if those microscopic pests evade our immune systems and cause disease. The innate immune response is always the first line of defense against intruders, while the adaptive immune response has two components: cellular and humoral. Both components of the adaptive immune response work in synergy to overcome pathogenic microorganisms.

- Remember that pathogenicity describes the ability of a microbe to cause disease, while virulence describes how sick an individual gets when infected with the organism. Diseases may be spread directly, by coughing or sneezing on your neighbor during class or while watching a movie. Microbes can also be spread indirectly by sneezing into your hands and wiping your hands with the bathroom towel at home. Then your brother or sister uses the towel to dry his or her mouth. The foundation has been laid in this chapter. Now it is time to go on to Chapter 2 and discuss medical microbiology.

Case Study

A 69-year-old male patient presents to the department of emergency medicine at a local hospital with a fever, cough, and low blood pressure. He had a dual kidney and liver transplant three months ago and was taking a medicine called tacrolimus, which suppresses cellular immunity (prevents T-cell activation) to prevent organ rejection. He was found to have cytomegalovirus (CMV) pneumonia. The donor of these organs tested positive for this virus but according to his family was not ill prior to his untimely death in an automobile accident. Why did the transplant recipient get sick from the virus but the organ donor was not ill? What broad category of immunity was suppressed in this transplant patient?

Chapter Review

Match the cellular component with its function.

1. _____ nucleus
2. _____ lysosome
3. _____ Golgi apparatus
4. _____ cell membrane
5. _____ pinocytic vesicles
6. _____ mitochondria
7. _____ cytoplasm

a. contains structures of the cell
b. forms a barrier and contains components of cell
c. brain of cell
d. powerhouse of cell
e. storage place
f. contains stored enzymes
g. bubbles in the cell membrane

Match the immune system component to its purpose.

8. __f___ mucous membranes
9. __d___ cilia
10. __g___ phagocytic cells
11. __e___ lysosomes
12. __a___ reticuloendothelial system
13. __c___ T cells and B cells
14. __b___ antibodies

a. spleen, liver, bone marrow, lymph nodes
b. immunoglobulins
c. specialized lymphocytes
d. "brooms" of the respiratory tract
e. contain enzymes that digest microbes
f. physical and chemical barrier to microbe entry
g. neutrophils, monocytes, macrophages

Answer the following questions and fill in the blanks as required.

15. What is a prion and what type of disease does it cause?

16. Discuss how microbes cause infections in humans.

17. Discuss the importance of normal flora.

18. _____ is the type of immunity that microbes encounter first.

19. _____ is a virus, substance, or other microorganism that causes disease.

20. Fever, redness, warmth, and swelling are produced by _____.

21. _____ and _____ are two types of cells formed from monocytes.

22. _____ are available to consumers in the form of foods (yogurt) and dietary supplements.

Classify the following routes of transmission.

23. _____ several people get a severe stomach illness after eating at a local restaurant

24. _____ you get sick after your friend sneezes without covering his mouth

25. _____ several people get an illness in a hospital and the common thread is they were all treated with the same piece of equipment

Additional Activities

1. Currently there is a "perfect storm" brewing in public health. Microbes are becoming more resistant to anti-infective agents (e.g., antivirals, antifungals, and antibiotics), and at the same time very few new anti-infective agents are being approved by the U.S. Food and Drug Administration to treat these resistant "bugs." At times, existing drugs end up in short supply because of drug manufacturers shifting production to more profitable medications. Although we will be discussing this in future chapters, research some of the reasons why drug resistance occurs and the dangers it poses.

2. Research the mandatory reporting of infections within your state. How do they relate to your surrounding states? Why are there differences?

3. Invite a medical technologist who works in a hospital microbiology lab to discuss bacterial resistance in your area.

Media Connection

Go to the accompanying online resources and have fun learning as you play games, view animations and videos, and take practice tests to help reinforce key concepts you learned in this chapter.

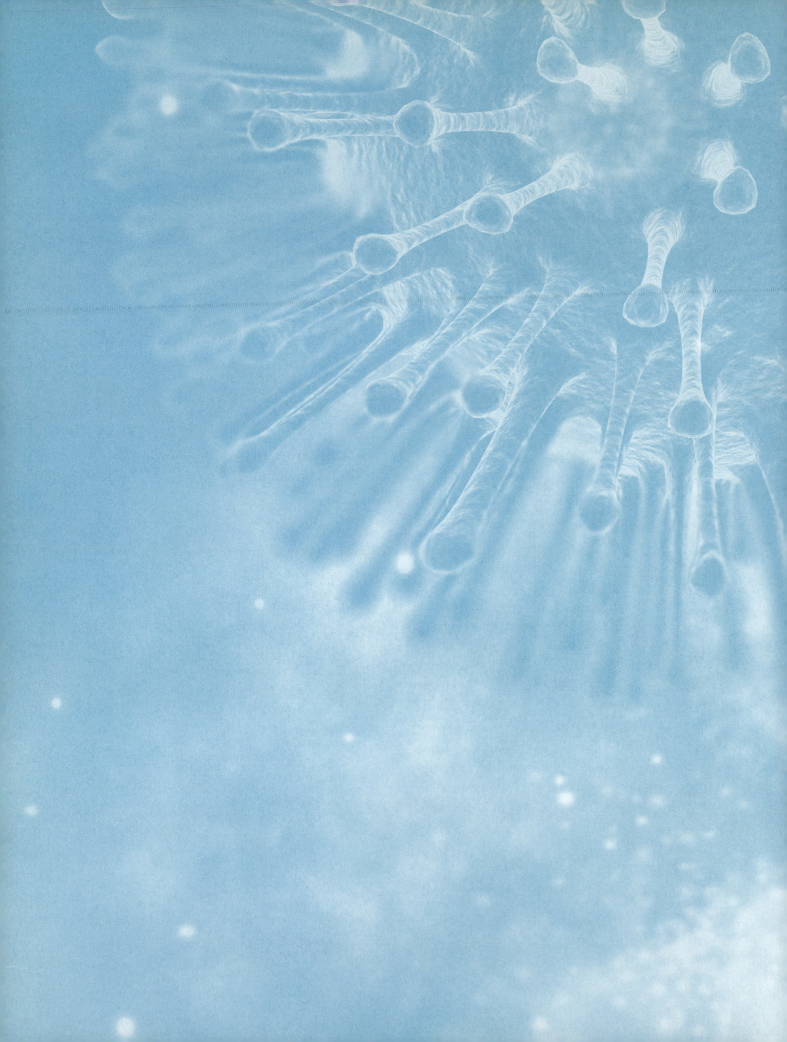

Medical Microbiology

OBJECTIVES

After studying this chapter, the learner will be able to:

- Differentiate various areas of medical microbiology specialization and study.

- Describe the history of microbiology.

- Describe the evolution of the "science" of microbiology.

- Discuss scientific principles of inquiry and research to include scientific reasoning and communicating results for public health.

- Contrast bacterial structure and morphology.

- Discuss the process and importance of bacterial staining.

- Describe the technique and importance of bacterial culture and sensitivity.

- Explain reasons for the development of antibiotic resistance.

KEY TERMS

acid-fast stain (Zeihl-Neelsen)

aerobic [air ROW bick]

anaerobic [an uh ROW bick]

antibiotic

asexual reproduction

automated

bacilli [bah SILL eye]

bactericidal
  [back TEER ih SIGH dul]

bacteriology

bacteriostatic
  [BACK teer ee oh STAT ik]

binary fission
  [BI nuh ree FISH un]

broad-spectrum drug

broth dilution

capsule

cerebral spinal fluid (CSF)

cocci [KOK sigh]

comparative research

culture and sensitivity test
  (C&S)

dependent variable

descriptive research

disk diffusion

empiric therapy

endotoxin

exotoxin

experimental research

flagella [fla JEL ah]

genus [JEE nus]

glycocalyx

Gram stain

health care–associated
  infections (HAIs)

(Continues)

KEY TERMS *(Continued)*

incubation

independent variable

infection control and
   prevention

medical microbiology

microbiology

morphology
   [more FALL oh gee]

mycology [my CALL uh jee]

narrow-spectrum drug

normal flora

opportunistic infections

parasitology
   [pair uh sigh TALL uh jee]

pathogenic [PATH oh JEN ick]

resistance

science

scientific inquiry

scientific hypothesis

scientific theories

serology

social ethics

species [SPEE seas]

spirilla [spih RILL uh]

spores

urinary tract infection (UTI)

virology [vear RALL oh jee]

virulence [VEAR you lence]

Introduction

In the next several chapters, we discuss the types of microbes that cause disease in humans, how they look under a microscope (also called **morphology**), what types of diseases they may cause in humans, and how we can treat these diseases with drugs. **Microbiology** is the study of these microscopic organisms. You learned about different types of microscopic cells in Chapter 1. Now we will focus on other microorganisms that can exist in the body and especially on those that can cause disease. Keep in mind from Chapter 1 that the majority of microorganisms are beneficial to the body and are known as **normal flora**. However, a small percentage can cause disease or be classified as **pathogenic**, and **virulence** is the potential ability for an organism to produce an infection. Some microorganisms such as *enterococcus* have a low virulence, while *Staphylococcus aureus* has a high virulence.

History of Microbiology

Antonie van Leeuwenhoek (LAY ven huck) is credited as one of the pioneers of the science of microbiology and, indeed, changing the way we look at the world. He was born in 1632 in the Netherlands and started as a tailor who was very interested in how his cloth was put together. He began looking at the various types of cloth with a magnifying glass. He was so curious, he became a lens grinder to make and improve on the magnifying glasses of his day. This soon led to his development of the microscope, where he viewed

---

morphology [more FALL oh gee]: the science of structure and form of organisms without regard to function

microbiology: the scientific study of microorganisms, that is, of bacteria, fungi, intracellular parasites, protozoans, viruses, and some worms

normal flora: mixture of bacteria normally found at specific body sites

pathogenic [PATH oh JEN ick]: productive of disease

virulence [VEAR you lence]: the relative power and degree of pathogenicity possessed by organisms

everything from a drop of water to a drop of blood and watched the "wee beasties" (what microorganisms were first called) with strange shapes swimming around. In a report to the Royal Society of Sciences, he wrote "the number of these animals in the plaque of a man's teeth, are so many that I believe they exceed the number of men in a kingdom." See Table 2-1 for some other important dates in the development of microbiology.

TABLE 2-1 Important Dates in the History of Microbiology and Antibiotic Development

Year	Accomplishment
Before 1660	Disease was associated with magic and mysticism, and no belief existed in microorganisms.
1660–1670s	Antonie van Leeuwenhoek developed a crude microscope with 200× magnification. He discovered tiny microbes, which he called "wee beasties." However, much of his discoveries went unnoticed for some time because van Leeuwenhoek kept to himself and did not share much of his knowledge of the construction of the microscope.
	In 1665, Robert Hooke published the first work of microscopic studies entitled *Micrographia*.
1800	Edward Jenner pioneered the smallpox vaccine.
1810	Nicolas Appert, the father of canning, developed a heating process to prevent spoilage of bottled fruit juices by microorganisms.
1830	German and French scientists concluded that yeast cells used in fermenting beers and wines are living microorganisms instead of chemical substances.
	Ignaz Semmelweis showed that childbed fever is transmitted by physicians. He began to use antiseptic procedures such as washing hands after examinations.
1850	Pasteur proved that bacteria cause wine spoilage.
1860 to 1890	Louis Pasteur discovered that fermentation is caused by living yeasts, discovered immunization techniques, and developed the rabies vaccine.
	Joseph Lister pioneered techniques for aseptic surgery.
	Albert Ludwig Neisser isolated the bacterium *Neisseria gonorrhoeae* from patients with gonorrhea.
	Robert Koch isolated the tubercle and cholera bacilli, developed pure culture techniques for microorganisms, and presented the germ theory of disease (proved that bacteria could be isolated and shown to cause disease).
	Christian Gram discovered and developed the Gram stain technique still used today.

(Continues)

TABLE 2-1 *(Continued)*

Year	Accomplishment
1870 to 1914	The "Golden Age of Microbiology." Most agents of bacterial disease were identified and cultivated. These include some of the following diseases: malaria, typhoid fever, diphtheria, pneumonia, meningitis, bubonic plague, and yellow fever.
1918	Worldwide epidemic of influenza killed millions.
1920s	Publication of the first edition of *Bergey's Manual of Determinative Bacteriology* for the classification of bacteria.
1928	Sir Alexander Fleming isolated and identified penicillin.
1930s	Ernst Ruska built first electron microscope.
1935	Sulfanilamide was discovered and developed. Sulfanilamide quickly became the principal agent for the treatment of war-related infections.
1940s	Zinder and Lederberg discovered process of bacterial transduction by viruses.
1945	Sir Alexander Fleming, Ernst Boris Chain, and Sir Howard W. Florey received the Nobel Prize for the discovery and development of penicillin. Since the 1940s, penicillin has remained an important antibiotic because of its low cost and the broad use of the thousands of penicillin derivatives.
1949	The first broad-spectrum antibiotic, chloramphenicol, was introduced.
1950s	The B-lactam nucleus of the penicillin molecule was identified and synthesized, thereby creating new penicillins.
1952	Selman Waksman received the Nobel Prize for the discovery and development of streptomycin. Erythromycin was also discovered.
1953	Tetracycline, a broad-spectrum antibiotic, was discovered.
1954	John F. Enders, Thomas H. Weller, and Frederick C. Robbins received the Nobel Prize for cultivation of the polio viruses.
1957	Amphotericin B, the drug of choice for serious systemic fungal infections, was introduced.
1958	Vancomycin, especially useful for severe staphylococcal diseases where penicillin allergy or resistance exists, was introduced.
1963	Ampicillin, a valuable agent against certain gram-negative rods and organisms of gonorrhea and meningococcal meningitis, was introduced.
1966	Gentamicin, one of the most popular of the aminoglycosides, was introduced.
1970s	Clindamycin, an alternative agent used when penicillin resistance is found, was discovered. Legionnaires' disease described during outbreak of pneumonia in Philadelphia.

(Continues)

TABLE 2-1 *(Continued)*

Year	Accomplishment
1971	Rifampin, a semisynthetic drug prescribed for tuberculosis and leprosy, was introduced.
1980s	The newer, second-generation of the quinolone drugs (ciprofloxacin, norfloxacin) was developed for clinical use. These second-generation quinolones have an expanded antibacterial spectrum that is active against most gram-negative bacteria.
	First cases of AIDS (acquired immunodeficiency syndrome) reported.
	Human insulin produced by genetically engineered bacteria.
	Drugs (AZT and protease inhibitors) introduced to treat AIDS.
1990s	Complete genome of the intestinal bacterium *Escherichia coli* coded with 4,403 genes.
	Human Genome Project completed. Determines the complete sequence of nucleotides in human DNA.
2000s	Linezolid and daptomycin were introduced to combat serious gram-positive infections such as methicillin-resistant Staphylococcus aureus (MRSA).

© 2016 Cengage Learning®.

Evolution of the "Science" of Microbiology

Once upon a time not so long ago, microbiology was not a science. Illnesses and infections were thought to be caused by an individual's bad behavior or social standing, for example. In fact, molds were often used to treat infections. This treatment was termed *mold therapy* and was based on folklore. Right in front of everyone's nose there were macroscopic, or large, examples of microbial growth such as bacterial or algae slimes containing billions of tiny organisms all living together, making them visible as a large group to the naked eye. However, the *individual* microscopic organisms could not be seen with the naked eye.

This all changed thanks to the work of the Dutch microscopist, Antonie van Leeuwenhoek, who ground his own lenses to make microscopes, thereby providing the ability to see these individual tiny microbes. In doing so, the science of microbiology started to take shape. **Science** is basically using a hunch to develop a theory on why things work the way they do. Van Leeuwenhoek used his microscopes to look at microorganisms in well water, rainwater, and seawater, among other things. He not only observed these microbes; he also described and drew them. His drawings clearly show that he observed bacilli, streptococci, and protozoa. This was a form of **descriptive research**.

science: knowledge about or study of the natural world based on facts learned through experiments and observation

descriptive research: used to describe characteristics of a population or phenomenon being studied. It does not answer questions about how/when/why the characteristics occurred

scientific inquiry: the activities through which individuals develop knowledge and understanding of scientific ideas, as well as an understanding of how scientists study the natural world

Even though these microorganisms were able to be seen, the connection between them and disease was not made until many years later. In fact, it was widely believed from the Middle Ages until just a few hundred years ago that life arose spontaneously from inanimate objects. The French Academy of Sciences offered a prize in the mid-1800s to anyone who could settle the controversy about whether life arose spontaneously. Louis Pasteur realized that if microbiology was to advance as a science, the idea that microorganisms arose spontaneously needed to be disproved. Pasteur, and others after him, used a method called **scientific inquiry** to disprove the theory of spontaneous generation. Scientific inquiry is a planned and deliberate investigation of the natural world.

Louis Pasteur used swan-necked flasks to show that heat-sterilized liquids could be kept sterile in an open flask as long as the part that was open to the air was twisted enough to allow any microbes that entered the flask to settle on the sides before reaching the liquid. He described his observations and wrote papers about his results to share his findings with others.

The science of microbiology needed two major developments to further advance: better microscopes and the ability to grow microorganisms in a controlled environment. Robert Hooke developed microscopes with more powerful magnifications. The introduction of staining procedures allowed the fine visualization of microbes. Robert Koch developed techniques to stain bacteria, including a special method to stain the microbe that causes tuberculosis. Science was used to discover the microbe that caused tuberculosis. However, it was **social ethics** that determined it was best to quarantine patients with tuberculosis in sanitariums so they would not infect other people. Further developments in the field of microscopy such as growing, categorizing, and visualizing microbes continued to develop.

social ethics: the philosophical or moral principles that, in one way or another, represent the collective experience of people and cultures

In 1788, an epidemic of smallpox broke out in the English county of Gloucestershire. A country doctor, Edward Jenner, decided to try to prevent his patients from becoming ill. Dr. Jenner had heard the "old wives' tale" that cowpox (disease in cows) protected against the disease in humans. So he decided to try an experiment. He inoculated a small boy with cowpox, and the boy became immune to smallpox. Modern day medial ethics would not have allowed this experiment to go forward since a human subject was used and would have required a review by an Institutional Review Board (IRB). This was **comparative research** because he injected the boy with cowpox and compared him with children who were not injected with cowpox instead of just observing what might happen if he became ill with cowpox. His hypothesis might have been something like, "I hypothesize that injecting subjects with cowpox will protect them from smallpox." Within a few years, vaccination became very common. The hypothesis that Dr. Jenner tested with his vaccination research was replicated numerous times by many

comparative research: a research methodology in the social sciences that aims to make comparisons across different countries or cultures

different researchers. From Dr. Jenner's research, the scientific theory of how immunity protects people from diseases was developed. Scientific theories are based on natural and physical phenomena and may be tested by many unaffiliated researchers.

Food for Thought

Milk Maids

Edward Jenner developed the first smallpox vaccine in the nineteenth century when he observed that milk maids did not acquire this disease. Milk maids were exposed to cowpox, a similar disease that affects cows, and thus the maids developed a cross-protective immunity to smallpox.

Another breakthrough development in microbiology further explains the difference between **scientific hypotheses** and **scientific theories**. During the 1840s in Vienna, a condition known as childbed, or puerperal, fever was a particularly terrible disease that affected many hospital patients. During a single month in 1856 in a Paris hospital, 31 mothers died from this disease. Ignaz Semmelweiss was a Hungarian doctor who was working at the Vienna General Hospital in 1844. In his first few months of practice, he heard that a very high death rate from this disease appeared to be concentrated in teaching wards where patients were frequently examined by both doctors and their students. Dr. Semmelweiss began to collect data and soon confirmed the old wives' tale that the highest rates of infection and death occurred in the teaching wards of the hospital. He hypothesized that the infection was being transmitted from doctors and students to patients. These health care professionals examined the wombs of patients without washing their hands, even after mortuary duty. To test this hypothesis he suggested that anyone examining patients should wash their hands first in chlorine water. The results of this simple experiment were phenomenal. Mortality rates went from 11% to 3% within a year. This was another type of comparative research because Dr. Semmelweiss was comparing death rates before and after instituting hand washing. He wrote a report based on his observations, which was largely ignored. Eventually, the view that infections were spread by some "organic particle" became widely accepted. To this day, hand washing, or the more modern term *hand hygiene*, is the single most important way to prevent the spread of infection.

Utilizing the knowledge that infections may be spread by airborne germs, English surgeon Joseph Lister, in the mid-1800s, decided to cover wounds with dressings containing chemicals that killed airborne germs.

scientific hypothesis: the initial building block in the scientific method. Many describe it as an "educated guess," based on prior knowledge and observation, as to the cause of a particular phenomenon

scientific theory: a well-substantiated explanation of some aspect of the natural world that is acquired through the scientific method and repeatedly tested and confirmed through observation and experimentation

experimental research: experiment where the researcher manipulates one variable, and controls/randomizes the rest of the variables

dependent variable: a variable (often denoted by *y*) whose value depends on that of another; what is being observed in an experiment

independent variable: a variable (often denoted by *x*) whose variation does not depend on that of another; what is being tested or changed in an experiment

Lister published his findings in a medical journal in 1867 that attracted immediate attention. The age of antiseptic surgery had begun. He may have hypothesized that germs in the air cause infections in wounds. This type of research is called **experimental research**, which is conducted by manipulating and controlling variables. The two most common types of variables are termed **dependent variables** and **independent variables**. The independent variable was the dressing soaked in a chemical, and the dependent variable was the infection rate. It may take a bit of thinking to keep these two types of variables straight. In general, the independent variable is what is being tested, changed, what is different between the groups (e.g., dressing soaked in chemical versus no dressing), or the "cause" of a change. The dependent variable is what is observed, measured, data that is collected, or the "effect" caused by the independent variable. With microbiology becoming a true science, this paved the way for it to evolve into an applied science in the medical field called *medical microbiology*.

Clinical Application

Modeling Disease Outbreaks and Communicating Public Health Data

The Centers for Disease Control and Prevention (CDC) monitors disease outbreaks and develops statistics, graphs, and models to help predict disease patterns and inform the public. One such example is their weekly report FLUVIEW represented in the illustration below:

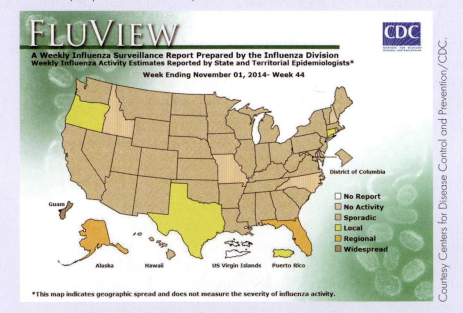

Courtesy Centers for Disease Control and Prevention/CDC.

This weekly communication and reporting of data can help track the emergence and spread of the flu. Notice in this report, we are just entering flu season and you can see there is at least some flu activity in all but four states. Also, notice the limitation of this model in that it does not indicate the influenza strain or severity level. Therefore, other reports, statistics, and graphs would need to be consulted to get the full picture. Given this model represents the beginning of flu season, can you predict what changes will happen in two weeks to this map?

Medical Microbiology

How do all of the microorganisms such as bacteria, fungi, viruses, and parasites relate to health care? Organisms from each of these groups have the potential to cause disease, but how can you systematically study and test for the multitude of organisms found in each of these categories? **Medical microbiology** is dedicated to collecting and identifying disease-producing (pathogenic) organisms and suggesting effective medical treatments. In most community hospitals, medical microbiology departments are housed within the laboratory department, also called division, of the hospital and are often under the direction of the pathology department. Medical microbiology laboratories in university hospitals are usually divided into departments, or sections, that specialize in the following areas:

Bacteriology: This is usually the largest department and is responsible for the growth, isolation, identification, and suggestions for optimal treatment of bacterial infections.

Virology: This department specializes in identification, study, and treatment of viral infections.

Mycology: This area focuses on the identification of fungi, including yeasts and molds that can cause infection.

Parasitology: This area is responsible for identifying specific parasites that may be inhabiting the host's body and adversely affecting physiological functions.

medical microbiology: a branch of medicine and microbiology that deals with the study of microorganisms including bacteria, viruses, fungi, and parasites that are of medical importance and are capable of causing infectious diseases in human beings

bacteriology: scientific study of bacteria

virology [vear RALL oh jee]: the study of viruses and viral diseases

mycology [my CALL uh jee]: the science and study of fungi

parasitology [pair uh sigh TALL uh jee]: the study of parasites and parasitism

Clinical Application

Health Care–Associated Infections (HAIs)

Health care–associated infections (HAIs) are infections that develop in patients who are seeking health care for other reasons. For example, a patient enters the hospital for gallbladder surgery and develops a postoperative wound infection. It is estimated by the Centers for Disease Control and Prevention (CDC, Figure 2-1) that 1 out of every 20 hospitalized patients will develop an HAI. It has been estimated by the CDC that the overall direct medical costs of these infections to U.S. hospitals in 2009 ranged from $35.7 billion to $45 billion. These infections can result in significant disability and even death. Hand hygiene is one of the most important ways health care professionals and patients can prevent HAIs. Hand hygiene consists of either washing visibly soiled hands with soap and water or using an alcohol-based hand rub when hands are not visibly soiled.

Health care–associated infections (HAIs): infections patients get while receitving medical treatment

Media Connection

To view videos on proper hand washing, go to the accompanying online resources.

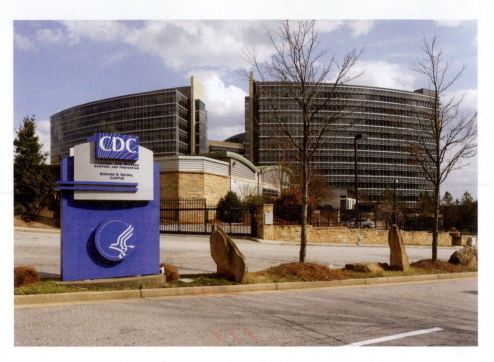

FIGURE 2-1 The Centers for Disease Control and Prevention in Atlanta, Georgia. © Katherine Welles/Shutterstock.com.

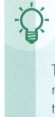 **Learning Hint**

Changing Terms for Changing Times

The older term for health care–associated infections was nosocomial infections. *Nosocomial* referred to hospital-acquired infections, but because infections can be spread in a variety of health care settings outside the hospital, such as nursing homes and dialysis centers, HAIs is becoming the more accepted term.

infection control and prevention: policies and procedures used to minimize the risk of spreading infections, especially in hospitals and human or animal health care facilities

opportunistic infections: any infection that results from a defective immune system that cannot defend against pathogens normally found in the environment

The microbiology department has responsibilities that go beyond isolation, identification of potential pathogens, and suggestion of possible treatments. This department works closely with the department of **infection control and prevention** to monitor for and prevent health care–associated infections (HAIs). These infections must be closely monitored to determine their origin and to prevent further spread, especially in an environment where patients may have compromised immune systems. These patients are very susceptible to **opportunistic infections** that will develop if their immune system and protective normal flora are compromised.

Other Fields and Applications of Microbiology

Even within the medical field, there are subspecialties of microbiology applied to specific areas. For example, the study of the specific antibodies in the blood

TABLE 2-2 Microbiology Fields/Disciplines

Discipline	Area of Study
Bacteriology	Bacteria
Mycology	Fungi
Parasitology	Parasitic protozoa and parasitic animals
Virology	Viruses
Phycology	Algae
Serology	Antibodies within blood and their indication of infection
Immunology	Body's defense against disease, especially at the cellular level
Epidemiology	Disease patterns such as frequency, distribution within a population, and spread of disease
Etiology	Study of causative agent of disease
Anti-infective drug development	Development of drugs used to treat infectious disease
Infection control and prevention	Hygiene issues and standards to prevent health care–acquired infections
Public health microbiology	Examples are sewage treatment, water purification, and insect control
Bioremediation	Use of microbes to remove pollutants
Pharmaceutical microbiology	Produce vaccines and antibodies
Recombinant DNA technology	Alteration of microbial genes to synthesize useful products or treat disease

© 2016 Cengage Learning®.

and how they indicate infection in response to a pathogen is termed **serology**. Microbiology is also used in industries such as pharmaceutical companies to manufacture vaccines. Table 2-2 lists some of the various fields of microbiology.

serology: the scientific study of fluid components of the blood, especially antigens and antibodies

Bacteriology

Let's take a more in-depth look at the four specialties of medical microbiology within the hospital, beginning with the largest: bacteriology. As mentioned earlier, bacteria are prokaryotic cells and are single-cell organisms that have no nucleus. See Figure 2-2A, which shows an example of a bacterial cell. Bacteria reproduce rather easily by a process called **binary fission**. During this process, a bacterial cell copies its DNA and other organelles within the cell, divides the cytoplasm, and splits in half. The ability of cells to make identical copies of themselves without the involvement of another cell is called **asexual reproduction**. In essence, two identical daughter cells result from a single parent cell (Figure 2-2B).

binary fission [BI nuh ree FISH un]: method of asexual reproduction in which DNA is replicated and the cell splits into two genetically identical daughter cells

asexual reproduction: without sex; a mode of reproduction in which offspring arise from a single parent and inherit the genes of that parent only, making the offspring a genetic copy

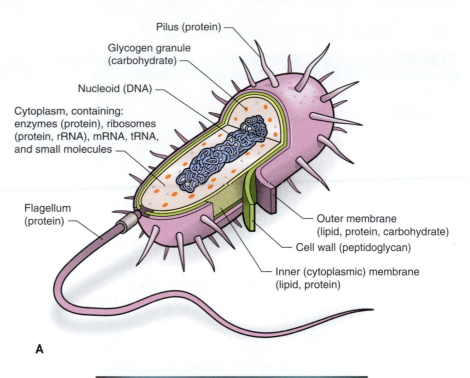

Pilus (protein)

Glycogen granule
(carbohydrate)

Nucleoid (DNA)

Cytoplasm, containing:
enzymes (protein), ribosomes
(protein, rRNA), mRNA, tRNA,
and small molecules

Flagellum
(protein)

Outer membrane
(lipid, protein, carbohydrate)

Cell wall (peptidoglycan)

Inner (cytoplasmic) membrane
(lipid, protein)

A

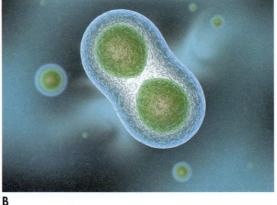

B

FIGURE 2-2 A. Structures of a bacterial cell. © 2016 Cengage Learning®.
B. Binary fission of *Staphylococcus aureus*. © iStock.com/Zinco79

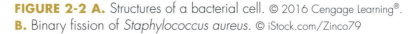

2-1
Stop and Review

1. _____ is the process used by bacteria to
reproduce.

2. The study of specific antibodies in the bloodstream and how they
react during infection is called _____.

3. _____ was a term previously used to
indicate infections acquired from hospitals. This term has been
replaced by the term *health care–associated infections*.

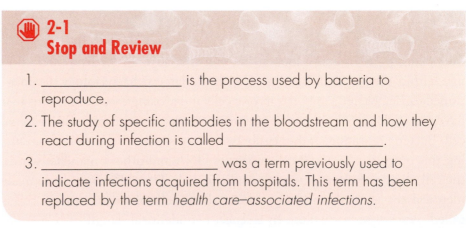

Food for Thought
Mythbuster

Do you think you can prevent the spread of infection using antibacterial products such as soaps or household cleaners? The Food and Drug Administration Nonprescription Drugs Advisory Committee voted unanimously in 2005 that there was a lack of evidence supporting any benefit from these generally more expensive products in our war against the spread of infection. In fact, too much hygiene may be harmful because killing normal flora can leave plenty of room for pathogens to move in.

Many bacteria live within the human body and are either harmless or serve a vital function that is essential for life. For example, normal intestinal bacterial flora helps to digest your food and synthesize vitamin K, which is vital to the blood clotting process.

Naming Bacteria

A binomial (two-name) nomenclature system is used to give names to various types of bacterial cells. The first name is the **genus** or family name (always capitalized), which represents a grouping of various bacteria that possess similar characteristics. The second name is the **species** name (always lowercase), which represents the specific characteristics of that particular bacterium. For example, *Staphylococcus aureus* and *Staphylococcus epidermidis* are both members of the family of bacteria that share the *Staphylococcus* characteristics that we will shortly learn. However, these are two distinct species (*aureus* and *epidermidis*) with unique characteristics that set them apart. As you may have noticed when writing the genus and species names, they should always be italicized.

genus [JEE nus]: in taxonomy, the classification between the family and the species

species [SPEE seas]: a category of classification for living organisms; group is just below the genus

Bacterial Structure and Morphology

As can be seen in Figure 2-2A, a bacterial cell contains a cell membrane, a cell wall, and no nucleus. However, it does contain a nucleus-like (nucleoid) region where the DNA is stored. Some bacteria can form a protective covering around the cell wall known as a **glycocalyx**. A glycocalyx comes in two forms: a **capsule** or a *slime layer*. Either can serve to increase microbial resistance to antibacterial agents. Although many bacteria have no independent forms of locomotion or movement, others do possess short fine filaments called cilia or longer whiplike structures called **flagella** that can

glycocalyx: a thin layer of glycoprotein and oligosaccharides on the outer surface of cell membranes that contributes to cell adhesion and forms antigens involved in the recognition of "self"

capsule: a sheath or continuous enclosure around an organ or structure

flagella [fla JEL ah]: threadlike structures that provide motility for certain bacteria and protozoa and for spermatozoa

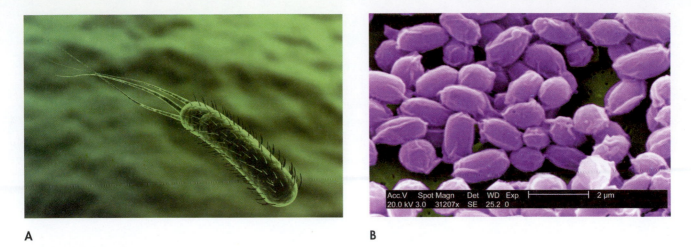

A   **B**

FIGURE 2-3 A. Bacterial flagella. © BioMedical/Shutterstock.com. **B.** Scanning electron micrograph of spores from the Sterne strain of *Bacillus anthracis* bacteria. Notice the wrinkled surface of the protein coat of these bacterial spores. These spores can live for many years, which enables the bacteria to survive in a dormant state. Source: CDC/Laura Rose. Photo credit: Janice Haney Carr.

spores: cells produced by fungi for reproduction; a resistant cell produced by bacteria to withstand extreme heat or cold or dehydration

provide motility. Certain types of bacteria can even go into a state of suspension or inactivity for long periods of time. These bacteria produce **spores**, which are highly resistant forms of the organism that develop in response to adverse environmental conditions. They can then regenerate and become active when the environmental conditions improve. Spores are extremely hard to kill and have been estimated to be able to remain in the dormant state for tens of thousands of years. See Figure 2-3 for examples of flagella and spores.

The morphology, or shape, of bacteria is an important diagnostic tool for identification. The three basic shapes are as follows:

Cocci: round or spherical shaped

cocci [KOK sigh]: a bacterial type that is spherical or ovoid

Bacilli: rod shaped

bacilli [bah SILL eye]: a genus of gram-positive, spore-forming, often aerobic, rod-shaped bacteria in the family *Bacillaceae* that exist singly or in chains and mostly inhabit soil or water

Spirilla: spiral shaped

Cocci

In addition to their basic round shape, cocci bacteria group together in distinct formations and can be named accordingly:

spirilla [spih RILL uh]: flagellated aerobic bacteria with an elongated spiral shape, of the genus *Spirillum*

- *Mono-* means spherical bacteria in single formation

- *Diplo-* refers to bacteria occurring in pairs

- *Strepto-* refers to a formation of bacteria in chain-like structures

- *Staphylo-* literally means "bunch" and refers to bacteria that group together in clusters like a bunch of grapes

Some bacteria with the diplococci shape have been associated with meningitis, pneumonia, and gonorrhea. *Streptococci* cause the familiar strep throat along with specific pneumonias, rheumatic fever, and some skin conditions like impetigo. *Staphylococcus epidermidis* is the normal flora on your skin and mucous membranes of the nose, throat, and intestines, where it does not normally present any problems. However, if you puncture your skin and allow this organism to enter the deeper tissue or bloodstream, a serious infection may result. Another species of the *Staphylococcus* family, *Staphylococcus aureus*, is pyogenic (pus producing) and can cause skin infections that result in abscesses, boils, and carbuncles. Figure 2-4 illustrates bacterial morphology.

Bacilli

The rod-shaped bacteria can possess flagella for motility and can also be found in pairs (diplobacillus) and chains (streptobacillus), as shown in Figure 2-4. *Escherichia coli*, or *E. coli* for short, is the needed normal flora in your intestinal tract. However, if it migrates to the urinary tract because of poor hygiene, it can cause a **urinary tract infection (UTI)**. If *E. coli* enters the bloodstream, it can result in a very serious infection called bacteremia. Bacteremia basically means the microorganisms are multiplying in the bloodstream, which should normally be sterile. Other bacillus-type diseases include typhoid fever, diphtheria, tuberculosis, botulism, and tetanus. Bacilli can form spores and therefore live for a long time in harsh environmental conditions (e.g., within the soil).

urinary tract infection (UTI): infection of the kidneys, ureters, or bladder by microorganisms that either ascend from the urethra or that spread to the kidney from the bloodstream

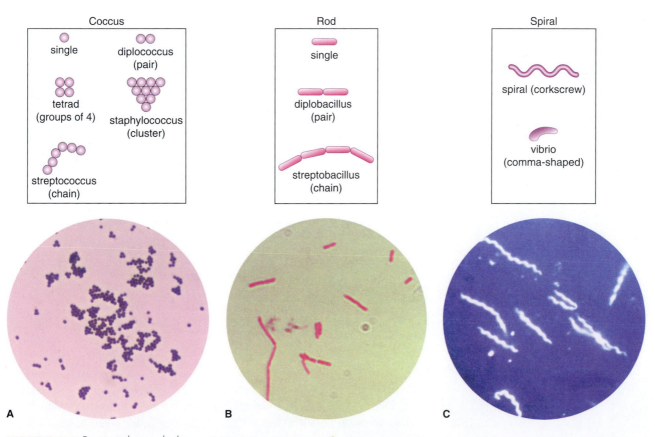

FIGURE 2-4 Bacterial morphology. © 2016 Cengage Learning®.

Spirilla

Spirochetes is another name for these tiny gram-negative organisms that look like corkscrews. Most of the spiral-shaped bacteria are mobile because of their shape (think of the movement produced by a spring coiling and un-coiling) and are responsible for diseases such as syphilis and Lyme disease.

Specimen Collection

Regardless of the specimen type that is collected, the following general guidelines should be maintained to ensure accurate results:

- Specimens ideally should be collected before antibiotics are begun

- Sterile supplies and collection containers should be used (see Figure 2-5 for examples of different transport media and specimen containers)

  ○ The specimen should be collected from the site of infection and not surrounding areas

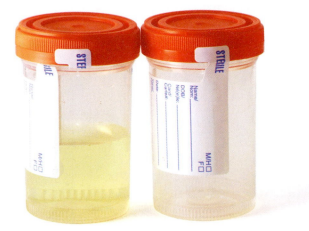

A

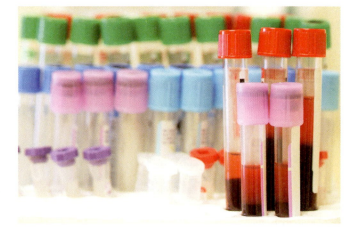

B

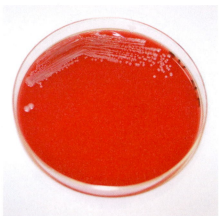

C

FIGURE 2-5 A. Urine specimen containers. © Sylvie Bouchard/Shutterstock .com. **B.** Blood specimen collection containers. © Marinerock/Shutterstock.com. **C.** Petri dish with sheep's blood agar culture media inoculated with *Yersina pestis* bacteria. Source: CDC/Megan Mathias and J. Todd Parker.

- Obtained specimen should be collected and placed in appropriate containers and/or transport media according to protocol

- Collect a sufficient amount of specimen for testing

- Appropriately label each specimen and transport to lab within an appropriate time

Safe collection and handling of specimens is critical for accurate results but also for the prevention of the spread of the disease to other patients or health care workers. One should always assume that all specimens potentially contain harmful pathogens and strictly follow the safety protocols of the institution.

Clinical Application
Specimen Collection

To assist in the diagnosis and treatment of the pathogen creating the disease, proper specimen collection procedures must be followed. The specimen collected can come from many body regions such as wounds; oral, nasal, or genital region; eyes; or ears. In addition, specimen collection can come from body fluids such as urine, blood, sputum, or **cerebral spinal fluid (CSF)**. See Table 2-3, which lists the specimen type or area along with collection considerations and possible pathogens that may be found.

Media Connection

To view a video on specimen collection and processing procedures, go to the accompanying online resources. More specific details on specimen collection will be given in Section II.

cerebral spinal fluid (CSF): The fluid surrounding the brain and spinal cord. A lumbar puncture or spinal tap can be performed to sample CSF fluid to test for the presence of microorganisms

Bacterial Staining

Once the specimen has been collected and processed by the microbiology laboratory, different dyes or stains to color the bacteria are used to make them easier to view under the microscope and to give important information about their classification and treatment. A *simple stain* would allow for contrast to better illustrate the structure and arrangement of bacterial cells.

2-2
Stop and Review

1. List and describe the four areas of medical microbiology.
2. _____ is the most effective way to prevent the spread of infection.
3. Describe the nomenclature system of naming bacteria.
4. Describe the morphology of bacteria.

TABLE 2-3 Sites of Specimen Samples and Potential Pathogens

Specimen Sample	Collection Site/Criteria	Some Possible Pathogens
Blood	Venipuncture or from an indwelling line using strict sterile technique	*Staphylococcus aureus* *Staphylococcus epidermidis* *E. coli* *Pseudomonas* species
Urine	Clean-catch midstream or from indwelling catheter	*E. coli* *Pseudomonas* species *Klebsiella-Enterobacter* species
Sputum	Collected from deep cough	*Streptococcus pneumoniae* *Staphylococcus aureus* *Haemophilus influenzae* *Legionella* species
Cerebrospinal fluid (CSF)	Lumbar puncture	*Streptococcus pneumoniae* *Haemophilus influenzae* *Neisseria meningitides*
Stool	Although sterile container not required, several specimens may be needed and must be sure not to be contaminated with urine	*Salmonella* species *Shigella* species *Giardia* species
Wound	May be aspirated (drawn) from pus-filled area with needle or placing a sterile swab deep within wound	*Staphylococcus aureus* *Streptococcus pyogenes* *E. coli* *Clostridium* species
Nasal	Sterile swab or thin wire in each nostril. Use separate swab per nostril	*Bordetella pertussis* *Staphylococcus aureus*
Throat	Use sterile tongue depressor and swab back of throat and tonsils making sure to avoid the cheeks	*Streptococcus pyogenes* or *group A strep*
Eyes and ears	Sterile swabs are mainly used	*Staphylococcus aureus* *Streptococcus pyogenes* *Haemophilus influenzae*

A *differential stain* would provide more information based on the composition of the bacterial cell wall. A common differential stain developed over 100 years ago, called the **Gram stain**, is still in use today.

The Gram stain technique places the bacteria on a slide and stains them with a purple stain called crystal violet. All organisms will take up this stain and therefore turn purple. Next, the slide is washed with water and then flooded with iodine solution (Gram's iodine) to help the stain adhere better. An alcohol decolorizing rinse is then applied that can wash away the stain depending on the type of bacteria. If the bacteria retain the purple color after the decolorizing rinse, they are called gram-positive or (gram +) bacteria. The slide is then counterstained with a red dye (usually safranin), and those bacteria that decolorized with the alcohol are now colored red or pink. These organisms that stain red or pink are called gram-negative (gram −) bacteria. See Figure 2-6.

Another type of differential stain used on the genus *Mycobacterium,* which is the causative agent of tuberculosis (TB) and leprosy, is the **acid-fast (Ziehl-Neelsen) stain**. Acid-fast organisms resist staining because of a glycolipid (sugar attached to a fat molecule) and a mycolic acid layer that make up the cell wall. Acid-fast bacteria appear red against a blue background because they retain the carbolfuchsin (red) stain that is first applied to them and do not take on the second methylene blue stain. Figure 2-7 illustrates some gram-positive and gram-negative organisms.

Gram stain: a method of differentiating bacterial species into two large groups (gram-positive and gram-negative) based on chemical and physical properties of their cell wall

acid-fast (Ziehl-Neelsen) stain: a bacterial staining procedure in which application of acid-alcohol does not cause decolorization, maintaining a dark stain

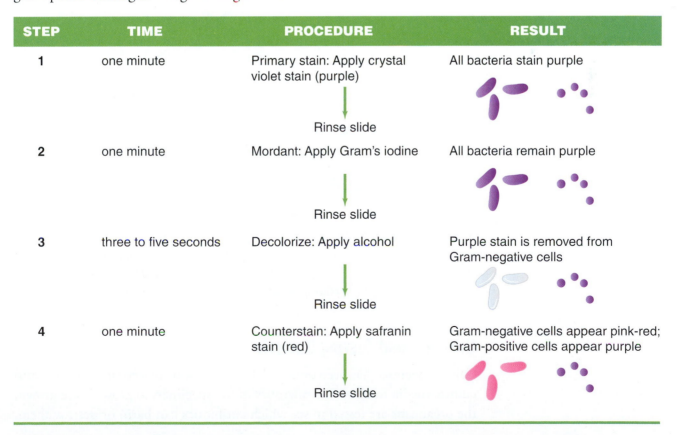

STEP	TIME	PROCEDURE	RESULT
1	one minute	Primary stain: Apply crystal violet stain (purple) ↓ Rinse slide	All bacteria stain purple
2	one minute	Mordant: Apply Gram's iodine ↓ Rinse slide	All bacteria remain purple
3	three to five seconds	Decolorize: Apply alcohol ↓ Rinse slide	Purple stain is removed from Gram-negative cells
4	one minute	Counterstain: Apply safranin stain (red) ↓ Rinse slide	Gram-negative cells appear pink-red; Gram-positive cells appear purple

FIGURE 2-6 Steps in the Gram stain procedure. © Cengage Learning®.

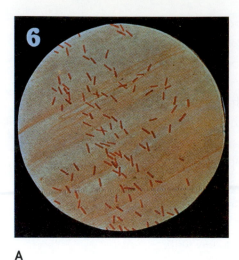

A

B

C

FIGURE 2-7 A. Gram negative *escherichia coli*. Source: Centers for Disease Control, Atlanta, GA. **B.** Gram positive *Staphylococcus* bacteria. Source: CDC/ Dr. Richard Facklam. **C.** Gram positive *streptococci*. © Cengage Learning®.

Clinical Application
The Cell Wall Makes a Difference

The cell wall in gram-negative organisms has three layers, and because many antibacterial agents work by destroying cell wall function, the tougher cell wall of the gram-negative organisms makes them harder to treat.

Growing and Testing Bacteria

Once a specimen has been obtained, it must now be placed (inoculated) onto culture media to allow the microbes in the specimen to grow. Once grown, the organisms are tested to see which antibiotics can harm or destroy them.

The combination of these two tests is called a **culture and sensitivity (C&S) test**. The culture media contain nutrients allowing the organism to grow in sufficient quantities to identify the organism. The sensitivity portion determines which antibiotics may work for treatment by subjecting the cultured organisms to various antibiotic agents to see which will harm or kill them.

Culturing

The culture is a group of microbes (colonies) growing in a nutrient-rich environment. Once collected, the specimen is placed on a culture medium that varies in composition with the needs of specific bacteria. Cultures are usually grown on a clear Petri dish to observe the culture growth without removing the lid to introduce other organisms (contamination). In Figure 2-8 you can also see bacterial colony growth on the nutrient-rich medium of the agar plate. Agar is a gelatin-like substance containing nutrients needed for microbial growth.

The first culture is called the primary culture, and results are usually available after 24–48 hours of **incubation** (growth in a controlled environment). The colonies are observed for differing characteristics, and if more than one organism is identified, it is considered a *mixed culture*. The mixed culture must now be separated into subcultures until each culture yields a *pure culture* containing only one microorganism species.

Most culture media contain simple nutrients such as water, carbon, hydrogen, nitrogen, oxygen, sulfur, calcium, potassium, and magnesium along with complex nutrients such as sugar, amino acids, and blood products. The media type can be a liquid broth, a semisolid, or a solid known as agar.

Inoculating the media means that the microbes from the original sampling instrument such as a swab must now be placed on the growth medium. It is often spread or streaked on the Petri dish or plate in a specific pattern that divides the plate into four quadrants (Figure 2-9). The culture plate

culture and sensitivity (C&S) test: a diagnostic lab procedure used to identify the type of bacteria or fungi and to determine which antimicrobials can successfully fight an infection by collecting urine, blood, or other body fluid and culturing it in a medium and analyzing for antimicrobial susceptibility

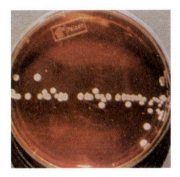

FIGURE 2-8 Agar culture with bacterial colonies. © Cengage Learning®.

incubation: the interval between exposure to infection and the appearance of the first symptom

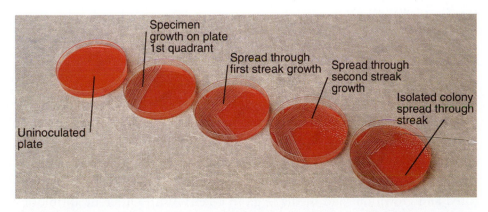

Specimen growth on plate 1st quadrant

Spread through first streak growth

Spread through second streak growth

Isolated colony spread through streak

Uninoculated plate

FIGURE 2-9 Streaking and inoculating patterns on blood agar. © Cengage Learning®.

Clinical Application
Choosing the Right Antimicrobial

Even though the term is a general term meaning "against life," *antibiotics* are used to treat bacterial infections only. You will shortly learn there are other specific antimicrobial agents to treat parasites (antiparasitic), viruses (antiviral), and fungi (antifungal).

It is best to collect the sample of material from the infected area before an antibiotic is started, or you may not be able to grow and identify the pathogen. In patient care situations, antibiotics are often started before the results of laboratory tests are available. For serious infections, it is important to start the right antibiotic as soon as possible, sometimes even before culture material is obtained, and to adjust the drug or dose once a more precise diagnosis is available.

is then placed in an incubator bottom up to prevent condensation from dripping onto the colonies. The incubator provides a stable temperature and humidity level for optimal growth.

Identification

Now that specific colonies of microorganisms have been isolated, initial examination and staining can be done to identify the unknown pathogen. Pathogens are identified by their appearance (morphology); growth requirements; biochemical tests; and, more recently, by their DNA. Preliminary, also called presumptive, identification of the organism usually takes 1 or 2 days to identify the microorganism family. Identifying the exact species of the organism may require additional hours or days after the presumptive identification.

Susceptibility Testing

After an organism is identified, its susceptibility to antibiotics may need to be determined to adjust or change antibiotic therapy if necessary. If a microorganism is susceptible to an antibiotic, the antibiotic has a better chance of fighting the infection than if it is not susceptible. There are several methods by which microbial susceptibility may be determined. We will review disk diffusion, broth dilution, and automated methods.

Disk diffusion (Bauer-Kirby test) is a classic laboratory technique that provides qualitative information about susceptibility. The bacteria are cultured and grown on solid media (e.g., in a Petri dish). Different antibiotic-containing paper disks are then placed on the "lawn" of bacteria. The bacteria

disk diffusion: test that uses antibiotic-impregnated wafers to test whether particular bacteria are susceptible to specific antibiotics

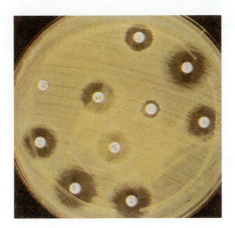

FIGURE 2-10 Disk diffusion showing culture lawn strewn with various antibiotic disks. Notice the bacteria are totally resistant to the antibiotic on the disk at the 10 o'clock position (no zone of inhibition). The other antibiotics have varying degrees of effectiveness; the ones with the largest zones of inhibition are the most effective. © Cengage Learning®.

will not grow near the specific antibiotic disks to which they are sensitive, and therefore there will be a zone of no growth surrounding those disks. The areas without bacterial growth, known as the "zone of inhibition," are measured and compared with established standards to determine whether it is sensitive (the antibiotic will work), intermediate (the antibiotic may or may not work), or resistant (the antibiotic will not work). See Figure 2-10. This method of testing is inexpensive and easy to perform, but it is labor intensive and cannot be used for slow-growing bacteria.

Broth dilution is a second, commonly used clinical method for determining bacterial sensitivity to an antimicrobial agent. This type of testing is more quantitative than the disk diffusion method; that is, it can identify more accurately the concentration or dosage of a drug needed to inhibit organism growth. The organism is placed in various test tubes containing defined concentrations of an antimicrobial agent (different drug doses) and a liquid growth medium. The test tubes are incubated for a designated amount of time and then visually inspected for organism growth. The test tube with the lowest concentration of antimicrobial agent that inhibits the growth of the organism is referred to as the *minimal inhibitory concentration, or MIC* (Figure 2-11).

Note that the MIC does not provide information about whether the organism is actually killed. The *minimum bactericidal concentration* or *MBC* determines this information. MBC determines its killing activity associated with an antimicrobial. The MBC is determined by taking a sample from each clear MIC tube and culturing it on agar plates. The concentration in which no significant bacterial growth is observed is the MBC (see Figure 2-11).

broth dilution: process of taking a known concentration and doing several serial dilutions to determine the lowest concentration needed to inhibit or kill bacteria

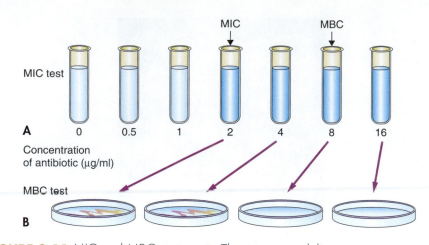

FIGURE 2-11 MIC and MBC testing: **A.** The minimum inhibitory concentration (MIC) is 2 micrograms/mL as shown in the middle tube. **B.** The minimum bactericidal concentration (MBC) is at 8 micrograms/mL where you see no growth in the agar plate. © 2016 Cengage Learning®.

If the MIC is identified at an antibiotic concentration that cannot be safely achieved in the patient, then the organism is considered resistant. If the MIC is identified at a clinically achievable level, the organism is considered sensitive. If the MIC is identified at a level that may or may not be clinically achievable, the organism is considered intermediate.

We are a society of automation, and antimicrobial susceptibility testing is no exception. The previously discussed methods are somewhat labor intensive and take more time than **automated** methods. There are several

automated: to install automatic procedures

empiric therapy: use of antimicrobials to treat an infection before the specific causative organism has been identified with laboratory tests

Clinical Application
Educated Guess

If a patient has an infection, especially if the infection is serious, antibiotics must be started quickly, and they must be the right antibiotics up front to prevent patient harm or death. Starting antibiotics before the actual organism is known is called **empiric therapy**. You can think of this as the best guess given the information/situation at hand. The clue to start the right antibiotic is provided to the clinician by the type or location of the suspected infection, the usual kind of bacteria found for that infection, and the local bacterial resistance patterns in the community where the patient and hospital reside. Once the organism has been identified and the susceptibility to antibiotics is known, the therapy may be modified based on this information if necessary. See Table 2-4, which shows common diseases or clinical situations along with the major suspected bacterial cause that would guide empirical therapy.

TABLE 2-4 Gram Stain Reaction of Medically Related Bacteria

Gram Positive (+)	Disease
Staphylococcus aureus	Skin and wound infections, pneumonia, septicemia
Staphylococcus epidermidis	Wound and HAI
Streptococcus pyogenes (group A strep)	Pharyngitis (acute sore throat)
Streptococcus pneumoniae (diplococci)	Pneumonia, meningitis
Bacillus anthracis	Anthrax
Clostridium tetani	Tetanus (lockjaw)
Gram Negative (−)	**Disease**
Escherichia coli (E. coli)	Urinary tract infections and sepsis
Neisseria species	Meningitis and gonorrhea
Haemophilus influenza	Sinusitis, pneumonia, otitis media (middle ear infection)
Vibrio species (bacilli)	Cholera
Salmonella species	Typhoid fever and food poisoning
Legionella (bacilli)	Pneumonia (Legionnaires' disease)
Shigella species (bacilli)	Dysentery

© 2016 Cengage Learning®.

companies that manufacture machines approved by the Food and Drug Administration (FDA), and this method of detecting antibiotic susceptibility is widely used in hospitals. These machines all use some form of optical detection to observe changes in bacterial growth. Trays or small cards are used to perform multiple antibiotic susceptibility tests at the same time against the pathogen. The results of this method of testing are usually reported in less than 24 hours. Microbiology laboratory computers are often linked with these machines so the clinical team can receive the susceptibility report quickly. Of course, we never get something for nothing. These machines are expensive and cannot detect certain forms of resistance in bacteria that are becoming more common.

Bacterial Disease

Although bacteria can cause disease directly by destroying infected tissue, many bacteria cause disease because of the release of toxins into the host body. The two types of toxins produced by bacteria are exotoxins and endotoxins. **Exotoxins** are proteins that can be secreted outside (exo) the cell by

exotoxin: a poisonous substance produced by certain bacteria

endotoxin: a lipopolysaccharide that is part of the cell wall of gram-negative bacteria released after the cell's death

both gram-positive and gram-negative bacteria. An **endotoxin** is the actual portion of the outer cell membrane that can be shed in small quantities by living bacteria or released in large quantities when bacteria are destroyed by antibiotics or immune system cells. Endotoxins are only found in gram-negative bacteria with one exception: *Listeria,* which is gram-positive.

Toxins can cause many problems including destruction of body tissues, destruction of blood cells, inhibition of ribosomes, fluid loss, high fever, decreased blood pressure, increased blood clotting, fluid in lungs, and paralysis. Signs and symptoms of bacterial infection may include high fever; rapid pulse and breathing; abnormal, often foul-smelling discharge from the infected area; and pain and swelling at the site of infection. Other symptoms depend on the location of the infection. Bacterial infections are treated with antibiotics—chemicals that can kill the prokaryotic bacteria without harming eukaryotic cells.

General Principles of Antibiotic Therapy

With the discovery of penicillin in the 1940s, the antibiotic era began. Antibiotic availability and widespread use have been both a tremendous benefit and a burden to medical care. The beneficial effects are clear in the number of lives that have been spared. The burden has presented itself with a vengeance in the last several decades with the evolution of pathogens that are able to resist the effects of many antibiotic agents.

antibiotic: a natural or synthetic substance that destroys microorganisms or inhibits their growth to prevent or treat infection in plants, animals, and humans

A chemotherapeutic substance derived from a living organism that kills microorganism growth is an **antibiotic**. *Antibiotic* is a general term derived from the Greek roots *anti-* ("against") and *bios* ("life"). The term *antibiotic* was meant to distinguish between chemical therapeutic agents and those that come from living organisms such as penicillin. Nowadays, drugs are made mainly in the lab, and the terms are used interchangeably. Traditionally, antibiotics refer to drugs for treating bacterial infections.

Antibiotic Classification

bacteriostatic [BACK teer ee oh STAT ik]: inhibiting the growth of bacteria

bactericidal [back TEER ih SIGH dul]: capable of killing bacteria

There are many ways to classify antibiotics. Antibiotics are classified as either bacteriostatic or bactericidal. **Bacteriostatic** agents inhibit the replication of microorganisms and prevent the growth of the organisms without destroying them. **Bactericidal** drugs actively kill bacteria. Most antibiotics are bacteriostatic at low concentrations, but at higher concentrations, bactericidal activity is more likely to be present.

Antibiotics can also be classified according to whether they are *broad spectrum* or *narrow spectrum*. Broad-spectrum antibiotics are effective against a wider range of bacteria than are narrow-spectrum antibiotics.

Another classification of bacteria is based on bacteria's need for oxygen. If a bacterium needs oxygen to survive, it is **aerobic**. If it does not, it is called **anaerobic**. Fewer antibiotic options are available to treat anaerobic infections, and those infections can be more serious. Remember that gram-negative infections, as a general rule, are harder to treat than gram-positive infections because of the gram negative microorganism's multi-layered cell wall.

The development of so-called "super-bacteria" has been facilitated by the widespread misuse of antibiotics for infections of viral origin (e.g., common colds and influenza) and the continued use of broad-spectrum agents in the treatment of infections caused by single organisms, in which case a narrow-spectrum agent would do. Use of an antibiotic effective against a wide range of microorganisms (**broad-spectrum drug**) can result in overkill if a drug effective against fewer microorganisms (**narrow-spectrum drug**) would be just as effective. Such use has resulted in selective evolution of bacteria that have developed **resistance** to certain antibiotics, leaving physicians with limited options for the management of some infections.

Resistance to antibiotics develops in many ways. One example is when the drug is destroyed by bacterial enzymes. Bacteria that produce the enzyme beta-lactamase can make the antibiotic penicillin group of drugs inactive. Another method for resistance to occur is when some organisms develop enzymes that bind to the drug and prevent the drug from attaching to the binding site of the bacteria.

Resistance also develops when patients do not finish an antibiotic treatment course. It is rather common for patients to stop taking the drug once they begin to feel better. Think about this possible mechanism for resistance to occur. If you discontinue use of an antibiotic as soon as you feel better, the drug may have just destroyed enough of the weaker pathogens to give you symptomatic relief. However, there are still some minimal pathogenic bacteria remaining that haven't yet been killed and therefore represent a stronger strain. Now that the antibiotic has been prematurely discontinued, these stronger pathogens can now multiply, and once they reach a certain level, the symptoms reappear. Now, however, when the drug is restarted it must contend with an overall stronger version of the pathogen.

aerobic [air ROW bick]: in the presence of oxygen

anaerobic [an uh ROW bick]: in the absence of oxygen

broad-spectrum drug: drug that acts on a wide range of disease-causing bacteria

narrow-spectrum drug: effective against specific families of bacteria

resistance: a lack of response of a pathogen to treatment such as antibiotic therapy

Media Connection

To view a video on antimicrobial resistance, go to the accompanying online resources. You can also visit http://www.fda.gov for more information. Click on the Animal & Veterinary tab at the top. Then click on the link for Safety & Health. Follow the link in the left navigation box to Antimicrobial Resistance. To the right you will see a Spotlight box with a link to an Animation of Antimicrobial Resistance.

2-3 Stop and Review

1. Contrast gram-negative and gram-positive bacteria.
2. A(n) _____ is the process of growing bacteria for purposes of identification. _____ testing is used to determine the susceptibility of the bacteria to various antibiotics.
3. Contrast bacteriostatic and bactericidal agents.
4. Why is it important to refrain from taking antibiotics for viral infections?

Chapter Summary

- This chapter laid the foundation for you to understand medical microbiology. Remember, the purpose of medical microbiology is to study microbes that produce disease.

- Within the medical microbiology umbrella, numerous specialty areas exist such as bacteriology, virology, parasitology, and so on. The hospital microbiology department generally works very closely with the infection control and prevention department to help identify and control infections.

- We discussed how organisms are identified and named. Organisms have two names: one each for genus and species. We presented the shape (morphology) and structure of bacteria and how this helps us to identify the organism prior to growing it.

- We elaborated on the basic principles of specimen collection. It should be clear that this is a very important function because patient care decisions are often based on specimens collected to assist in the diagnosis of infectious diseases.

- Once the specimen is collected, we discussed how it is processed by the microbiology laboratory including staining the collected material, identifying the bacteria causing disease, and then finally methods for detecting bacterial susceptibility.

- Antibiotics that inhibit the growth of bacteria are called bacteriostatic, and those that result in cell death are termed bactericidal.

- We finished with a discussion of bacterial resistance, which no chapter on medical microbiology would be complete without. Although we cannot stop the development of resistance, the principles discussed in this chapter concerning the stewardship of antimicrobials should help readers assist in the proper use of these important medications in the hope that resistance can be delayed.

Case Study

An 89-year-old gentleman presents to the emergency room with a chief complaint of cough, shortness of breath, and fever with shaking chills. You are the allied health professional assisting the emergency room team in his care. His chest x-ray is suggestive of pneumonia (lung infection). Sputum and blood cultures are obtained, and the emergency room physician orders an antibiotic to be given STAT (immediately). The microbiology lab Gram stains the sputum culture and reports that they see many gram-positive diplococci. What organism is the likely cause of this patient's pneumonia? Why is it important to start the right antibiotic as soon as possible?

Chapter Review

Match the organism with its morphology.

1. _____ *Staphylococcus aureus*
2. _____ *E. coli*
3. _____ Enterococci
4. _____ Legionella
5. _____ *Haemophilus influenzae*
6. _____ *Streptococcus pneumoniae*
7. _____ *Clostridium tetani*

a. gram-positive coccobacillus
b. gram-positive diplococci
c. gram-negative bacilli
d. gram-positive cocci

Match the specimen sample with the pathogen that may be found.

8. _____ Blood
9. _____ Cerebrospinal fluid
10. _____ Urine
11. _____ Lung
12. _____ Stool
13. _____ Throat
14. _____ Wound

a. *Streptococcus pneumoniae*
b. *Staphylococcus aureus*
c. *Giardia*
d. *E. coli*
e. *Neisseria meningitidis*
f. *Clostridium* species
g. *Streptococcus pyogenes*

Answer the following questions and fill in the blanks as required.

15. What is the difference between an endotoxin and an exotoxin?

16. Discuss the difference between MIC and MBC.

17. Discuss the signs and symptoms of a bacterial infection.

18. _____ is the study of parasites.

19. _____ and _____ are two structures that help bacteria move.

20. If bacteria require oxygen to exist, then they are called _____.

21. _____ may be secreted by both gram-negative and gram-positive bacteria, but _____ is mainly secreted by gram-negative bacteria.

22. If bacteria are not sensitive to a particular antimicrobial or class of antimicrobials, they are called _____.

23. The _____ variable is what is being tested or changed and the _____ variable is what is observed or measured.

Match the term with its definition.

24. _____ scientific inquiry

25. _____ comparative research

26. _____ descriptive research

27. _____ experimental research

a. adding to the body of knowledge by making careful observations

b. adding to the body of knowledge by manipulating and controlling variables

c. planned and deliberate investigation of the natural world

d. assessing the results of different situations, therapies, or conditions

Additional Activities

1. Contact your local hospital's microbiology department and see if its employees would be willing to provide you with the hospital's antibiogram. This document, often produced as a pocket card that clinicians can carry in their lab coats, will give you clues as to how well certain antibiotics work in your local area. If you are unable to obtain an antibiogram from a hospital, see if you can find one on the Web. Find a common pathogen such as *E. coli* and look at the susceptibility of the organism to various antibiotics.

2. Research the history of the development of antibiotics. What was the first class of antibiotics that was available? Were these antibiotics bacteriostatic or bactericidal against pathogens?

3. Invite a pharmacist who works in a hospital to discuss how bacterial resistance is affecting the care of patients in your area.

Media Connection

Go to the accompanying online resources and have fun learning as you play games, view animations and videos, and take practice tests to help reinforce key concepts you learned in this chapter.

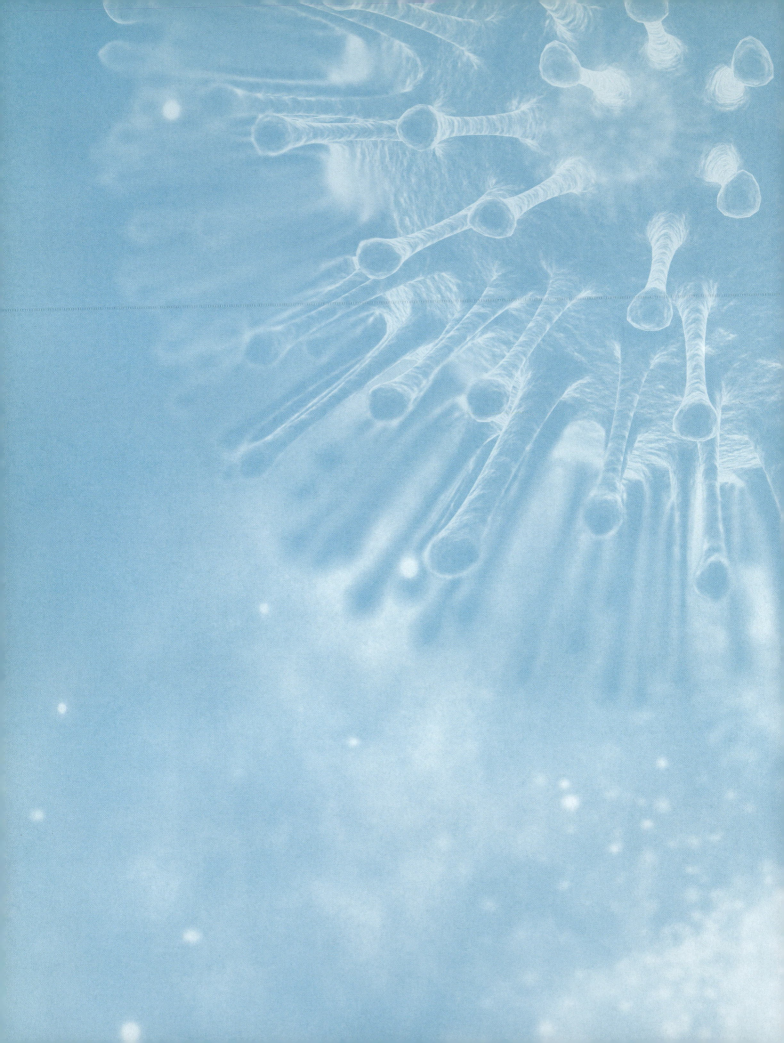

More Medical Microbiology Specialties

OBJECTIVES

After studying this chapter, the learner will be able to:

- List and define additional areas of medical microbiology specialization and study to include virology, mycology, and parasitology.

- Differentiate among parasites, fungi, viruses, and prions.

- Relate diseases caused by parasites, fungi, viruses, and prions.

- Describe medical treatments for microbial infections related to parasites, fungi, viruses, and prions.

KEY TERMS

acquired immunodeficiency syndrome (AIDS)

amebiasis
   [ah me BUY uh sis]

artificial immunity

Aspergillus

blastomycosis
   [blas toe my KOH sis]

capsid

coccidioidomycosis
   [KOK sid ee oy dough my KOH sis]

dermatophytes
   [der MAT uh fites]

dimorphic
   [di MORE fic]

Ebola virus

ectoparasites
   [eck toe PAIR uh sites]

ergosterol

Giardia
   [jee ARE dee uh]

helminths
   [HELL minths]

hepatitis C virus (HCV)

histoplasmosis
   [his toe plaz MO sis]

hookworm

human immunodeficiency virus (HIV)

immunization

influenza

latency

malaria

molds

mucormycosis
   [mu core my KOH sis]

mycology
   [my CALL uh jee]

natural active immunity

(Continues)

KEY TERMS *(Continued)*

parasitology
[pair uh sigh TALL uh jee]

pinworm

prion [PRI on]

protozoa
[pro tah ZOE uh]

**respiratory syncytial
virus** [sin SISH ul]

**severe acute respiratory
syndrome (SARS)**

spores

tapeworm

vaccines

viral load

virology [vear RALL oh jee]

virus

yeasts

Introduction

In this chapter, we continue to explore the various medical microbiology subspecialties beyond bacteriology. We visit the exciting fields of virology, mycology, and parasitology. Next, we discuss the microbes responsible for disease in humans. You will notice, with the exception of treatments for the virus responsible for causing acquired immunodeficiency syndrome (AIDS), the drugs used to treat diseases caused by these microbes are not as numerous as those for bacterial infections. Finally, we finish the chapter with some information concerning diseases caused by infectious particles called prions.

We discussed bacteria in Chapter 2, and our focus in this chapter turns to viruses, molds and yeasts, parasites, and prions. As you will soon see, when a virus invades the body it often produces disease and then the body's immune system either eliminates or controls it. Some viruses may remain dormant in our body and sometimes cause disease later in life (e.g., shingles after you have had chickenpox). Yeasts or molds may set up residence in humans after treatment with antibiotics has wiped out their normal flora. This may cause serious disease, especially in patients with compromised immune systems. Parasites are microbes that live on or in another organism. Prions infect the nervous system in humans, and when symptoms of this infection are present, death usually occurs within a year.

Virology

virology [vear RALL oh jee]:
the study of viruses and viral diseases

Viruses are the most common infectious agents in humans and **virology** is the branch of science that studies them. Viruses (from a Latin term meaning "poison") are infectious particles that have a core containing genetic material (codes to replicate) surrounded by a protective protein coat called a **capsid**. A **virus** is an obligate parasite, which means it can only replicate in a living host cell. This makes it difficult to eradicate the virus without harming the host cell. Because this is a different situation than with bacteria, different drugs are needed to treat viruses than bacteria. Viruses come in all shapes and sizes and are so small (0.02–0.03 microns) that they can only be seen under a powerful electron microscope. They contain no organelles and are basically a protein coat that covers a single strand or strands of DNA or RNA (Figure 3-1).

Viruses are classified by whether they contain RNA or DNA. RNA viruses cause diseases such as influenza, polio, acquired immunodeficiency syndrome (AIDS), rabies, and encephalitis. DNA viruses cause the common cold, cold sores, warts, and infectious mononucleosis.

Viruses cause disease in two ways: directly, by shutting down a cell or destroying the cell outright (cell lysis); or indirectly, by reproducing within the cell and then bursting out of the host cell to go and infect other cells. Diseases caused by viruses (e.g., influenza) may make a host more susceptible to other infectious diseases by making a favorable environment for the development of secondary bacterial or fungal infections. For example, influenza (the flu) rarely kills people. The leading cause of death as a result of the flu is bacterial pneumonia, which can easily infect lung tissue damaged by the flu virus.

Signs and symptoms of viral infection include low-grade fever (although it may also be high sometimes), muscle aches, and general fatigue, although some viral infections may cause no symptoms. Most viruses will be destroyed by the immune system within a few days of infection. The typical treatment

capsid: the protein covering around the central core of a virus that protects the nucleic acids in the core and promotes attachment of the virus to susceptible cells

virus: a pathogen composed of nucleic acid within a protein shell that can grow and reproduce only after infecting a host cell

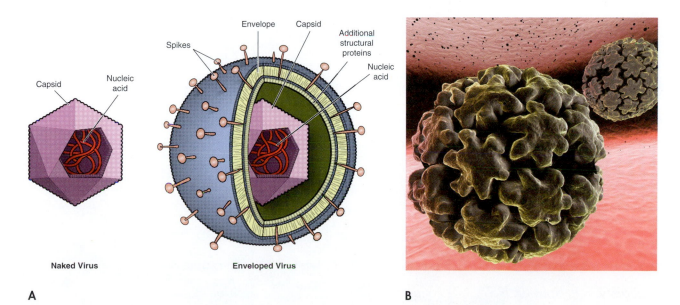

A **B**

FIGURE 3-1 A. Schematic representation of a virus. © 2016 Cengage Learning®. **B.** The human papillomavirus (HPV). © Michael Taylor/Shutterstock.com.

natural active immunity: an active immunity acquired by experiencing and having recovered from a disease

artificial immunity: deliberate exposure of antigen to develop immunity such as in immunizations

immunization: the protection of individuals or groups from specific diseases by vaccination or the injection of immune globulins

vaccine: any suspension containing antigenic molecules derived from a microorganism, given to stimulate an immune response to an infectious disease

for some viral infections is rest, fluids, and treatment of symptoms to keep the patient comfortable.

You can acquire immunity in several different ways. **Natural active immunity** is acquired in the course of daily life. When you catch a virus or a bacterium, your immune system fights it off, and memory cells are created for the next meeting. Anybody old enough to have had the chickenpox as a child (before the vaccine became available) is usually protected from a second round of chickenpox. **Artificial immunity** is acquired during **immunizations**, and the immunity produced may be either *active* or *passive*.

Vaccines have become the mainstay preventative treatment of many of the viral infections such as influenza, measles, mumps, polio, hepatitis A and B, and rubella. For example, getting a measles vaccine exposes you to small amounts of weakened virus, not enough to make you sick, but enough for your immune system to be alerted and create memory cells. If you meet the virus later in life, you will be able to fight it off and not become ill. See Table 3-1, which gives common viruses, their resulting condition, and if vaccines exist. Immunity achieved through vaccination is called *artificial active immunity*.

TABLE 3-1 Virus, Resulting Disease, and Artificial Immunization Status

Virus	Disease	Immunization Exists
Rhinovirus or *coronavirus*	Common cold	No
Influenza A,B	Viral flu	Yes
Hepatitis A virus (HAV)	Hepatitis A	Yes
Hepatitis B virus (HBV)	Hepatitis B	Yes
Hepatitis C virus (HCV)	Hepatitis C	No
Varicella zoster virus	Chickenpox and shingles	Yes
Epstein Barr virus (EBV)	Infectious mononucleosis	No
Human immunodeficiency virus (HIV)	Acquired immunodeficiency syndrome (AIDS)	No
Human papillomavirus (HPV)	Genital, common, and plantar warts	Yes
Herpes simplex virus-1	Fever blisters, genital herpes	No
Herpes simplex virus-2	Genital herpes, fever blisters	In progress
Respiratory syncytial virus (RSV)	Croup, bronchitis	No

Food for Thought

Where Viruses Can Hide

Herpes and HIV can inhabit host cells in the body and remain undetectable for a long period of time. They can then resurface after the initial transmission and cause disease at a later point in time.

If you dissect this term, it means that an "artificial" vaccine induces our immune systems to "actively" produce an immune response. As of the writing of this text, vaccines were being tested for the Ebola virus that was severely affecting West Africa and had cases spread for the first time to the United States.

Artificial passive immunity involves the administration of antibodies that have already been produced from either humans or animals. This type of immunity offers short-term protection only, so it is rarely recommended. It may be used in either people with deficient immune systems who cannot produce their own antibodies or occasionally for health care workers, international travelers, or pregnant women.

Only recently have more antiviral drugs become available for diseases such as the HIV and hepatitis C viruses. Viral infections are classified by their severity, length of time present, and body parts affected. Infections such as the common cold and influenza can be acute and quickly resolve in 7–14 days, or they can be slow and have a progressive course, as with HIV. Viral infections can be local and just affect the respiratory tract, for example, or generalized and spread throughout the bloodstream. Some viruses can be dormant and then under certain conditions reproduce again. This is called **latency** and implies that a disease may surface years after transmission or after the initial breakout.

latency: state of being concealed, delayed, dormant, or inactive

Viral Identification

Several methods exist to isolate and identify viruses and are often done at large medical laboratories. Identification can be accomplished by the following methods:

Cell culture: Viruses are grown in a layer or suspension of living tissues (because they require a host cell) and then are identified under electron microscopy because of their very small size. Figure 3-2 contrasts the relative size of viruses, bacteria, and human cells. This technique is usually only performed in university research laboratories or at the Centers for Disease Control and Prevention (CDC).

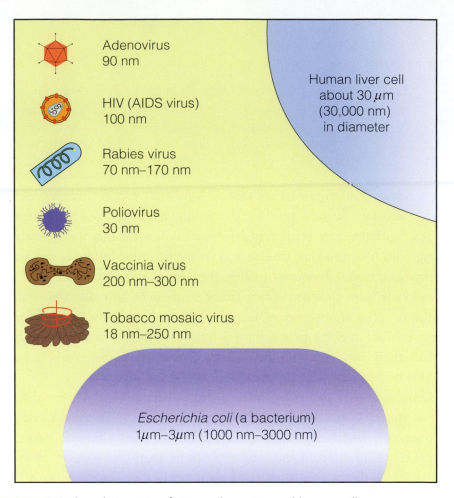

Adenovirus
90 nm

HIV (AIDS virus)
100 nm

Rabies virus
70 nm–170 nm

Poliovirus
30 nm

Vaccinia virus
200 nm–300 nm

Tobacco mosaic virus
18 nm–250 nm

Human liver cell
about 30 μm
(30,000 nm)
in diameter

Escherichia coli (a bacterium)
1μm–3μm (1000 nm–3000 nm)

FIGURE 3-2 The relative size of viruses, bacteria, and human cells. © 2016 Cengage Learning®.

Direct detection: The viral antigen is detected in the specimen showing that the patient was exposed to the virus. There are several methods for direct viral detection. They include:

- Isolation in cell culture

- Electron microscopy examination of specimen

- Immunofluorescence staining of specimen and microscopic examination

- Enzyme immunoassay (detects presence of antigen)

- Polymerase chain reaction (detects presence of DNA)

Multipathogen detection systems: These testing systems can test for numerous viral pathogens at the same time. Two systems are currently approved by the Food and Drug Administration in the United States for clinical testing. See Table 3-2 for an explanation of how these systems work. These tests may help clinicians reduce the unnecessary use of

TABLE 3-2 How Multipathogen Viral Detection Systems Work

Step 1. A health care professional collects a sample from the patient's nose, throat, sinuses, or lungs.
Step 2. The viral RNA is used to produce DNA, which is more stable for testing.
Step 3. The DNA is "amplified" by making multiple copies using PCR (polymerase chain reaction) technology.
Step 4. The "amplified" DNA is mixed with short sequences of DNA from each virus the test can identify. This "TAGS" the viral DNA.
Step 5. Color-coded beads are added that bind to the TAGS.
Step 6. Samples are then placed in an instrument, and the color-coded beads are read and analyzed by lasers.
Step 7. The lasers identify the color of a bead, which is specific to a particular virus. If a particular virus is present, a signal is generated.
Step 8. If a signal is generated, software analyzes the signal and identifies the virus.

*For a video demonstrating Luminex Corporation's multipathogen detection system, visit http://www.luminexcorp.com.
© 2016 Cengage Learning®.

antibiotics. If you can determine a patient has a viral instead of a bacterial infection, then you can withhold antibiotics, hopefully contributing to a reduction in resistance.

Serodiagnosis: Virus antibodies are detected in serum by special serology testing. There are several serology techniques that can be used depending on the suspected antibodies. Because serology tests are labor-intensive, they have been largely replaced when possible by newer tests such as the ELISA (enzyme-linked immunosorbent assay) and EIA (enzyme immunoassay) which detect specific viral proteins.

If a patient is infected with HIV, hepatitis B, or hepatitis C, the amount of virus circulating in the bloodstream can be counted or quantified. This is called the **viral load**. The higher the viral load (e.g., the amount can be in the millions), the more likely the patient will be ill from the virus. Once treatment is started, the viral load can be followed because it should decrease over time to undetectable levels if the therapy is successful. Unfortunately, this does not mean the patient is virus free. Residual virus can hide within the cells and not circulate, or our current detection methods are just not sensitive enough to detect small amounts of virus still circulating in the blood.

viral load: a measure of the total body burden of viral particles present in human blood; the greater the number, usually, the sicker the patient

Antiviral Agents

Antiviral agents can also help in the treatment of **influenza**. "The flu" is a common viral respiratory infection caused by different strains of the influenza

influenza: an acute contagious respiratory infection marked by fever, chills, muscle aches, headache, prostration, runny nose, watering eyes, cough, and sore throat

Clinical Application
Antiviral Therapy

Antivirals do not typically cure the disease but lessen the severity or keep the infection under control. Herpes can be treated with antiviral medications. Herpes simplex is a DNA virus that can cause the vesicular skin eruption most people know as fever blisters or cold sores. It can also cause genital herpes, which can be spread by sexual contact with an infected person. Other organ-system infections caused by the herpes simplex virus-1 include the eye, skin, central nervous system (encephalitis), and rarely the liver. The main drugs to lessen the severity of herpes are acyclovir (Zovirax), famciclovir (Famvir), and valacyclovir (Valtrex). These drugs interfere with viral DNA and inhibit viral replication.

virus. Certain patients are at higher risk for complications from influenza. These include the elderly, diabetics, and patients with cardiac, renal, and respiratory problems. Influenza agents include amantadine (Symmetrel), rimantadine (Flumadine), zanamivir (Relenza), and oseltamivir (Tamiflu). Zanamivir and oseltamivir are active against influenza types A and B, whereas amantadine and rimantadine are only active against type A influenza.

Respiratory syncytial virus (RSV) is a pathogen causing bronchiolitis and pneumonia and is a major cause of acute respiratory disease in children. Ribavirin is an antiviral with inhibitory activity against respiratory syncytial virus (RSV), influenzas A and B, and herpes simplex. Although its actual mechanism is not known, it inhibits essential nucleic acid formation in viral particles. It is generally reserved to treat infections in children who are immunocompromised with severe RSV lung disease.

Acquired immunodeficiency syndrome (AIDS) used to be a progressively fatal disease of the immune system caused by the retrovirus **human immunodeficiency virus (HIV)**. AIDS is the most advanced stage of HIV infection and is diagnosed when a patient's CD4 (infection-fighting white blood cells of the immune system) T cells decline to less than 200 cells/mm^3 or the patient has an AIDS-defining disease. New treatments for HIV infection prevent the progression of the infection to AIDS. Treatment of HIV infection or AIDS comprises several different drugs to suppress the virus. HIV cannot be cured with treatments available today. In general, most patients are treated with three drugs. Three-drug treatment regimens are required to keep the virus suppressed and to delay the development of drug resistance. It is helpful to think of each drug as the leg of a stool containing three legs. If the patient stops taking one of the medicines or the virus becomes resistant to it (a leg of the stool falls off), then the virus can increase in number and

respiratory syncytial virus (RSV) [sin SISH ul]: virus that causes infection of the lungs and breathing passages

acquired immunodeficiency syndrome (AIDS): a late-stage infection with the human immunodeficiency virus (HIV)

human immunodeficiency virus (HIV): a retrovirus of the subfamily *Lentivirus* that causes acquired immunodeficiency syndrome (AIDS)

TABLE 3-3 Antiretrovirals

Drug Class	Representative Drugs
Entry and Fusion Inhibitors	enfuvirtide, maraviroc
Integrase Inhibitors	raltegravir
Non-nucleoside Reverse Transcriptase Inhibitors	delaviridine, efavirenz, etravirine, nevirapine, rilpivirine
Nucleoside Reverse Transcriptase Inhibitors	abacavir, lamivudine, zidovudine, tenofovir, emtricitabine, stavudine
Protease Inhibitors	atazanavir, darunavir, ritonavir, fosamprenavir, lopinavir, tipranavir

© 2016 Cengage Learning®.

the patient's immune system begins to fail. The drugs used to treat HIV infection are termed *antiretrovirals* (Table 3-3). In addition, several HIV vaccines are undergoing clinical testing.

Hepatitis C virus (HCV) infection in humans is usually without symptoms during the initial or acute stage of the infection, and almost all infected patients progress to a chronic infection because our bodies are unable to clear the virus. Most patients with chronic infection do not have symptoms either, which is why all health care workers must follow strict infection control practices (discussed in chapters to follow) to prevent exposure to blood and accidental needlesticks. Chronic HCV infection can progress to liver cirrhosis and liver cancer. HCV virus has six genetically distinct types labeled Genotypes 1–6. Genotypes are the genetic makeup of an individual organism. Genotypes 1 and 4 are more resistant to treatment with ribavirin and peginterferon alone. Recently, new medicines have been approved to treat HCV, and they are used individually or as add-on therapy to peginterferon and ribavirin. These new treatments have proven effective in eradicating the virus in patients who did not have a response to older therapies or in patients with Genotypes 1 and 4, which as mentioned above, are more difficult to treat. Telaprevir and boceprevir are two protease inhibitors recently approved as add-on therapy to peginterferon and ribavirin. Sofosbuvir is a polymerase inhibitor which is the newest addition to the anti-HCV drug lineup. It may be used in combination with other anti-HCV medicines to treat Genotypes 1–6.

In 2003, an outbreak of a disease known as **severe acute respiratory syndrome (SARS)** made headlines across the globe. The disease was first reported in Asia but rapidly spread to North America, South America, and Europe. This viral respiratory illness was identified as a SARS-associated coronavirus. According to the World Health Organization more than 8,000 people globally were sickened resulting in 774 deaths. Eight of these deaths occurred in the United States in people who had recently traveled to

hepatitis C virus (HCV): a small enveloped, positive-sense single-stranded RNA virus of the family *Flaviviridae* responsible for hepatitis C disease in humans

severe acute respiratory syndrome (SARS): a highly contagious, potentially lethal viral respiratory illness characterized by a fever, cough, difficulty breathing, or hypoxia

another part of the world with SARS. The illness is characterized by fever, headache, body aches, and dry cough. SARS is spread by respiratory droplets when an infected person coughs or sneezes or by touching a surface or object containing these droplets. More recently, in 2012 a viral respiratory illness called Middle East Respiratory Syndrome (MERS) was reported in Saudi Arabia. In 2014 the first imported case of MERS in the United States was confirmed in a traveler from Saudi Arabia. Thirty percent of the people infected with this virus die, and therefore the spread of this virus as well as other deadly viruses such as Ebola are a concern worldwide.

Ebola virus disease, also known as Ebola hemorrhagic fever (EHF) is a disease with a high mortality rate. Signs and symptoms of fever, sore throat, muscle pain, and headache begin between 2 days and 21 days after contracting the virus. Severe vomiting, diarrhea, and rash can follow with the possibility of internal and external bleeding. Death can occur due to dehydration, electrolyte imbalance, kidney or liver failure and low blood pressure. Treatment consists of supportive therapies such as oral rehydration or intravenous fluids. The largest outbreak to date is the 2014 West African outbreak that has resulted in the spread of the disease to other countries to include the United States.

Ebola virus: causative microorganism of Ebola hemorrhagic fever (EHF), a disease with a high mortality rate

3-1
Stop and Review

1. Why is it important to treat HIV infection with at least three medications at once?
2. Why is it important to identify a virus as the cause of illness?
3. _____ is a serious complication that may occur if a patient with HCV infection is left untreated.
4. _____ are generally only cultured in research laboratory settings or the CDC.

parasitology [pair uh sigh TALL uh jee]: the study of parasites and parasitism

protozoa [pro tah ZOE uh]: unicellular protists with animal-like behavior

helminth [HELL minths]: a wormlike animal; any animal, either free-living or parasitic belonging to the phyla *Platyhelminthes*, *Acanthocephala*, *Nemathelminthes*, or *Annelida*

Parasitology

Parasitology is the branch of science that studies parasites, A parasite can be a one-celled (unicellular) or multicellular organism that lives in or on another organism or host at the host's expense. Some parasites can cause illnesses that vary in severity from mild to life threatening. Parasites can exist in many areas of the human body to include blood, bone marrow, liver, spleen, urinary tract, intestines, skin, hair, and so on. The three main classes of parasites that cause disease in humans are **protozoa**, **helminths**, and *ectoparasites*.

Parasites are identified by not only their name but also at their specific stage of development as follows:

Trophozite: motile, multiplying form (feeding and growing stage)

Cyst: dormant form

Ova: eggs of specific parasites

Larvae: immature form of the parasite

Adult: mature form of parasite

Stool specimens are tested for ova and parasites as are urine, vaginal secretions, blood, and areas of the skin. See Figure 3-3, which shows a tapeworm with ova (eggs).

Protozoa

You need a microscope to see these one-celled organisms (see Figure 3-4 from the CDC website showing *Entamoeba histolytica*). They can live without a human host, but the environment in humans allows them to multiply and survive. Most protozoan infections are caused by ingestion of contaminated water, directly through the skin or from insect bites. Many of these protozoans are parasites, actually taking up residence in the human body and living off its cells. Most protozoans that infect humans cause disease. Symptoms of protozoan infections vary widely depending on the type of protozoan infection. Many are very serious diseases that cause long-term debilitating illness, such as malaria, which is transmitted by mosquitoes. Others are relatively mild illnesses, like "beaver fever" caused by *Giardia*, a protozoan that lives in streams and water supplies contaminated by fecal matter. Table 3-4 shows some common protozoans, mechanism of transmission, and disease or condition.

Media Connection

To view videos on proper sampling and handling of stool specimens, please go to the accompanying online resources.

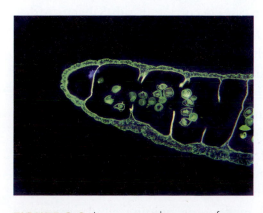

FIGURE 3-3 A segmented portion of a tapeworm with ova (eggs) contained within the segments. © Jubal Harshaw/Shutterstock.com.

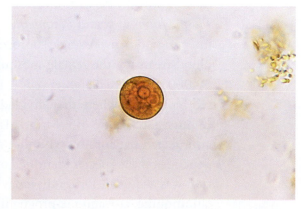

FIGURE 3-4 The protozoa *Entamoeba histolytica* cyst. Source: CDC/Dr. L.L.A. Moore, Jr.

TABLE 3-4 Common Protozoans and Disease

Protozoans	Route of Transmission	Specimen for Testing	Disease or Condition
Giardia lamblia	Drinking or eating food or water contaminated with feces	Feces	Severe diarrhea
Entamoeba histolytica	Drinking or eating contaminated food or water	Feces	Amoebic dysentery
Plasmodium	Bite of infected mosquito	Blood	Malaria

© 2016 Cengage Learning®.

Giardia [jee ARE dee uh]: a genus of protozoa that are pear shaped, have two nuclei and four pairs of flagella, and inhabit the small intestine of humans and other animals to which they attach and absorb nourishment

amebiasis: an infection of the intestines caused by the parasite *Entamoeba histolytica* invading the colon causing colitis, acute dysentery, or long-term (chronic) diarrhea; may also spread to other areas of the body

malaria: a febrile hemolytic disease caused by infection with protozoa of the genus *Plasmodium*

Giardia is one of the most common parasites to infect human gastrointestinal (GI) tracts. It is spread either by person-to-person, food, or water transmission to human hosts. Once it takes up residence in the human GI tract, a patient can either exhibit mild or no symptoms or it can cause sudden watery, foul-smelling diarrhea, nausea and vomiting, and/or abdominal gas, cramps, and bloating. Treatment consists of fluids, electrolytes, and antimicrobials such as metronidazole or tinidazole.

Amebiasis is caused by *Entamoeba histolytica*. Most infections are without symptoms, but it may cause mild to severe diarrhea or abscesses in the lungs, brain, heart, and liver. It is rarely seen in developed countries such as the United States. The diagnosis may be made by examining the stool of an infected patient for cysts (infective form) or trophozoites (invasive disease form). Metronidazole for 7 to 10 days is recommended as a treatment for *Entamoeba histolytica*.

Malaria is a serious and sometimes fatal disease caused by the bite of a mosquito carrying the *Plasmodium* species. Symptoms of malaria initially mimic the "flu" with fever and chills. If left untreated, severe complications and even death can occur. In 2010, approximately 655,000 people died from malaria worldwide with most of the cases occurring in sub-Saharan Africa. *Plasmodium vivax* and *Plasmodium falciparum* are the most common species infecting humans. A single sporozoite (form of the parasite injected into the bloodstream by the female mosquito) invades a liver cell and can produce 30,000 to 40,000 daughter cells within 6 days. These parasites invade human red blood cells where they divide into 8–24 offspring, which cause the cell to burst. See Figure 3-5. Malaria is diagnosed by viewing the parasites from an infected patient's blood under a microscope. Drug treatment of malaria depends on the species identified and the part of the world where the infection was acquired. Drugs that may be used alone or in combination include chloroquine, atovaquone-proguanil, mefloquine, quinine, clindamycin, and doxycycline. Some of these medications may be recommended to prevent malaria in travelers visiting countries where malaria is common.

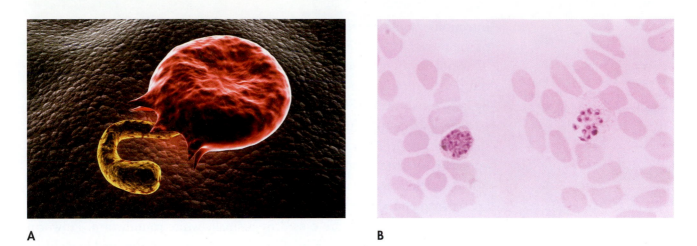

A   **B**

FIGURE 3-5 A. Digital image of malarial parasite in red blood cell. © RAJ CREATIONZS/Shutterstock.com.
B. A photomicrograph of red blood cells with two cells infected with the plasmodium parasite. The one on the right has mature forms within it that are ready to be liberated. Source: CDC/Dr. Mae Melvin

Helminths

These large organisms can be viewed without help from a microscope. They are similar to protozoa in that they can survive either in nature or in humans equally well. The three main groups of helminths are tapeworms (beef or pork tapeworm), flukes (*Schistosoma mansoni*), and roundworms (hookworms and pinworms) (Table 3-5).

Infections caused by pork or beef tapeworm occur worldwide. **Tapeworm** infections are more common in underdeveloped countries in areas with poor sanitation. Individuals infected with tapeworms can have symptoms ranging from none to mild digestive symptoms such as abdominal pain, sick stomach, and loss of appetite. Depending on the type of tapeworm infection, some patients can develop blindness or even seizures. All tapeworm

tapeworm: species of worms of the class Cestoda, which are intestinal parasites of humans and animals

TABLE 3-5 Main Helminth Groups

Helminths	Route of Transmission	Specimen for Testing	Disease or Condition
Beef or pork tapeworm (*Taeniasis*)	Eating raw or undercooked beef or pork	Examine stool samples for eggs	Taeniasis or cysticercosis (larval cysts infect brain and other tissues)
Hookworm	Soil larvae can penetrate bare feet	Feces (identification of eggs)	Iron deficiency/anemia
Pinworm	Ingestion of pinworm eggs	"Tape test"—cellophane tape picks up eggs around skin of anus	Anal itching

hookworm: a parasitic nematode belonging to the family *Strongyloidea* that can cause hookworm disease

pinworm: any of numerous long, slender nematode worms that parasitize humans

infections should be treated with either praziquantel or niclosamide because of the possibility of the patient developing seizures without treatment.

Hookworm infections are common in subtropical and tropical countries but uncommon in the United States. Infection is most commonly acquired by individuals walking barefoot through fecally contaminated soil. Once the parasite gains entry through the skin, it migrates through the body, eventually setting up residence in the GI tract. Once there it can cause nausea, vomiting, diarrhea, and abdominal pain. Chronic infection results in nutritional deficiencies and anemia from blood loss. Albendazole or mebendazole are recommended for treatment.

Pinworm infections are caused by a small, white roundworm. Pinworm infection can affect anyone, but infections are usually concentrated in children and institutionalized individuals. Anal itching that is most intense at night is the most common symptom of pinworm infection. This is caused by the female depositing her eggs around the skin surrounding the anus. Pinworm infestation is diagnosed by "the tape test." As soon as a person or child awakens, a piece of cellophane tape is placed firmly around the anal skin. Eggs, if present, will be collected on the tape and can be viewed under a microscope. Albendazole, mebendazole, or pyrantel pamoate are medications that can be used to treat pinworm infection. Pyrantel pamoate is available without a prescription. See Figure 3-6, which shows various examples of helminths.

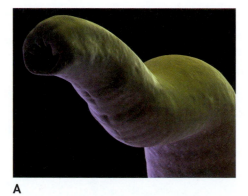
A

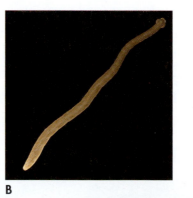
B

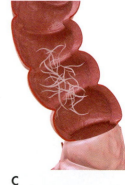
C

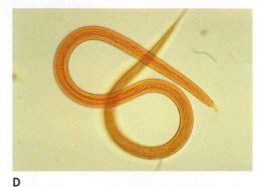
D

FIGURE 3-6 Examples of helminths. **A.** Hookworm. © Sebastian Kaulitzki/Shutterstock.com. **B.** Tapeworm. © 3drenderings/Shutterstock.com. **C.** Adult pinworms in the intestine. © Sebastian Kaulitzki/Shutterstock.com. **D.** Roundworm (*Ascaris lumbricoides*). Source: CDC/Dr. Mae Melvin

Clinical Application
The Importance of Good Water

Guinea worm disease is caused by the parasite *Dracunculus medinensis*. It infects people who drink water from ponds containing the Guinea worm larvae. The larvae grow, in a body cavity after penetrating the stomach, to full-size adults that are about 2–3 feet long and as wide as a cooked spaghetti noodle in about 10–14 months. The mature worm bursts through the patient's skin usually on the feet or hands causing pain (Figure 3-7).

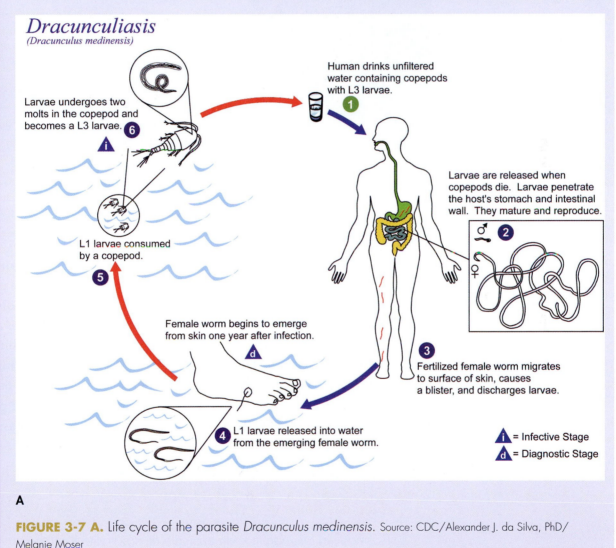

Dracunculiasis
(Dracunculus medinensis)

Larvae undergoes two molts in the copepod and becomes a L3 larvae. **6** **i**

Human drinks unfiltered water containing copepods with L3 larvae. **1**

Larvae are released when copepods die. Larvae penetrate the host's stomach and intestinal wall. They mature and reproduce. **2**

L1 larvae consumed by a copepod. **5**

Fertilized female worm migrates to surface of skin, causes a blister, and discharges larvae. **3**

Female worm begins to emerge from skin one year after infection. **d**

L1 larvae released into water from the emerging female worm. **4**

i = Infective Stage
d = Diagnostic Stage

A

FIGURE 3-7 A. Life cycle of the parasite *Dracunculus medinensis*. Source: CDC/Alexander J. da Silva, PhD/ Melanie Moser

(Continues)

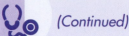 *(Continued)*

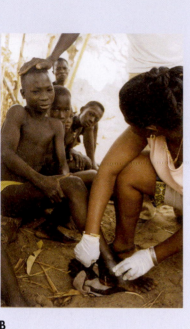

FIGURE 3-7 B. Young girl with painful Guinea worm disease. Source: CDC/The Carter Center. Photo credit: E. Staub

B

Ectoparasites

ectoparasites [eck toe PAIR uh sites]: any parasite that thrives on the skin; such as fleas, lice, maggots, mites, or ticks

Ectoparasites (external parasites) are a class of parasites with hard segmented bodies such as fleas, ticks, bed bugs, and mosquitoes. These parasites generally feed on blood from humans or other animals and can transmit diseases in the process. For example, mosquitoes can transmit malaria, which is a protozoan parasite. Rocky Mountain spotted fever is acquired from the bite of a tick and if untreated can be fatal in up to 20%–60% of cases. Bed bugs are an example of a class of ectoparasites that do not transmit disease but do feed on the blood of humans causing a variety of negative economic and public health consequences. See Figure 3-8 for various examples of ectoparasites.

3-2 Stop and Review

1. *Plasmodium falciparum* is an example of a parasite from the broad category called _____.
2. Iron deficiency anemia may be caused by _____, which is a parasitic infection of the helminth class of parasites.
3. _____ are a type of ectoparasite that do not cause disease in humans but may be detrimental to hotel occupancy rates.

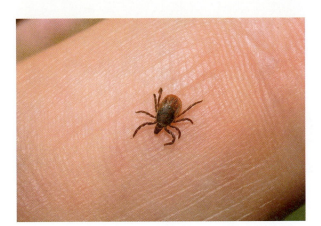

A

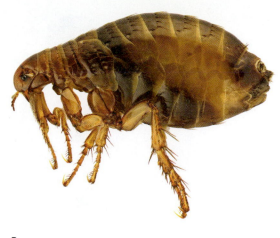

B

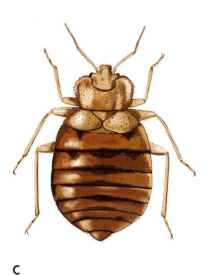

C

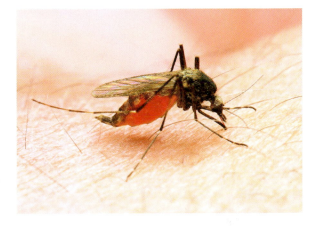

D

FIGURE 3-8 A. Tick crawling on human skin. © Roman Prokhorov/Shutterstock.com. **B.** Flea. © Cosmin Manci/Shutterstock.com. **C.** Bed bug. © Artur Tiutenko/Shutterstock.com. **D.** Mosquito. © Kletr/Shutterstock.com.

Mycology

Mycology is the study of fungi. A fungus is reproduced by spores, has a rigid cell wall, and has no chlorophyll (Figure 3-9). Fungi include mushrooms, yeasts, and molds. Fungi have **ergosterol** instead of the cholesterol in human cells. Antifungals work by preventing the making of ergosterol, which is a building block for the cell membranes. Fungal infections are most likely to develop in patients with an impaired immune system. In addition, antibiotics or steroids can destroy the body's natural flora or weaken the immune system, which can result in an opportunistic fungal infection. Fungal infections are identified by microscopic observation and

mycology [my CALL uh jee]: the science and study of fungi

ergosterol: the primary sterol found in the cell membrane of some fungi; it stabilizes the membrane, as does cholesterol in human cells

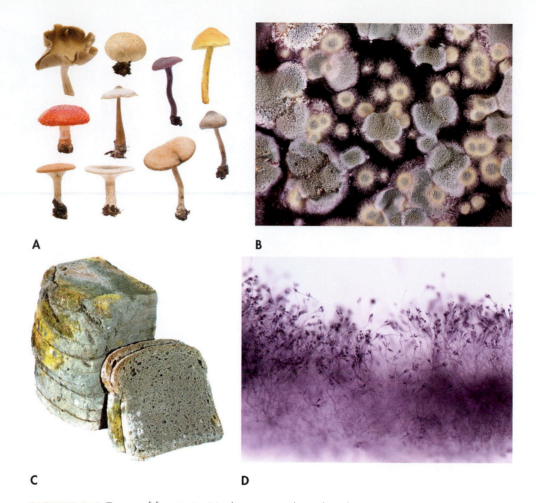

A

B

C

D

FIGURE 3-9 Types of fungi. **A.** Mushrooms and toadstools. © Christopher Elwell/
Shutterstock.com. **B.** Grass mold. © Sarah2/Shutterstock.com. **C.** Mold on bread. © RoyStudio.eu/
Shutterstock.com. **D.** Penicillin. © Christopher Meade/Shutterstock.com.

spores: cells produced by
fungi for reproduction; a
resistant cell produced by
bacteria to withstand extreme
heat or cold or dehydration

biochemical reaction testing. In addition, molds are identified by the spores
they produce.

Fungal infections can be caused by the inhalation or ingestion of
fungal spores or the entrance of spores through open wounds. **Spores** are
tiny bodies resistant to environmental changes, meaning they can stay
dormant until conditions are just right. Most fungal spores do not cause
disease in otherwise healthy individuals, although fungal infections of
the skin, such as athlete's foot and jock itch, are common (Figure 3-10).
Many fungal infections are opportunistic, causing disease in individuals
with compromised immune systems or other underlying disease. Symptoms of fungal infection vary widely depending on the location of the

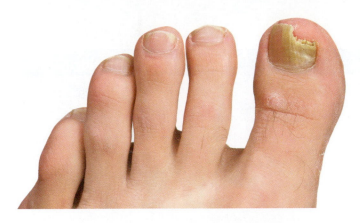

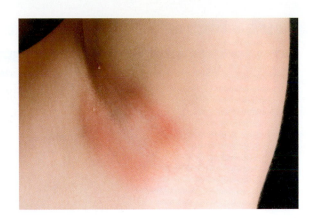

A

B

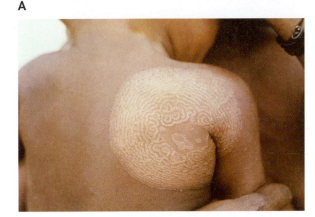

FIGURE 3-10 Examples of various fungal diseases.
A. Toenail fungus. © deepspacedave/Shutterstock.com.
B. Yeast infection of armpit. © Rob Byron/Shutterstock.com.
C. Tinea imbricata, a fungal infection called "Tokelau."
Source: CDC/K. Mae Lennon, Tulane Medical School; Clement Benjamin

C

infection. Fungal infections can be difficult to treat because many of the more serious infections are found in patients with weakened immune systems.

There are many different ways to organize a discussion of fungi. We have decided to use the broad categories of yeasts and molds and discuss common fungi that cause human disease under each category. We also provide a brief overview of antifungal treatments.

Yeasts

Yeasts are single-celled, microscopic organisms that cannot manufacture their own food. Therefore, they thrive on organic matter found in living organisms for food. One of the most important yeast species in humans is *Candida*. It can either colonize our bodies, or *Candida* can cause infections ranging from local mucous membrane infections (oral thrush)

yeast: any of several unicellular fungi, for example, *Candida*, that reproduce by budding

TABLE 3-6 Infections Caused by *Candida* Species

Type of Infection	Risk Factors	Clinical Presentation
Thrush (infection in the mouth, oropharyngeal candidiasis)	AIDS, dentures, antibiotic use, inhaled steroids	Cottony feeling in mouth, loss of taste, pain when eating
Esophagitis (inflammation of the esophagus)	AIDS or HIV infection	Pain upon swallowing
Vulvovaginitis (inflammation of the vagina)	Elevated estrogen, diabetes, steroids, antibiotics, oral contraceptives	Redness, swelling, white curd-like discharge
Invasive *Candida* infections (blood, bone, eye, spleen, liver, brain, kidney, bladder)	Central venous catheter, intravenous nutrition, antibiotics, immunosuppression (e.g., organ transplant, steroids)	Depends on organ involved Eye—decreased vision Bone—pain Blood—fever, low blood pressure

© 2016 Cengage Learning®.

dermatophytes [der MAT uh fites]: fungal parasites that grow in or on the skin

to life-threatening bloodstream and multisystem organ infections. See Table 3-6 for a list of infections caused by *Candida* species.

Most of you will be familiar with infections caused by **dermatophytes**. These fungal species cause skin or nail infections. They can secrete an enzyme called keratinase that can digest skin keratin resulting in scaling of the skin, loss of hair, and thickening of the nails. Table 3-7 lists common dermatophyte infections. These infections are usually easy to diagnose based on visual inspection of the affected body area. In addition, simply scraping the area, dissolving these scrapings in potassium hydroxide, and observing the specimen under the microscope for branched hyphae can aid in the diagnosis. A topical cream, ointment, or shampoo (Can you determine which dermatophyte infection would be treated by using a shampoo?) containing ketoconazole or another imidazole works for most dermatophyte infections with the exception of nail infections. Nail infections usually are treated with terbinafine or itraconazole taken by mouth for 12 weeks or longer.

Cryptococcus neoformans is a yeast that infects the brains of severely immunocompromised patients (e.g., AIDS) causing a life-threatening condition known as meningitis (inflammation of brain membrane covering, or meninges). Symptoms of a brain infection are headache, stiff neck, and change in mental status (patient doesn't respond or is not himself or herself). It can also infect the lungs where it causes pneumonia resulting in

TABLE 3-7 Common Dermatophyte Infections

Dermatophytes	Disease/Condition	Clinical Presentation
Tinea corporis (body)	Ringworm	Ring shape with red-raised border
Tinea cruris	Jock itch	Itchy red patches on the groin and/or scrotum
Tinea pedis	Athlete's foot	Cracking and peeling of skin between toes
Tinea capitis	Cradle cap (occurs primarily in children)	Red scaly lesions with loss of hair
Tinea unguium	Onychomycosis (nail infection)	Thickened, discolored, brittle nails

© 2016 Cengage Learning®.

fever, cough, and shortness of breath. The diagnosis can be made based on patient history, radiology studies (e.g., chest x-ray or CT scan of the brain), culture, or testing for the cryptococcal antigen using an antibody test. The initial treatment is with amphotericin B and flucytosine for brain infections followed by fluconazole for 10 weeks or longer. Severe lung infections are treated with a similar regimen. For milder lung infections, fluconazole may be used for 6 to 12 months. Amphotericin B and flucytosine can be toxic, and patients need to be monitored carefully for kidney injury and suppression of the bone marrow.

Histoplasma capsulatum, Blastomyces dermatitidis, and *Coccidioides immitis* are so-called **dimorphic** fungi because, depending on their growing conditions, they can appear either as unicellular yeasts or molds forming hyphae and spores. All three of these infections are acquired by inhaling spores. **Histoplasmosis** is caused by inhaling spores from soil where bats and birds have been roosting. **Coccidioidomycosis** is also known as San Joaquin Valley fever and is generally found in people who live in or travel to the southwestern United States. Figure 3-11 shows a positive skin test for coccidioidomycosis. **Blastomycosis** is commonly found in people living on the Canadian border surrounding the Great Lakes and in the south central, southeastern, and midwestern United States. All of these lung infections can either cause few, if any, symptoms or can spread to other organs resulting in death especially in immunocompromised individuals. Severe infections are often treated with amphotericin B, but milder infections may respond to fluconazole or itraconazole.

dimorphic [di MORE fic]: occurring in two distinct forms

histoplasmosis [his toe plaz MO sis]: a systemic fungal respiratory disease caused by *Histoplasma capsulatum*

coccidioidomycosis [KOK sid ee oy dough my KOH sis]: infection with the pathogenic fungus, *Coccidioides immitis,* whose spores, when inhaled, may cause the development of active or subclinical infection

blastomycosis [blas toe my KOH sis]: a rare infection caused by inhalation of the fungus *Blastomyces dermatitidis* which may produce inflammatory lesions of the skin or lungs or a generalized invasion of the skin, lungs, bones, central nervous system, kidneys, liver, and spleen

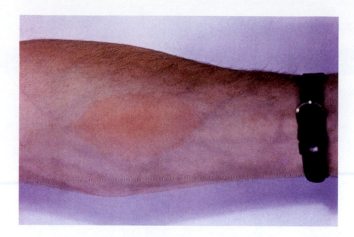

FIGURE 3-11 Positive skin test for the presence of *Coccidioides* antigen showing exposure to the fungal organism. Source: CDC/Dr. Lucille K. Georg

Molds

mold: one of the parasitic or saprophytic fungi that grow in a mycelium pattern; a fuzzy coating due to growth of a fungus on the surface of decaying vegetable matter or on an inorganic object

Aspergillus: a genus of fungi comprising more than 600 species of molds, some of which can cause human disease

Molds are multicellular colonies of intertwined hyphae that form tiny knobs at their tips. When these tiny knobs rupture, they release thousands of spores into the air. Molds require food (e.g., old bread), air, warmth, moisture, and darkness to grow and thrive. If you take away one of the growth requirements, you stunt or inhibit the growth of the mold. We will discuss a few species of molds that are likely to be encountered in clinical practice.

Aspergillus is a potential cause of disease in humans that is found throughout our environment. It can be found in the soil of potted plants, compost piles, and even in hospitals where outbreaks of infection have been reported during hospital construction projects. This mold can cause an allergic reaction when its spores are inhaled into the lungs. This is an allergic reaction and not a true infection. At times the body can wall off the organism in the lungs creating a fungus ball in a lung cavity that resembles tuberculosis. In severely immunocompromised patients (especially those with very low white blood cell counts), infection can start in the lungs but quickly can spread to

Learning Hint

What's in a Name?

Later in this book, we talk more about specific infectious diseases and drugs used to treat them. This can get quite overwhelming, but sometimes the drug names give you a hint. For example, any drug that ends in "azole" is used to treat fungal infections. Examples include fluconazole, itraconazole, and miconazole.

the blood and other organs resulting in death if not recognized and treated immediately. Diagnosis is made by examining tissue specimens and/or body fluids. Recommended treatment for infections caused by *Aspergillus* consists of possible surgical excision of infected material along with voriconazole or alternatively amphotericin B.

Mucormycosis is a life-threatening disease that is caused by one of three different types of saprophytic (loves dead or decaying material) molds: *Rhizopus, Rhizomucor,* or *Mucor.* These organisms are found worldwide in decaying material and soil. Poorly controlled diabetics and patients with certain blood cancers are prone to this rare disease. It starts in the nasal passage where it invades blood vessels causing tissue fed by this blood supply to die. This dead tissue or "food" for the mold sets up optimal growing conditions. The infection spreads rapidly causing facial pain, fever, and headache. The tissue invaded by the mold looks black because it is dead. Death from this disease occurs in 80%–90% of patients. Treatment is surgery to cut away the dead tissue and amphotericin B. Figure 3-12 shows examples of disease-producing molds.

mucormycosis [mu core my KOH sis]: an invasive and frequently fatal infection with fungi of the family *Mucoraceae* and the class *Zygomycetes*

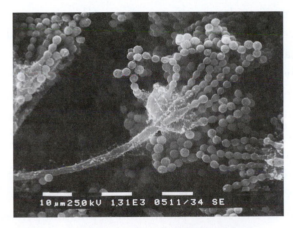

A

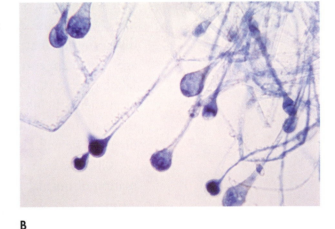

B

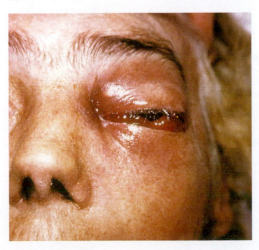

C

FIGURE 3-12 Examples of disease-producing molds. **A.** *Aspergillus.* Source: CDC/Robert Simmons. Photo credit: Janice Haney Carr **B.** *Mucor* fungus. Source: CDC/Dr. Lucille K. Georg **C.** Patient with mucormycosis. Source: CDC/ Dr. Thomas F. Sellers/Emory University

3-3 Stop and Review

1. _____ is a very common fungi that may cause thrush or vulvovaginitis.

2. *Tinea unguium* may infect the nail beds causing a disease called _____, which is very difficult to treat.

3. What types of disease may be caused by *Aspergillus*? What types of patients are the most susceptible to infections with *Aspergillus*?

Prions

prion [PRI on]: a small proteinaceous infectious particle that is believed to be responsible for central nervous system diseases in humans and other mammals

Prions are infectious agents that are in a class all by themselves. They are unique in that they are infectious proteins that *lack* nucleic acid. Another distinguishing feature is their resistance to a number of routine sterilization techniques. They can infect the nervous systems of humans or animals. They cause certain cellular proteins to fold in an abnormal way, thus disrupting their structure and function. This causes progressive brain damage. There are currently five prion-related diseases in humans: Creutzfeldt-Jakob disease (CJD), variant Creutzfeldt-Jakob disease (vCJD), Gerstmann-Straussler-Scheinker syndrome, fatal familial insomnia, and kuru. Wasn't that a mouthful? Because CJD is probably the most well known of the prion diseases, we will discuss it in a little more detail.

CJD has been recognized since the early 1920s and is caused by the formation of normal proteins into abnormal prions. This worldwide disease is estimated to occur at a rate of 1 to 2 cases per million population per year. The majority of CJD (85%) occur sporadically but 5%–15% of patients develop CJD from their ancestors (Gerstmann-Straussler-Scheinker syndrome and fatal familial insomnia). The disease is categorized by loss of intellectual functions (dementia), disorientation, impaired memory, difficulty with

Clinical Application
Spread of rare but deadly disease

Over 250 cases of accidental transmission of Creutzfeldt-Jakob disease have been reported worldwide. Most of these cases were caused by corneal or dura mater grafts (tissue grafts used in brain surgery), contaminated human growth hormone medicine, or contaminated brain surgery equipment.

walking and balance, and twitching of the extremities (myoclonus). In general, the affected individual is dead within a year of diagnosis. A diagnosis of CJD is based on signs, symptoms, and the presence of the abnormal prion proteins in the cerebrospinal fluid, but a definitive diagnosis requires testing of brain tissue. There is no known treatment for this devastating condition.

Chapter Summary

- This chapter focused on the nonbacterial forms of microorganisms that can produce disease. Our discussion began with a review of viral species that cause disease in humans.

- Remember that viruses are essentially pieces of genetic material that lack the capability to reproduce without a host cell. Because they are hard to grow in a laboratory, their presence is usually detected by looking for antibodies our bodies produce to fight the virus, viral antigens, or the nuclear thumbprint of the virus (detect viral DNA or RNA).

- Until recently, antiviral drug development has lagged behind antibiotic development. New options for the treatment of hepatitis C and HIV infections have provided clinicians and patients with new weapons to fight these infections.

- Parasites are similar to viruses in that they need a host to live in or on. We discussed three broad categories of disease-causing parasites including protozoa, helminths, and ectoparasites.

- Mycology is the study of fungi. We reviewed common fungi that cause disease in humans such as *Candida* sp., for example.

- It is important to recall that serious fungal infections are most likely to develop in patients with an impaired immune system.

- Finally, we finished the chapter with a section on prions. Fortunately the disease burden caused by these infectious proteins is uncommon.

Case Study

A 59-year-old male is admitted to the hospital for pneumonia. He has a past medical history of AIDS and has been taking Atripla for his HIV disease. You were an excellent student, and you recall when you studied medical microbiology that the HIV virus is always treated with at least three medications. In a panic, you look up this medication and then realize it is a combination of three antivirals (efavirenz, tenofovir, and emtricitabine) all combined into one pill.

The hospital pharmacy does not have this drug because it is costly and they do not have many HIV/AIDS patients admitted to the hospital. They dispense two of the medications, but they do not have the third one so it is placed on hold. The patient is discharged after a 5-day hospital stay and resumes his Atripla upon discharge. Was it a good idea to hold one of his antivirals? What would be your concern? What could have been done differently?

Chapter Review

State whether the following diseases are caused by bacteria, fungi, parasites, or viruses.

1. _____ Ringworm
2. _____ Fever blisters
3. _____ Thrush
4. _____ Giardiasis
5. _____ Cryptococcal meningitis
6. _____ Influenza

7. _____ Shingles
8. _____ Liver cancer
9. _____ Pinworm
10. _____ Bloodstream infection with *Candida*
11. _____ Athlete's foot

Answer the following questions and fill in the blanks as required.

12. List some possible treatments for the following microbes.
    Giardia
    Hepatitis C virus
    HIV
    Candida species
    Aspergillus

13. Why do we need to use at least three medicines to treat HIV infection?

14. Why should you not use antibiotics on the common cold?

15. Describe the two ways that viruses cause disease.

16. List and describe the stages of development of a parasite.

17. _____ is a common respiratory virus that causes seasonal outbreaks. Vaccination is an important way of preventing this infection.

18. _____ is acquired during vaccinations and may be either active or passive.

19. _____ is one of the most common human parasitic infections.

20. Mycology is the study of _____.

21. _____ is a common species of yeast that may cause infections ranging from thrush to life-threatening bloodstream infections.

22. _____ may cause an allergic reaction when the spores of this organism are inhaled into the lungs.

23. _____ is a life-threatening fungal infection that may occur in diabetics who have poor control of their blood sugar.

Additional Activities

1. Antiviral drug development continues to provide additional options to treat viral infections like HIV and hepatitis C. Research treatments for other viral diseases. When might they become available? (Hint: visit the website www.clinicaltrials.gov.)

2. Research and then discuss the pros and cons for universal HIV testing. What are the laws concerning HIV testing in your state?

3. Invite a medical technologist to discuss testing for viruses, parasites, and fungi. Ask him or her to explain the difficulties in identifying viruses in comparison to bacteria.

4. Play "name that organism." Using the list of diseases and causative agents in this chapter, develop a game to identify organisms and their corresponding disease. Research more to add to the list.

Media Connection

Go to the accompanying online resources and have fun learning as you play games, view animations and videos, and take practice tests to help reinforce key concepts you learned in this chapter.

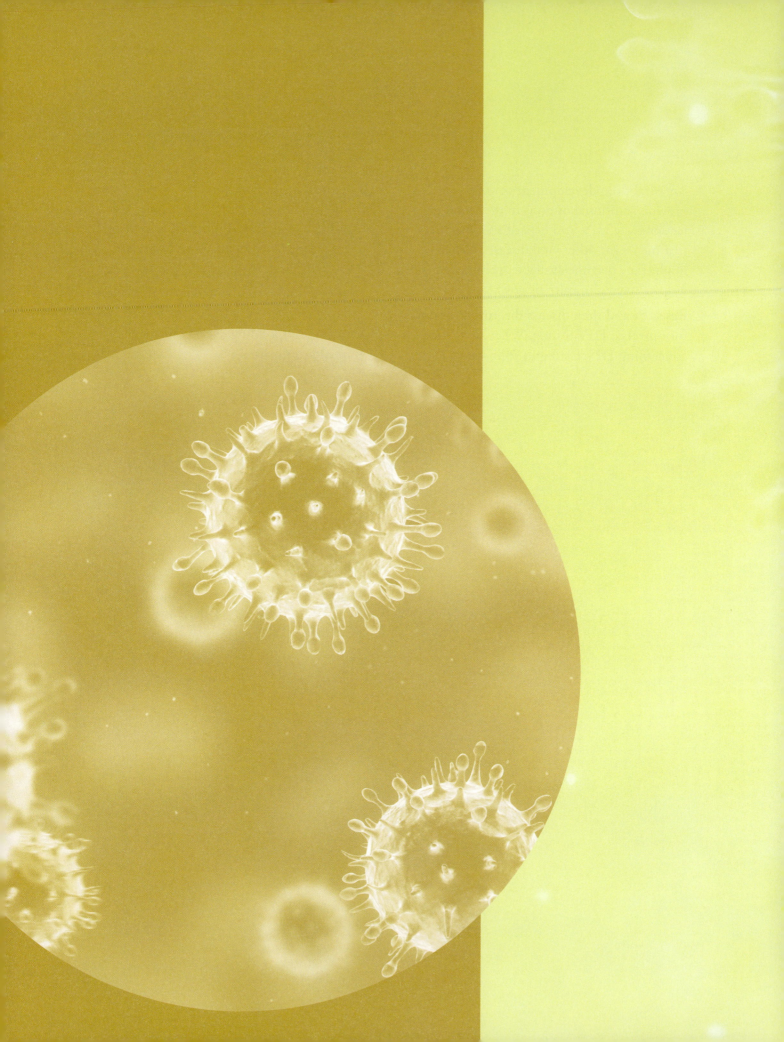

SECTION II

Microbiology in Practice

Now that you are familiar with the background and science of microbiology, it is time to put this knowledge to work and understand how to prevent the spread of infectious diseases. We will discuss the principles and practice of infection control including the chain of infection and how to disinfect and sterilize instruments. Next we tackle topics that in sum will help us protect patients and ourselves from acquiring infections from other people and our environment. We show you how infections are spread and what types of isolation are used to help prevent the spread of specific types of infections. We discuss the use of personal protective equipment (including a suit that makes you look like you

are ready to walk on Mars). Finally, we discuss infectious waste disposal and how to properly obtain samples for culture from wounds, urine, blood, and lung secretions. In this section, we discuss the most important way of controlling the spread of infectious diseases. Can you guess what that may be? If you guessed proper hand hygiene, you are correct! Washing our hands correctly and frequently is the most important way we can prevent the spread of infections. Hopefully we will convince you to become a champion of hand hygiene because this simple way of preventing infection is so simple it can be overlooked in the busy health care environment.

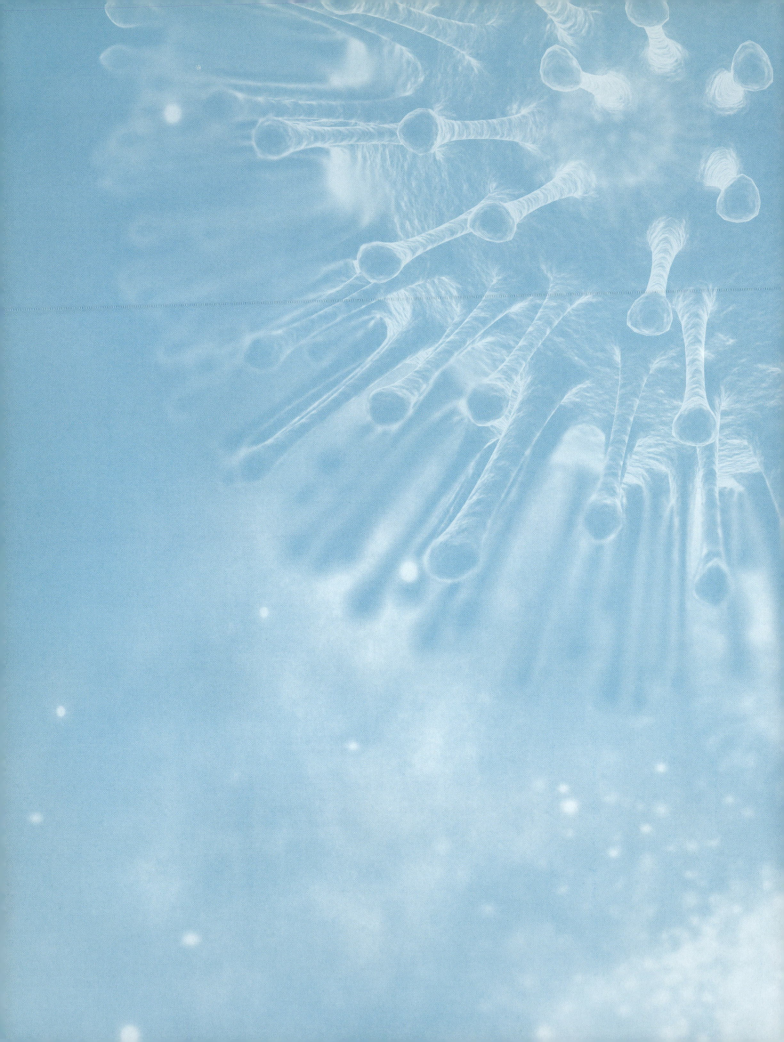

CHAPTER 4

Infection Prevention

OBJECTIVES

After studying this chapter, the learner will be able to:

- Define the basic terms related to infection control.

- Discuss the chain of infection.

- Contrast germicidal susceptibility of various microorganisms.

- Discuss issues to consider when killing microorganisms.

- Describe the different methods used to disinfect and sterilize medical equipment to include heat, pasteurization, boiling water, steam, liquid compounds, radiation, and gas sterilization.

KEY TERMS

acetic acid [uh SEE tic]

autoclave

bacteriostatic
[BACK teer ee oh STAT ik]

Centers for Disease Control and Prevention (CDC)

chain of infection

chlorine

cleaning

contamination

decontamination

denatured

disinfection

ethanol
(ethyl alcohol)

ethylene oxide (ETO)

gamma irradiation

germicidal
[JUR muh side ul]

glutaraldehydes
[glue tuh RAL duh hides]

health care–associated infections (HAIs)

hydrogen peroxide

infection

infection control and prevention

inflammation

isopropyl
[eye sah PRO pil]

nosocomial infections
[nos uh KOH mee al]

pasteurization
[PASS tuh rise aye shun]

phenols [FEE nawls]

portal of entry

quaternary ammonium compounds
[KWOT er ner ee uh MOH nee uhm]

sanitization

spores

standard precautions

sterilization

vegetative organisms

Introduction

In this chapter we learn the language of infection prevention. We start by discussing the concept of the chain of infection and then continue by defining basic infection prevention terminology. Finally, we finish by taking a look at various methods used to disinfect and sterilize instruments and our environment.

To help protect the health of your patients, coworkers, and yourself, you need to have a basic understanding of **infection control and prevention**. As a general term, infection prevention includes policies and procedures designed to monitor and control the transmission of communicable diseases. This also includes professionals who are involved with conducting infection prevention activities with other health care professionals, government agencies, and voluntary organizations. At the staff level, infection prevention includes education and performing basic procedures such as cleaning, sanitization, sterilizing, isolation procedures, and hand hygiene as well as performing various diagnostic and therapeutic procedures you will learn in upcoming chapters in a manner that protects patients and staff from the spread of infection.

The **chain of infection**, a cycle or pathway of infection, begins with the creation of a source of infection, continues with the transportation of a given pathogen, and ends with the entry into the body (also known as the **portal of entry**). Our goal, then, is to prevent the spread of infection by breaking the chain of infection at some point along the way. Figure 4-1 illustrates the chain of infection.

Our patients may already be compromised because of the nature and severity of their disease(s) that have weakened their immunity. Possibly, their immune systems are impaired as a result of chemotherapy or antirejection drugs used for organ transplants. They may be susceptible to exposure to organisms as a result of various procedures performed on them that breach their normal defenses such as the use of urinary catheters, bronchoscopy, or hip replacement surgery.

infection control and prevention: policies and procedures used to minimize the risk of spreading infections, especially in hospitals and human or animal health care facilities

chain of infection: process that begins when an agent leaves its reservoir or host through a portal of exit, and is conveyed by some mode of transmission, then enters through an appropriate portal of entry to infect a susceptible host

portal of entry: the area in which a microorganism enters the body such as cuts, lesions, injection sites, or natural body orifices

Food for Thought

Expanding Infection Prevention Outside the Hospital

Over the past several decades, health care delivery has been shifting from hospitals to outpatient settings such as physician offices and clinics, ambulatory surgery centers, and the home. More than 75% of all operations are now performed in outpatient surgery centers. The focus of infection prevention and control has traditionally been on hospitals. However, outbreak reports have described transmission of numerous microorganisms in outpatient settings.

Media Connection

To view an animation on the chain of infection, visit the accompanying online resources.

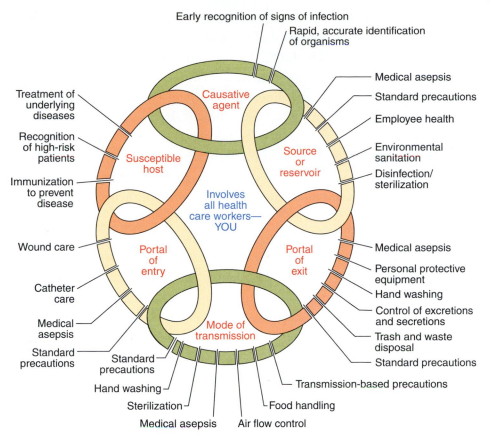

Early recognition of signs of infection

Rapid, accurate identification of organisms

Treatment of underlying diseases

Recognition of high-risk patients

Immunization to prevent disease

Wound care

Catheter care

Medical asepsis

Standard precautions

Causative agent

Susceptible host

Involves all health care workers— YOU

Portal of entry

Source or reservoir

Portal of exit

Mode of transmission

Medical asepsis

Standard precautions

Employee health

Environmental sanitation

Disinfection/ sterilization

Medical asepsis

Personal protective equipment

Hand washing

Control of excretions and secretions

Trash and waste disposal

Standard precautions

Transmission-based precautions

Standard precautions

Hand washing

Sterilization

Medical asepsis

Air flow control

Food handling

FIGURE 4-1 Components of the chain of infection with ways it can be broken.
© Cengage Learning®.

Basic Definitions

Before we go any further, it's important to learn a few basic terms; we have already discussed some of them. **Vegetative organisms** are organisms that are actively growing. **Spores** are a dormant and protective state of an organism. Spores are resistant to external environmental effects that would ordinarily damage or destroy that organism. In this form, they are very hard to kill.

Denatured means "structurally altered." When this is done to a substance or organism, it usually results in its death. **Contamination** is the presence of microorganisms without tissue reaction. **Infection** is the presence of microorganisms with a tissue reaction. **Inflammation** is a tissue's reaction to injury that may, or may not, be a result of infection. The term **nosocomial infections** (means "our house") has been replaced by the **Centers for Disease Control and Prevention (CDC)** with a more generic term called **health care–associated infections (HAIs)**. This change in

vegetative organisms: microorganisms that can grow and reproduce in rich, moist soil where many nutrients are available

spores: cells produced by fungi for reproduction; a resistant cell produced by bacteria to withstand extreme heat or cold or dehydration

denatured: to deprive a substance of its natural qualities

contamination: the presence of extraneous, especially infectious, material that renders a substance or preparation impure or harmful

infection: a disease caused by microorganisms, especially those that release toxins or invade body tissues

inflammation: A localized reaction that produces redness, warmth, swelling, and pain as a result of infection, irritation, or injury

nosocomial infections [nos uh KOH mee al]: infection resulting from treatment in a hospital or a health care service unit; older term that is replaced with health care–associated infections (HAIs) by the Centers for Disease Control and Prevention (CDC)

Centers for Disease Control and Prevention (CDC): federal agency under the Department of Health and Human Services that serves to protect public health through the control and prevention of disease

health care–associated infections (HAIs): infections patients get while receiving medical treatment

standard precautions: guidelines recommended by the Centers for Disease Control and Prevention for reducing the risk of transmission of bloodborne and other pathogens in hospitals; the standard precautions synthesize the major features of universal precautions (designed to reduce the risk of transmission of bloodborne pathogens) and body substance isolation (designed to reduce the risk of pathogens from moist body substances) and apply them to all patients receiving care in hospitals regardless of their diagnosis or presumed infection status

cleaning: the process of physically removing all foreign material from an object

sanitization: the process whereby pathogenic organisms are reduced to safe levels on inanimate objects, thereby reducing the likelihood of cross-infection

decontamination: the process of making a person, object, or environment free of microorganisms, radioactivity, or other contaminants

disinfection: using specialized cleansing techniques that destroy or prevent growth of organisms capable of infection

germicidal [JUR muh side ul]: preventing infection by inhibiting the growth or action of microorganisms

terminology recognizes that infections can be acquired not just in hospitals but in nursing homes, dialysis facilities, and outpatient surgical centers to name a few. The CDC does so much more than just updating terminology. Just one example is the development of **standard precautions** which are a set of guidelines for reducing the risk of transmission of bloodborne and other pathogens in hospitals.

There are several different levels of microorganism removal. **Cleaning** is the *physical* removal of all foreign matter such as dirt, blood, and sputum that may allow the growth of an organism. Cleaning exposes the surface to more intensive cleaners, or chemicals, by scrubbing with hot water and soaps or detergents. **Sanitization** is a general term for any process that reduces the total bacterial contamination to a level in which an object may be handled safely. **Decontamination** is the process used to remove contaminants by chemical or physical means. **Disinfection** is the process that eliminates vegetative, pathogenic microorganisms from an inanimate object. There are several levels of disinfectants.

- *Low-level disinfectants* are **germicidal** (*cide* means killing action) that can kill some but not all vegetative bacteria and fungi and denature some viruses.

- *Intermediate-level disinfectants* are germicidal agents that can kill all gram-negative bacteria and fungi but have variable success against spores and their ability to denature certain viruses.

 Food for Thought

Agencies Looking out for You

The National Healthcare Safety Network (NHSN) was established by the Centers for Disease Control and Prevention (CDC) to integrate all former surveillance systems including the National Nosocomial Infection Surveillance System (NNISS). Currently more than 3,000 facilities report data on health care–associated infections (HAIs) and other personnel and patient safety-related data. The Centers for Medicare and Medicaid Services (CMS) is now mandating participation in NHSN to incentivize health care facilities to decrease and prevent the occurrence of HAIs. In other words, a hospital will get more money from Medicare if it can decrease its health care–associated infection rates. States vary in their requirements for hospitals to report HAIs, and currently 22 states require hospitals to report HAIs using the CDC's NHSN system.

TABLE 4-1 Germicidal Susceptibility of Various Microorganisms

Microorganism	Germicidal Susceptibility		
	High	**Intermediate**	**Low**
Bacteria			
Endospores	Killed	Not killed	Not killed
Vegetative cells[a]	Killed	Killed	Killed
Myobacterium tuberculosis[b]	Killed	Killed	Not killed
Fungi	**Killed**	**Killed**	**Some killed**
Viruses			
Naked and small	Killed	Some killed	Some killed
Enveloped and medium sized	Killed	Killed	Killed

[a]Vegetative cells of most bacteria.
[b]Because of its resistance, the bacterium that causes tuberculosis is considered separately.
© 2016 Cengage Learning®.

- *High-level disinfectants* are capable of killing all microorganisms except their spores.

- **Sterilization** is the complete destruction or inactivation of all forms of microorganisms.

  Table 4-1 shows germicidal susceptibility to different levels of disinfectants.

Media Connection

To view videos on sanitizing an exam room and equipment and on disinfecting equipment and cleanup, visit the accompanying online resources.

sterilization: a technique for destroying microorganisms on inanimate objects using heat, water, chemicals, or gases

4-1 Stop and Review

1. Differentiate between the following terms: cleaning, sanitization, disinfection, and sterilization.

2. _____ is the new term that replaces nosocomial infections. These are infections acquired in health care settings.

3. The _____ of _____ is a cycle or pathway of infection that begins with the creation or source of infection and ends with pathogen entry into the body.

Issues to Consider When Killing an Organism

We need to have the ability to kill microorganisms, or at the very least, keep them from reproducing. To accomplish this, there are several things that we need to consider. First, the initial number and type(s) of organisms we have to kill may dictate what methods and procedures we need to utilize. In addition, some species can exist in protective spores and can't always be destroyed by means such as chemicals or dry heat. Some species even exist in different environments that require special techniques. For example, rough surfaces must be first physically cleaned to expose all of the surfaces to disinfecting or sterilizing substances, or they will not be as effective. We must also consider factors when choosing the type of agent chosen for infection control. The length of time the killing agent is used and its intensity are other considerations to accomplish our goal of sterilization.

Environmental issues such as temperature is another factor. Generally, killing action increases as the temperature increases. For example, in some situations, a 10°F temperature increase can double the killing rate.

Methods Used to Disinfect and Sterilize

There are several methods used to disinfect and sterilize medical equipment and facilities. We will present an overview of each of the following methods:

- Heat
- Pasteurization
- Boiling water
- Steam and pressure
- Various liquids and compounds
- Gas sterilization
- Radiation

Heat

The application of heat to disinfect and sterilize is very common. Generally, the higher the temperature used, the less time is needed to disinfect or sterilize. Heat causes the denaturing (breaking down and unraveling long protein chains) of proteins and leads to cellular coagulation. While dry heat is fairly effective, the use of steam is more so due to its greater heat capacity because water molecules are involved. Steam can be even more effective if it is pressurized such as in an autoclave, as you will soon see.

While not as effective as steam heat, dry heat is used on objects that moist heat could damage such as oils, powders, or dressings. Glassware is normally sterilized by using dry heat. In the extreme form, incineration is used to destroy and thus "sterilize" disposable objects.

Pasteurization

Pasteurization is the use of water heated enough to kill vegetative cells and denature most viruses such as HIV. Equipment is immersed in 70°C water for 30 minutes. The object must then be dried and packaged in a sterile manner.

Boiling Water

Immersion in boiling water for at least 15 minutes will kill most bacteria and inactivate most viruses, but it is ineffectual against many bacterial and fungal spores. As a result, this method cannot be considered a true sterilizing process, but it does greatly reduce the number of pathogens when no other method is available. Altitude does play a factor in the effectiveness of using boiling water, so for every 1,000 foot increase of altitude, the boiling time must be increased by 5 minutes.

Steam and Pressure

These two methods of heat and pressure are effectively combined when using an **autoclave** (Figure 4-2). This is the most efficient method of sterilizing. Items are usually packaged with a heat-sensitive indicator before being placed in an autoclave. This way you will know if the item has been heated sufficiently to be sterilized. This method can kill bacteria, fungi, spores, and

pasteurization [PASS tuh rise aye shun]: partial sterilization of foods at a temperature that destroys harmful microorganisms without major changes in the chemistry of the food

autoclave: a strong, pressurized, steam-heated vessel often used for laboratory experiments, sterilization, or cooking

Learning Hint
The Relationship between Altitude and Pressure

Keep in mind that barometric pressure decreases as you rise in altitude, so the pressure on water is less at higher altitudes. It can therefore boil at lower temperatures. This is why, when people "can" certain foods for preservation, they must heat the jars in a pressure cooker and adjust the time for their altitude to properly kill the organisms that could grow in the jar and infect or poison them at a later date when they open the jar to consume the contents. This is also why it takes a lot longer than 10 minutes to make a hard-boiled egg at high altitudes.

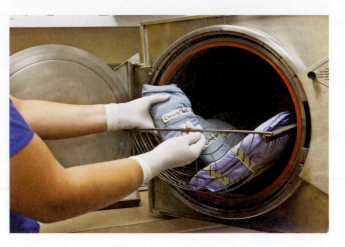

FIGURE 4-2 An autoclave that uses steam and heat to sterilize medical equipment. ©iStock.com/DenGuy.

denature viruses. The downside to this method is that it can melt some plastics and rubber and corrode some metals. It also cannot be used on oils and waxes because steam cannot penetrate those substances.

Various Liquids and Compounds

There are many types of liquids and compounds used in infection prevention and control and each has specific advantages, disadvantages, and indications for clinical use.

Alcohol

If you have ever gotten an injection at the doctor's office, then you are familiar with the use of alcohol as a disinfectant. Your skin was rubbed with a small patch soaked in alcohol, which cleaned your skin and removed any fats and lipids. Alcohol disorganizes the cell's lipid structures of the cell membrane and denatures the cellular proteins. Alcohol is effective against gram-positive, gram-negative, and acid-fast bacteria. Although alcohol is effective against some viruses, such as HIV, it is not sporicidal. Alcohol is also somewhat irritating to the skin and can damage some plastics and rubber materials. There are two forms of alcohol commonly used. **Ethanol** (ethyl alcohol) is most effective when used at a 90% concentration. **Isopropyl** alcohol is most effective when used at a 70% concentration (Figure 4-3).

Acetic Acid

Acetic acid, commonly known as vinegar, has traditionally been used as a food preservative because it inhibits the growth of many bacteria (**bacteriostatic**, static = inhibits growth or reproduction) and fungi. Acetic acid's action is

ethanol (ethyl alcohol): a primary alcohol formed by microbial fermentation of carbohydrates or by synthesis from ethylene; excessive ingestion results in acute intoxication, and ingestion during pregnancy can harm the fetus; also known as alcohol

isopropyl [eye sah PRO pil]: a colorless, flammable, water-soluble liquid; used chiefly in the manufacture of antifreeze and rubbing alcohol and as a solvent

acetic acid [uh SEE tic]: a clear, colorless organic acid, CH_3COOH, with a distinctive pungent odor, used as a solvent and in the manufacture of rubber, plastics, acetate fibers, pharmaceuticals, and photographic chemicals. Also known as vinegar

bacteriostatic [BACK teer ee oh STAT ik]: inhibiting the growth of bacteria

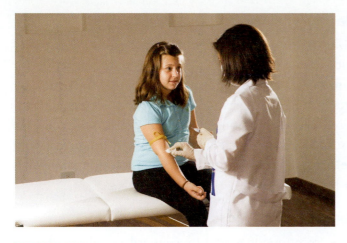

FIGURE 4-3 Caregiver swabbing a patient with isopropyl before injection. © Orange Line Media/Shutterstock.com.

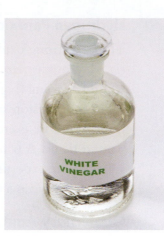

FIGURE 4-4 White distilled vinegar. © Pat_Hastings/Shutterstock.com.

caused by its acidity that denatures the cell's proteins. Normally, a 1.25% acetic acid solution is utilized for disinfecting by combining 1 part vinegar (5% strength acetic acid) with 3 parts water. White distilled vinegar is preferred over brown apple cider vinegar (Figure 4-4).

Phenols

Phenols are a result of coal tar distillation and are used because they cause cell leakage and inactivate enzymes in the cell membrane. This group has some virucidal properties but is not sporicidal. This class of liquids is commonly used for cleaning instruments and for general housekeeping activities, but contact with skin should be avoided. An example of a phenol is phenylphenol.

phenols [FEE nowls]: extremely poisonous compounds that are caustic and disinfectant; used as a pharmaceutical preservative and in dilution as an antimicrobial and topical anesthetic and antipruritic

Chlorine

If you have ever gone swimming in a public swimming pool or hot tub, you are probably already familiar with this substance. **Chlorine**, in both its gaseous and liquid forms, is very effective against most bacteria, viruses, and fungi but is not sporicidal at room temperature. As a liquid, it is widely used in the dairy and food industry and is commonly used in hospitals and public buildings as a sanitizer. It is highly corrosive to some metals and cannot be used on rubber.

chlorine: a chemical element with the atomic number 17; a disinfectant, decolorant, and irritant poison used for disinfecting, fumigating, and bleaching

A common and very effective liquid form of chlorine is household bleach. In a 1:50 diluted bleach solution, it is effective against gram-negative bacteria, bacterial spores, and bacteria that cause tuberculosis with a 10-minute exposure time. A 1:10 solution is recommended to clean up blood spills. Hexachlorophene is a chlorinated disinfectant, without the chlorine smell, commonly called Phisohex.

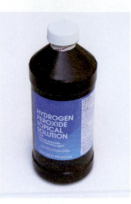

hydrogen peroxide:
a colorless, heavy, strongly oxidizing liquid capable of reacting explosively with combustibles and used principally in aqueous solution as a mild antiseptic, a bleaching agent, an oxidizing agent, and a laboratory reagent

quaternary ammonium compounds [KWOT er ner ee uh MOH nee uhm]:
a group of compounds used as disinfectants that are bactericidal to many organisms

glutaraldehyde [glue tuh RAL duh hide]: a disinfectant used in aqueous solution for sterilization of non–heat-resistant equipment; also used as a tissue fixative for light and electron microscopy

Hydrogen Peroxide

This is a strong oxidizer that is as effective as chlorine against most bacteria. **Hydrogen peroxide** in a 3% solution is used as a mild antiseptic for wound cleaning (Figure 4-5). It is commonly used in cleaning tracheostomy tubes and incision sites as well as surgical devices and contact lenses. Caution should be exercised because a stronger solution can actually damage wound tissue. A 6% solution is bactericidal, virucidal, and fungicidal with a 10-minute exposure at room temperature. This same solution strength is sporicidal if given a 6-hour exposure.

Quaternary Ammoniun Compounds

Quaternary ammonium compounds act by causing cell membrane loss of semipermeability leading to lysis and denaturing of the cell's proteins. They are bactericidal to many organisms, especially gram-positive bacteria, but are ineffective against the bacillus spores that cause tuberculosis, bacterial spores, enteroviruses, hepatitis B, and some fungi.

Glutaraldehydes

This group of disinfecting and sterilizing agents is widely used for cleaning surgical instruments and equipment parts. **Glutaraldehydes** are bactericidal, tuberculocidal, fungicidal, and virucidal with a 10- to 30-minute exposure and sporicidal in approximately 10 hours. Its action is through interrupting metabolism and reproduction. Caution must be taken when using this group because it can cause irritation to skin, mucous membranes, and eyes. It also can damage some rubbers and plastics and can corrode some steels. It is important to rinse, dry, and package cleaned objects in a sterile or clean manner after soaking in a glutaraldehyde solution. Figure 4-6 shows the effects or non-effects of the liquid agents chlorine, hexachlorophene, phenylphenol, and quaternary ammonium on various pathogens.

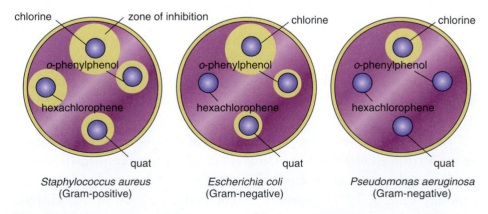

FIGURE 4-6 Comparing the effectiveness of four germicides on various pathogens.
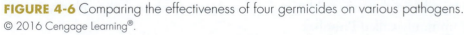

Gas Sterilization

Gas sterilization is a common method used in hospitals to sterilize equipment.

Ethylene oxide

Ethylene oxide (ETO) is extensively used in gas sterilization. ETO interrupts the normal metabolism and reproduction of organisms. Proper sterilization with gas is dependent on the following:

ethylene oxide (ETO): a colorless flammable gas with a slightly sweet odor and taste that is used to sterilize objects

- Gas concentration

- Humidity

- Temperature

- Time

A typical setup for effective sterilization would then be a gas concentration of 450 mg of ETO/L of air, 50°C–60°C, and 30% relative humidity at a pressure of 5 to 7 psi (pounds per square inch) for 1.5–6 hours of exposure.

The object to be sterilized is usually packaged with an indicator tape to ensure that there was exposure to the gas. This does not guarantee sterility so a biological indicator of a specific organism is used daily to ensure sterilization is occurring (the biological indicator, a bacteria culture, dies).

Although the use of ETO is very effective, there are some cautions. There is a mandatory airing time of at least 24 hours in a well-ventilated area that is necessary to get rid of any residual gas. This gas can be toxic to humans. If objects made of PVC have been previously gamma irradiated, they may react with ETO to form thylene chlorhydrin, which can be a skin irritant. Also, if an object to be sterilized contains water, it will react with ETO to form ethylene glycol (antifreeze), which is potentially poisonous.

🤚 4-2
Stop and Review

1. A(n) _____ degree Fahrenheit increase in temperature may result in a doubling of the microorganism kill rate.

2. _____ is the process by which heated water is used to kill vegetative cells and denature viruses.

3. When used as a disinfectant, _____ alcohol is most effective at a 70% concentration, while _____ alcohol is most effective at a 90% concentration.

Radiation

In addition to gas and liquid agents, ultraviolet and gamma radiation can be used as disinfectants.

Ultraviolet

Something as simple as sunlight can have some bactericidal action. Ultraviolet rays can be used for disinfection where UV rays damage the bacteria's DNA. UV rays generated by mercury vapor lamps can be used in closed areas to disinfect, as in operating rooms and nurseries.

Gamma

gamma irradiation: a type of radiation therapy that uses short wavelengths of light that ionize water molecules for sterilization

Gamma irradiation uses very short wavelengths of light that ionize water molecules thus inactivating DNA molecules. This form of sterilizing is highly efficient, does not generate excessive heat, and items can be prepackaged and sealed. The disadvantages of this method are that sterilization can take up to 48 to 72 hours, it may cause polyvinyl chloride (PVC) to release chlorine gas, and currently can only be used on a large-scale level. Thus it is quite expensive to set up. See Table 4-2 for a synopsis of the various treatments to control microorganisms.

TABLE 4-2 Examples of Methods of Sterilization and Disinfection, Modes of Actions, and Practical Uses

Treatment	Effect	Mode of Action	Uses
Physical Methods			
Heat			
Dry heat	Sterilizes.	Denatures protein.	In the laboratory, used to sterilize dry materials that can withstand high temperature and any materials damaged by moisture.
Moist heat	Sterilizes.	Denatures protein.	In the laboratory, used to sterilize liquids and material easily charred. Used in food canning.
Pasteurization	Kills certain microorganisms.	Denatures protein.	Eliminates pathogens and slows spoilage of milk and dairy products, wine, and beer (canned, evaporated, or condensed milk is sterilized).

(Continues)

TABLE 4-2 *(Continued)*

Treatment	Effect	Mode of Action	Uses
Physical Methods			
Radiation			
UV light	Sterilizes.	Damages DNA.	In the laboratory, sterilizes surfaces.
X-rays and gamma rays	Sterilizes.	Strips electrons from atoms.	Used to sterilize plastic equipment and surface of fresh fruits and vegetables.
Chemicals			
Phenols	Kills most microorganisms.	Denatures protein.	Germicides.
Phenolics	Kills most microorganisms.	Denatures proteins and disrupts plasma membrane.	Disinfectants, antiseptics.
Alcohols	Kills most microorganisms.	Denatures proteins and disrupts plasma membrane.	Disinfects surfaces, including skin and thermometers.
Hydrogen peroxide	Kills many microorganisms.	Oxidizes vital biochemicals.	Mild skin disinfectant.
Surfactants			
Soap detergent	Washes away microorganisms.	Physically removes microbes.	Disinfects surfaces, including skin, bench tops.
Quaternary ammonium salts	Kills microorganisms.	Disrupts membranes.	Widely used sterilizing agents.
Alkylating Agents			
Formaldehyde and glutaraldehyde	Kills microorganisms.	Inactivates enzymes by adding alkyl groups.	Preserves tissues, prepares vaccine, sterilizes surgical instruments.
Ethylene oxide (ETO)	Kills microorganisms.	Inactivates enzymes by adding alkyl groups.	Gas used to sterilize heat-sensitive materials and unwieldy objects in hospitals.

© 2016 Cengage Learning®.

Media Connection

Go to the accompanying online resources to view additional videos on infection control procedures, pathogens, and controlling diseases.

4-3 Stop and Review

1. Why is the use of an autoclave more effective than boiling water?
2. What are the four factors that determine the effectiveness of ETO sterilization?
3. Give the mode of disinfectant action for the following:

   Alcohol

   Quaternary ammonium

   Glutaraldehydes

   Phenols

Chapter Summary

- Now you should have a better handle on the language of infection prevention. We began this section by discussing the meaning of infection prevention and how putting these principles into practice helps protect ourselves, our co-workers, and most importantly, our patients.

- Remember, our goal is to prevent infections from ever occurring, but once an infection occurs, the goal would be to prevent the spread.

- We illustrated how infections occur, using the concept of chain of infection, and where a health care professional might intervene to break this chain and prevent the spread of infection.

- We defined basic infection prevention terms such as *vegetative organisms, spores, denaturing, contamination,* and *infection.*

- Microorganisms may be removed from environmental objects by cleaning, sanitization,

  decontamination, or disinfection. Decontamination refers to removal of contaminants by chemical or physical means, while disinfection is a process to remove pathogenic microorganisms from inanimate objects.

- We presented methods used to disinfect and sterilize medical equipment. You now know that common household bleach can bleach your clothes and be used to clean up blood spills in a 1:10 dilution.

- Many of the other liquid disinfectants are common household products you were probably familiar with, but now you have an understanding of how they work.

- Finally, we completed our infection prevention journey by discussing methods to disinfect our environment and instruments we may use in patients to diagnose and treat disease.

Case Study

A 25-year-old male who works as a landscaper cut his right forearm while using hedge trimmers. The owner of the company drives him to a local urgent care center where you are employed. He is immediately taken to an exam room, and the blood-soaked towel that was wrapped around his arm is removed. The bleeding has not stopped and about 2 tablespoonfuls of blood has spilled onto the floor. It was decided to transfer the patient to a hospital emergency room because of the depth and location of the cut. After the patient is transferred, one of your coworkers is about to clean up the blood spill with Lysol. Is this the appropriate action to take? What would you recommend to clean up the blood spill?

Chapter Review

Match the term with its description.

1. _____ chain of infection
2. _____ vegetative organisms
3. _____ spores
4. _____ denatured
5. _____ contamination
6. _____ health care–associated infections
7. _____ nosocomial infections
8. _____ sanitation
9. _____ disinfection
10. _____ sterilization

a. dormant, protective state of organism
b. presence of organisms in absence of infection
c. infections occurring in health care setting
d. reduction in bacterial load to safe level
e. the spread of infectious diseases
f. elimination of vegetative organism from object
g. complete destruction of all microorganisms
h. actively growing organism
i. old term for HAIs
j. structural alteration of substance or organism

Define the following.

11. Low-level disinfectants _____

12. Intermediate-level disinfectants _____

13. High-level disinfectants _____

Fill in the blanks.

14. _____ irradiation is highly efficient, and items can be prepackaged and sealed.

15. Ethylene oxide is used extensively in _____ sterilization.

16. _____ disinfectants may cause irritation to skin, mucous membranes, or eyes.

17. Hydrogen peroxide is used as a 3% solution for mild antisepsis and _____.

18. Household bleach is used in a(n) _____ dilution to clean up blood spills.

19. _____ rays work to disinfect operating rooms and nurseries by damaging bacterial DNA.

20. If ethylene oxide comes into contact with water, it forms _____, which is also known as antifreeze.

21. _____ is more effective than dry heat for sterilization because water molecules increase heating capacity.

22. _____ compounds cause cell lysis by disrupting cell membrane semipermeability.

23. Ethanol and isopropyl are two kinds of _____.

Additional Activities

1. Look up the infection rates of hospitals in your area at www.hospitalcompare.hhs.gov. You can find information concerning bloodstream and urinary tract infections caused by the insertion of catheters in veins and the bladder, respectively. How do the rates compare? Would this affect your choice of hospitals in case you need health care?

2. The infections discussed in the previous question are called catheter-associated bloodstream infections and catheter-associated urinary tract infections. Research how to prevent these infections at www.cdc.gov. Explain how these prevention efforts might break the chain of infection.

3. Invite an infection prevention specialist who works in a hospital infection control department to discuss infection prevention efforts at their hospital.

4. Visit the central sterile supply department at your local hospital. Take a tour of their facility and ask them to demonstrate the different methods of disinfection and sterilization of instruments used at the hospital.

5. Have each student bring in an empty bottle of a commonly used cleaning agent. Divide the class into groups and have each group analyze the active ingredients in the cleaning products brought in by their group. Use the classification scheme discussed in this chapter to sort the cleaning products into their respective cleaning agent category (e.g., alcohols, phenols, etc.).

Media Connection

Go to the accompanying online resources and have fun learning as you play games, view animations and videos, and take practice tests to help reinforce key concepts you learned in this chapter.

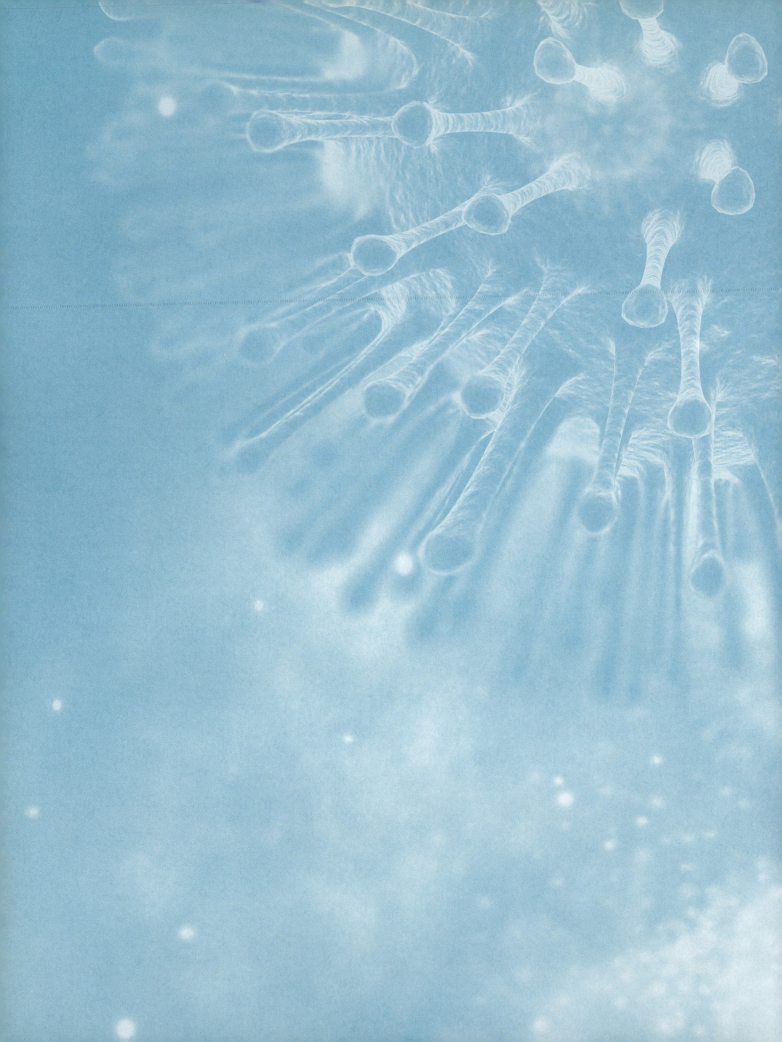

CHAPTER 5

Protecting Patients and Ourselves

OBJECTIVES

After studying this chapter, the learner will be able to:

- Describe the various portals of entry and related microorganisms and diseases.

- Contrast the different routes of transmission of infection.

- List and define the types of precautions that are used in the health care environment.

- Explain the importance of proper hand hygiene.

- Describe standard precautions.

- Differentiate contact, droplet, and airborne precautions.

- List the various types of personal protective equipment and when it would be appropriate to wear the equipment.

- Describe safe injection practices.

- Explain safe handling of potentially contaminated surfaces or medical equipment.

- Describe OSHA regulations as they pertain to health care workers.

KEY TERMS

airborne precautions

Bloodborne Pathogen Standard

contact precautions

direct contact

droplet precautions

eye protection

face masks

fomite [FO might]

gloves

gowns

hand hygiene

indirect contact

Occupational Safety and Health Administration (OSHA)

personal protective equipment (PPE)

reservoir of infection

(Continues)

KEY TERMS *(Continued)*

resident flora

route of transmission

sharps container

standard precautions

transient flora

transmission-based
precautions

vectors

Introduction

Occupational Safety and Health Administration (OSHA): a government agency in the Department of Labor that strives to maintain a safe and healthy work environment

In this chapter we use our newly acquired knowledge of infection prevention and learn how something as simple as washing our hands correctly can help us break the chain of infection and protect ourselves and patients from acquiring microorganisms. We learn about standard and transmission-based precautions to prevent the spread of infection. Finally, we talk about the protections afforded us by the **Occupational Safety and Health Administration (OSHA)** regulations, how they protect us from acquiring pathogens from body fluids, and what to do in the event of an exposure to these fluids.

In Chapter 4 we introduced you to the basic vocabulary of infection prevention and control and discussed the chain of infection and methods to disinfect and sterilize the environment and equipment used in health care. With that as a background, you are ready to learn how we might protect patients and ourselves from infections. Have you ever walked through a hospital and noticed a sign hanging outside a patient room that listed some type of precaution? Did you wonder why the health care workers were putting on gloves and gowns before entering the room with the precaution sign? What is all the fuss about hand hygiene? During your hospital visit, did you notice if the health care workers washed their hands before and after patient contact? This chapter will answer these questions and more as we expand our infection prevention knowledge. Hopefully, the proper ways to perform hand hygiene will have "rubbed off" on you as a side effect of reading and studying this chapter.

Portals of Entry

Portals of entry are a limited number of openings by which infectious agents can gain access to the body (Figure 5-1). These portals can include the respiratory tract, mucous membranes, gastrointestinal tract, genitourinary tract, breaches in the skin, and wounds. Normally, pathogens entering one of these portals are stopped by the body's defense system, or at most, they create only a local infection. However, depending on the type of organism and the patient's

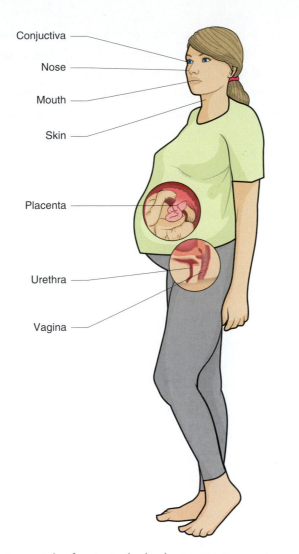

Conjuctiva

Nose

Mouth

Skin

Placenta

Urethra

Vagina

FIGURE 5-1 Major portals of entry to the body. © 2016 Cengage Learning®.

immune system, that invader may be able to spread systemically and establish infections in various parts of the body with potentially deadly results.

It is interesting to note that some individuals may only be *carriers* of a disease and possess no disease symptoms. That individual would then become what is known as a **reservoir of infection** and thus spread the disease to others.

reservoir of infection: a continuous source of infectious disease; people, animals, and plants may be reservoirs of infection

Food for Thought
Typhoid Mary

The classic example of a disease carrier occurred in the early 1900s when Mary Mallon, a cook, spread typhoid fever from one community to another but never became ill with the symptoms of the disease herself. She came to be known as "Typhoid Mary."

fomite [FO might]: object that may harbor microorganisms and is capable of transmitting them

In addition to humans, reservoirs of infection may include animals, the environment, and **fomites**. Fomites are nonliving objects such as clothing, towels, and medical instruments that may harbor and transmit diseases.

Quite often, hospital procedures cause breaches in the natural defenses of the body. Surgical procedures that create deep wounds, such as hip replacement surgery, have the potential to deposit pathogens deep within the body. Once deposited, the wound is stitched up, sealing the pathogens inside where they can grow, colonize, and spread throughout the body via the circulatory and lymphatic systems. The insertion of an artificial airway to facilitate the use of a mechanical ventilator bypasses the natural defenses of coughing and the natural mucus removal by the cilia in the airways. This makes an individual more prone to respiratory infections. Table 5-1 lists the portals of entry and examples of related microorganisms and their diseases.

TABLE 5-1 Portals of Entry with Examples of Related Microorganisms and Diseases

Portal of Entry	Microorganism	Microorganism Type	Disease Produced
Skin	Staphylococcus aureus	Bacteria	Impetigo
	Papillomavirus	Virus	Warts
	Trycophyton	Fungus	Ringworm
Wound	Clostridium tetani	Bacteria	Tetanus
	Rabies virus	Virus	Rabies
Respiratory tract	Bordetella pertussis	Bacteria	Whooping cough
	Influenza	Virus	Influenza
	Blastomyces dermatitidis	Fungus	Blastomycosis
Gastrointestinal tract	Clostridium difficile	Bacteria	Diarrheal illnesses (often accompanied with pseudomembranous colitis)
	Polio	Virus	Polio
	Giardia lamblia (G. duodenalis)	Protozoan	Giardiasis
Genitourinary tract	Treponema pallidum	Bacteria	Syphilis
	Herpes simplex virus type II	Virus	Genital herpes
	Candida albicans	Fungus	Vaginitis

Routes of Transmission

So how do pathogens find their way inside us and cause infections? While we already discussed these concepts in Section One, a brief review is warranted to apply this knowledge to actual procedures. The avenues that pathogens can use are known as the **route of transmission**. These routes include contact, common vehicle, airborne, and vector routes of transmission. Some of these routes can even be further divided.

route of transmission: the passing of a communicable disease from an infected host individual or group to a nonspecific individual or group, regardless of whether the other individual was previously infected

Contact

The contact route can be subdivided into direct contact and indirect contact as follows:

Direct Contact

Direct contact is the spread of infective agents to an individual directly from a contaminated source. Shaking dirty hands and then rubbing your eyes or kissing an individual with an open sore on the lip are examples of direct contact spread of pathogens.

direct contact: mutual touching of two individuals or organisms; many communicable diseases may be spread by direct contact between an infected and a healthy person

Indirect Contact

Indirect contact spread involves an infected individual and an object improperly cleaned that is then used on, or by, another individual. A clinical example would be performing a bronchoscopy on an individual to examine his or her lungs for tuberculosis. *Mycobacterium tuberculosis* is found, and a sputum sample is taken to culture. The bronchoscope is then removed and improperly cleaned for use on the next patient, leaving *Mycobacterium tuberculosis* in and on the bronchoscope. The next patient has the bronchoscope inserted into his lungs, and the *Mycobacterium tuberculosis* organisms fall off the bronchoscope, deposit in his lungs, and begin to grow.

indirect contact: transmission achieved through some intervening medium, such as prolongation of a communicable disease through the air or by means of fomites

Common Vehicle

The common vehicle route occurs when there is a contamination of a specific substance such as tainted blood supplies or *Escherichia coli* in hamburger that is transported and consumed by a number of individuals. It is relatively easy to recognize this one: You usually see it occurring within a specific time frame, many individuals are affected at the same time, a patient history work-up of each individual reveals the consumption of the same or very similar substance, and a specific pathogen is identified in most, if not all, of the cases.

Airborne

Because we normally inhale between 10,000 and 20,000 liters of air per day with between 10,000 to 1,000,000 microorganisms riding those volumes, it shouldn't be a shocker that your respiratory tract is a main portal of entry for a variety of pathogens. These pathogens are spread as a result of the aerosol generated from a sneeze or cough and can float around in the air for some time before being inhaled by another person. As you can see from Figure 5-2, an uncovered sneeze has the potential to spread a multitude of aerosol particles leading to the potential infection of others.

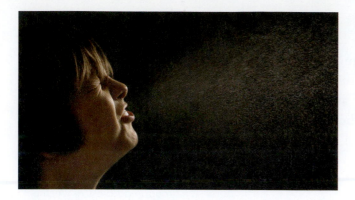

FIGURE 5-2 A sneeze propels aerosols containing microorganisms. Can you now understand why it is important to properly contain a sneeze? © iStock.com/ mammamaart.

Vector

vectors: carriers of disease

Vectors are organisms that carry a disease agent to the host (the victim). Figure 5-3 illustrates a variety of disease-carrying arthropod vectors. The vector doesn't need to develop the disease to be able to spread it to a human. It can merely serve as a reservoir of infection. Mosquitoes are frequently the vectors for the spread of diseases such as malaria and West Nile virus. Vector transmission can occur in two ways: either biological or mechanical.

Biological

A *biological* form of vector transmission occurs when the vector (in this case a mosquito) ingests blood from an infected source, flies to a human and bites that individual. Some of that tainted blood from the previous bite is injected into the fresh bite on that human. Now the pathogen can begin to grow in the new host, as in malaria or the West Nile virus.

Mechanical

The *mechanical* spread of infection by a vector occurs when the pathogen is located on the outside of the vector's body. A common example would be flies

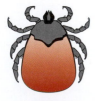
Tick

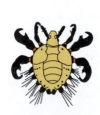
Louse

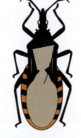
Reduviid Bug

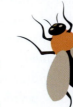
Mosquito

Deer Fly

Flea

FIGURE 5-3 Various arthropod vectors. © 2016 Cengage Learning®.

walking over fresh feces with pathogens attaching to their little "feet." They then fly away to a nearby picnic table where there is a big bowl of uncovered potato salad and begin walking around on it. As they continue to walk around, the pathogens on their "feet" begin to slough off, contaminating the potato salad. If it is a nice warm day, the number of pathogens begins to grow, waiting for someone to consume them. Another related term to review is *parasite*. Remember that a parasite is any organism living within, on, or at the expense of another organism or host. Table 5-2 shows various routes of transmission and related parasitic diseases. Figure 5-4 shows examples of various types of parasites.

🤚 5-1
Stop and Review

1. The respiratory tract, mucous membranes, gastrointestinal tract, genitourinary tract, breaches in the skin, and wounds are all potential _____ into our bodies for microorganisms.

2. _____is the spread of infective agents to an individual directly from a contaminated source.

3. Mosquitoes are a good example of _____, which are organisms that carry a disease-causing agent to a host.

TABLE 5-2 Common Parasites and Their Mechanism of Transmission and Related Disease or Condition

Parasite	Route of Transmission	Specimen for Testing	Disease or Condition
Giardia lamblia	Drinking or eating contaminated feces	Feces	Severe diarrhea
Entamoeba histolytica	Drinking or eating contaminated food or water	Feces	Amoebic dysentery
Hookworm	Soil larvae can penetrate bare feet	Feces	Iron deficiency/anemia
Pinworm	Ingestion of infected food, or soiled bedding or clothing; common in children	Feces	Anal itching
Plasmodium	Bite of infected mosquito	Blood	Malaria

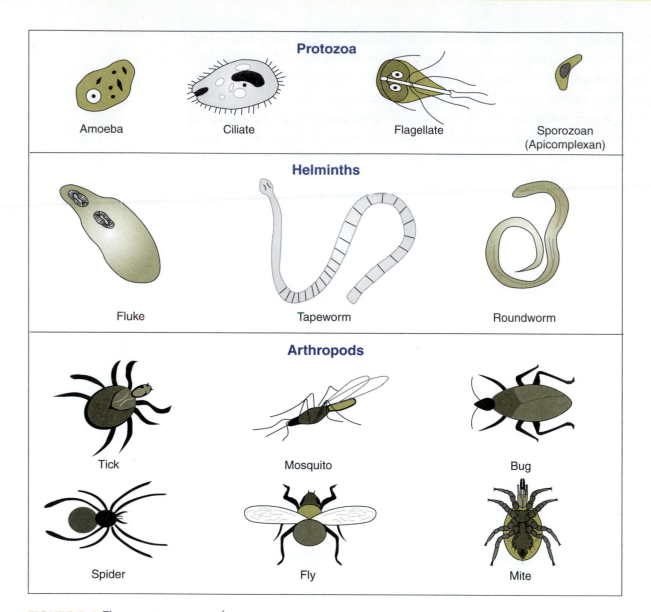

FIGURE 5-4 Three major groups of parasites. © Cengage Learning®.

Hand Hygiene

hand hygiene: the removal of visible soil and the removal or killing of transient microorganisms from the hands accomplished by using soap and running water or an alcohol-based hand rub

Now that you know the routes of transmission, we need to spend some time explaining the importance of **hand hygiene** because it is one of the simplest and most important ways to prevent the spread of infection. There are two types of flora on our hands. The first type is called **resident flora**, and they are microorganisms found just beneath as well as on top of the outermost layer of skin cells (stratum corneum). Coagulase-negative staphylococci (e.g.,

Staphylococcus epidermidis and *Staphylococcus hominis*) are the predominant microbes followed by coryneform bacteria (e.g., *propionibacteria, corynebacteria*). The predominant fungal species is *Pityrosporum*. The resident flora prevents our skin from becoming contaminated with other microbes by antagonizing other microorganisms and competing for food. Those of you with brothers and sisters who remember competing with them for food and space as you were growing up know what we mean. These organisms are difficult to remove by hand washing but are generally not pathogenic (disease-causing) unless they enter a sterile body cavity in a person with a weakened immune system (immunocompromised).

The second type of flora is called **transient flora**. This type is often acquired by health care workers during direct contact with patients or contaminated surfaces surrounding patients. The hands of some health care workers may become persistently colonized by disease-causing organisms such as *Staphylococcus aureus*, gram-negative bacilli, or yeast. Fortunately, this type of flora is easier to remove with routine hand hygiene.

There is substantial evidence that routine hand hygiene reduces the transmission of health care–associated pathogens (transient flora) resulting in fewer health care–associated infections. Observational studies of hand

resident flora: species of microorganisms that are always present on or in the body and are not easily removed by mechanical friction

transient flora: microorganisms that may be present in or on the body under certain conditions and for certain lengths of time; they are easier to remove by mechanical friction than resident flora

Clinical Application
Basics of Hand Washing

Arguably, the easiest, most cost-effective way to prevent the spread of infection is hand washing. However, there is a correct way to wash your hands:

- Remove all jewelry from your hands.
- Crank out enough paper towel to dry your hands but don't tear it off.
- Turn on the water as hot as tolerable.
- Wet hands and apply soap.
- Work the soapy water over your hands, between fingers and around nails.
- Continue this action for at least 25–30 seconds (sing "Happy Birthday to You" or "Row, Row, Row Your Boat" if you prefer, twice).
- Rinse with water, positioning your hands so the water flows from above the wrists, downward and over the hands, then fingers.
- Tear off the paper towel and dry hands.
- Use the paper towel to turn off the water. Note that some texts will recommend using a new clean towel.
- Discard the towel into the trash can.

(Continues)

(Continued)

See Figure 5-5 for the proper hand washing procedure.

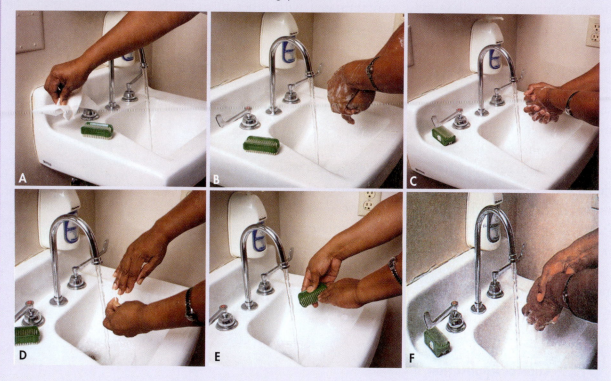

FIGURE 5-5 Proper technique for hand washing. **A.** Use a dry towel to turn the faucet on. **B.** Point the fingertips downward and use the palm of one hand to clean the back of the other hand. **C.** Interlace the fingers to clean between the fingers. **D.** The blunt end of an orange stick can be used to clean the nails. **E.** A hand brush can also be used to clean the nails. **F.** With the fingertips pointing downward, rinse the hands thoroughly. © Cengage Learning®.

hygiene practices document on average about 40% compliance with hand washing. Why are health care workers so noncompliant with hand hygiene? The list of reasons are many, but now that you know how important proper hand hygiene is to prevent the spread of infection to yourself and your patients, hopefully you will be a role model for your peers when it comes to hand hygiene.

Alcohol-based, antiseptic hand sanitizers are useful when full hand washing cannot be performed. Just be sure to use the same hand cleaning action as described above. Continue that action until the sanitizer has evaporated and your hands are dry (Figure 5-6).

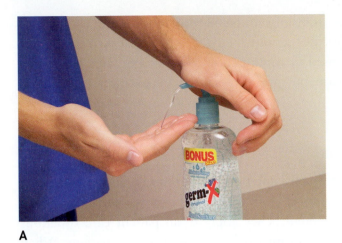

A

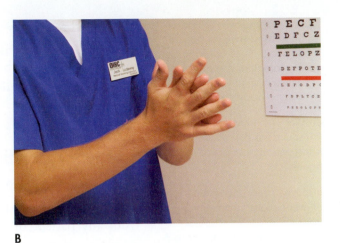

B

FIGURE 5-6 Using alcohol-based, antiseptic hand sanitizers. **A.** Apply the appropriate amount of alcohol-based hand rub. **B.** Rub your hands together until all the hand rub is absorbed/evaporated. Be sure to rub between your fingers. © Cengage Learning®.

Learning Hint

See It in Action

For additional educational resources concerning hand washing, visit the World Health Organization's website at www.who.int, and search for hand washing. You may also view a video on proper hand washing on the accompanying online resources.

Fundamental Principles of Infection Prevention and Control

There are two broad categories of precautions that apply to patient care. **Standard precautions** are the minimum standards that should be applied to all patients in any health care setting. Standard precautions assume that any patient could have an infection or microorganisms that could be transmitted to other patients or you, the health care professional. The other type of precaution is called **transmission-based precautions**. These are used on top of standard precautions in patients with known or suspected colonization or infection of easily transmissible or important pathogens (e.g., multidrug-resistant bacteria). These are used in addition to standard precautions when standard precautions alone are insufficient to interrupt the route of pathogen transmission.

standard precautions: guidelines recommended by the Centers for Disease Control and Prevention (CDC) for reducing the risk of transmission of bloodborne and other pathogens in hospitals; the standard precautions synthesize the major features of universal precautions (designed to reduce the risk of transmission of bloodborne pathogens) and body substance isolation (designed to reduce the risk of pathogens from moist body substances) and apply them to all patients receiving care in hospitals regardless of their diagnosis or presumed infection status

transmission-based precautions: safeguards designed for patients documented or suspected to be infected with highly transmissible or epidemiologically important pathogens for which additional precautions beyond standard precautions are needed to interrupt transmission in hospitals

contact precautions: a type of isolation used when a patient is infected with or carrying an epidemiologically important organism that can be spread by body-to-body contact

droplet precautions: measures to reduce the risk of droplet transmission of infectious agents

airborne precautions: set of precautions to prevent transmission of infectious agents that remain infectious over long distances when suspended in the air

personal protective equipment (PPE): Specialized clothing or equipment worn by employees for protection against health and safety hazards and designed to protect many parts of the body, for example, eyes, head, face, hands, feet, and ears

The three types of transmission-based precautions are (1) **contact precautions**, (2) **droplet precautions**, and (3) **airborne precautions**. Remember, these may be used in combination for microbes with more than one route of transmission but are always used in addition to standard precautions.

Standard Precautions

These are used to protect yourself and patients and should be used whenever there is a possible exposure to blood, body fluids, or any other excretions from any patient or equipment. They apply to all patient care situations regardless of suspected or confirmed infection status of the patient. When practiced properly, they are designed to prevent the spread of infections among patients and to protect health care personnel from acquiring infections from patients. Standard precautions include the following activities: (1) hand hygiene, (2) use of **personal protective equipment (PPE)** (e.g., face masks, gowns, and gloves), depending on what you might be exposed to, (3) cough etiquette and respiratory hygiene, (4) safe injection practices, and (5) safe handling of potentially contaminated surfaces or equipment in the patient care environment.

Hand Hygiene

It seems like we are beating this topic to death, but hopefully you know by now how important it is to prevent infection. As discussed before, hand washing should be performed before and after patient contact even if gloves are worn. Alcohol-based rubs are preferred unless the hands are visibly soiled or the patient has diarrhea. In these cases, wash your hands using soap and water. The following situations are times when hand hygiene is indicated.

Antimicrobial soap and water should be used:

- Before eating

- If hands are visibly soiled

- After using the restroom

- If exposure to spore-forming organism (e.g., *Clostridium difficile*) is suspected

Alcohol-based hand rubs should be used in all other situations as follows, unless hands are visibly soiled:

- Before and after direct patient contact

- Before donning sterile gloves

- After removing gloves

- Before inserting invasive devices (e.g., bladder catheter)

- After contact with patient's intact skin

- After contact with objects and equipment in the patient's immediate vicinity

- When moving from a contaminated body site to a clean body site during patient care

Personal Protective Equipment (PPE)

This is specialized clothing worn by the health care worker to protect against acquiring microorganisms. The type of personal protective equipment needed is based on the type of patient contact and the potential for exposure to blood or body fluids. Perform hand hygiene immediately before and after using personal protective equipment. Some examples of PPE follow with explanations:

- **Gloves** are worn when touching blood, body fluids, mucous membranes, non-intact skin, or contaminated medical equipment. Do not wear the same pair of gloves for more than one patient.

- **Gowns** are worn to protect your skin and clothing during any activity that may generate splashes or spray of blood, body fluids, secretions, or excretions. Do not wear the same gown to care for more than one patient and remove the gown before leaving the room.

- **Face masks** and **eye protection** (or a face shield) must be worn to protect your eyes, nose, and mouth during any activity that could cause a splash of blood, body fluids, secretions, or excretions. Personal eyeglasses are not considered adequate protection.

You can view video demonstrations of donning and removing personal protective equipment and proper hand hygiene at http://www.cdc.gov.

gloves: sterile or clean fitted coverings for the hands, usually with a separate sheath for each finger and thumb

gowns: a robe or smock worn in operating rooms and other parts of hospitals as a guard against contamination

face masks: a personal protective device (PPE) to shield the facial area from contamination

eye protection: recommended safety glasses, chemical splash goggles, or face shields to be used when handling a hazardous material

5-2
Stop and Review

1. Why is it important to properly wash your hands?

2. When is it important to wear a gown when caring for a patient?

3. What method of hand hygiene (soap and water versus alcohol-based hand rub) should be used when caring for a patient with diarrhea?

Media Connection

To view videos on proper removal of gloves and gowns, sterile gloves, and field and other infection control precautions, visit the accompanying online resources.

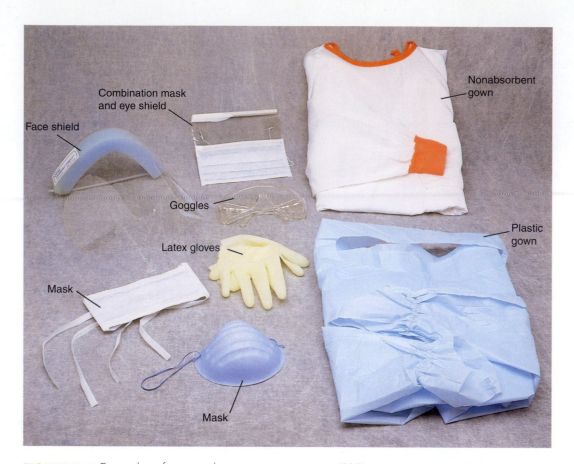

FIGURE 5-7 Examples of personal protective equipment (PPE). © Cengage Learning®.

Figure 5-7 shows some examples of PPE, and Figure 5-8 presents an example of a standard precautions chart.

Cough Etiquette and Respiratory Hygiene

We must be vigilant for individuals with signs and symptoms of respiratory illness such as cough, runny nose, fever, and congestion. Signs should be posted in clear view of patients and visitors to self-report symptoms during the patient registration process. It is useful to make sure the reception area is stocked with tissues and no-touch waste cans for disposal of used tissues.

Another simple and effective way to prevent the spread of pathogens is to cover your mouth when coughing or sneezing. In the past it was suggested that you cover your mouth with your hand. This, however, is somewhat counterproductive especially if you cover a sneeze with your hand and then shake someone else's hand, turn a doorknob, or pick up a ketchup bottle to squeeze some on your fries. You've just spread the pathogens that your hand captured! It is better to use a tissue or cough/sneeze into the crook of your elbow if no tissue is available. Don't forget to perform hand hygiene after contact with respiratory secretions whether it be your own or your patient's.

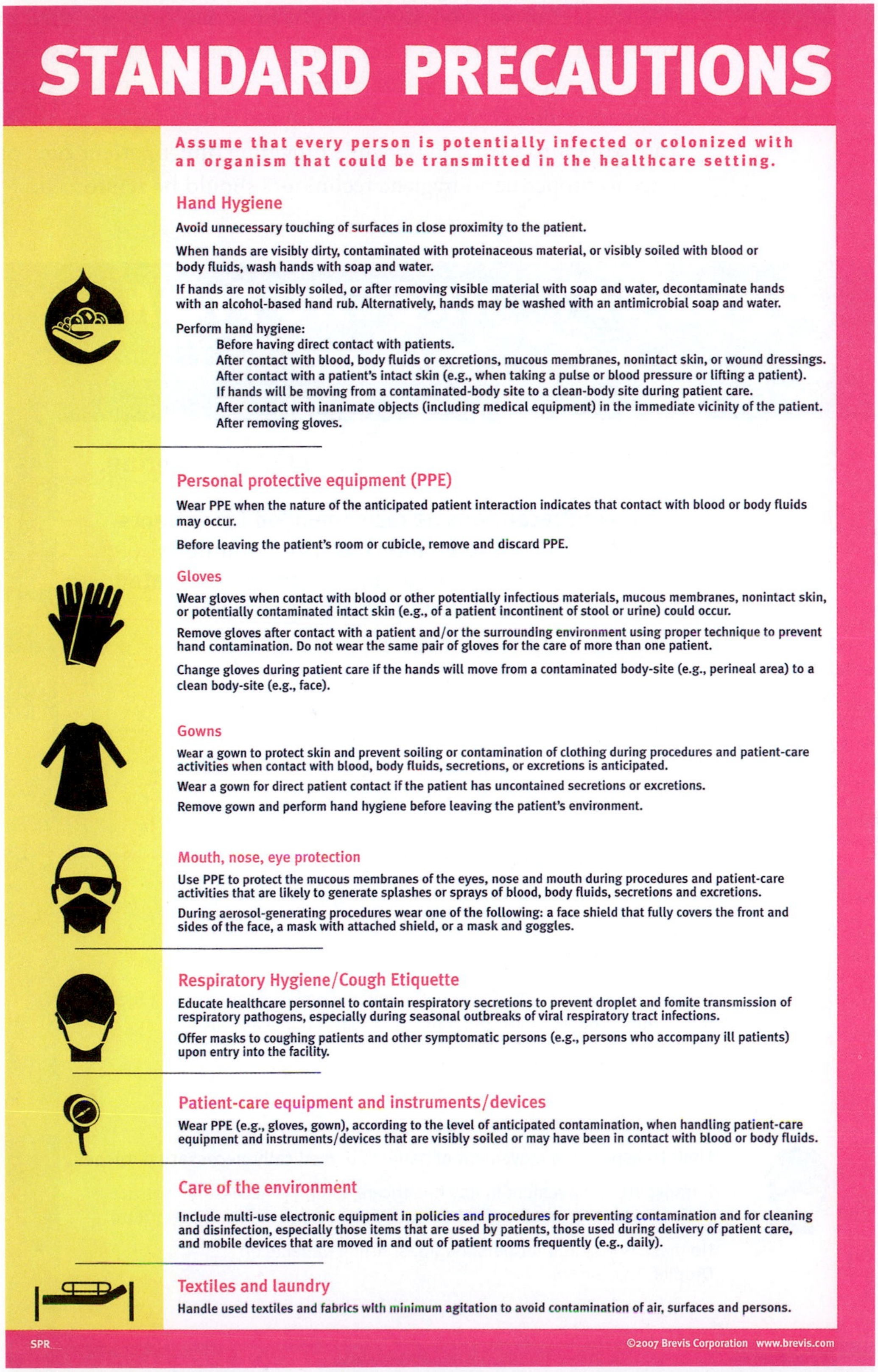

STANDARD PRECAUTIONS

Assume that every person is potentially infected or colonized with an organism that could be transmitted in the healthcare setting.

Hand Hygiene

Avoid unnecessary touching of surfaces in close proximity to the patient.

When hands are visibly dirty, contaminated with proteinaceous material, or visibly soiled with blood or body fluids, wash hands with soap and water.

If hands are not visibly soiled, or after removing visible material with soap and water, decontaminate hands with an alcohol-based hand rub. Alternatively, hands may be washed with an antimicrobial soap and water.

Perform hand hygiene:
  Before having direct contact with patients.
  After contact with blood, body fluids or excretions, mucous membranes, nonintact skin, or wound dressings.
  After contact with a patient's intact skin (e.g., when taking a pulse or blood pressure or lifting a patient).
  If hands will be moving from a contaminated-body site to a clean-body site during patient care.
  After contact with inanimate objects (including medical equipment) in the immediate vicinity of the patient.
  After removing gloves.

Personal protective equipment (PPE)

Wear PPE when the nature of the anticipated patient interaction indicates that contact with blood or body fluids may occur.

Before leaving the patient's room or cubicle, remove and discard PPE.

Gloves

Wear gloves when contact with blood or other potentially infectious materials, mucous membranes, nonintact skin, or potentially contaminated intact skin (e.g., of a patient incontinent of stool or urine) could occur.

Remove gloves after contact with a patient and/or the surrounding environment using proper technique to prevent hand contamination. Do not wear the same pair of gloves for the care of more than one patient.

Change gloves during patient care if the hands will move from a contaminated body-site (e.g., perineal area) to a clean body-site (e.g., face).

Gowns

Wear a gown to protect skin and prevent soiling or contamination of clothing during procedures and patient-care activities when contact with blood, body fluids, secretions, or excretions is anticipated.

Wear a gown for direct patient contact if the patient has uncontained secretions or excretions.

Remove gown and perform hand hygiene before leaving the patient's environment.

Mouth, nose, eye protection

Use PPE to protect the mucous membranes of the eyes, nose and mouth during procedures and patient-care activities that are likely to generate splashes or sprays of blood, body fluids, secretions and excretions.

During aerosol-generating procedures wear one of the following: a face shield that fully covers the front and sides of the face, a mask with attached shield, or a mask and goggles.

Respiratory Hygiene/Cough Etiquette

Educate healthcare personnel to contain respiratory secretions to prevent droplet and fomite transmission of respiratory pathogens, especially during seasonal outbreaks of viral respiratory tract infections.

Offer masks to coughing patients and other symptomatic persons (e.g., persons who accompany ill patients) upon entry into the facility.

Patient-care equipment and instruments/devices

Wear PPE (e.g., gloves, gown), according to the level of anticipated contamination, when handling patient-care equipment and instruments/devices that are visibly soiled or may have been in contact with blood or body fluids.

Care of the environment

Include multi-use electronic equipment in policies and procedures for preventing contamination and for cleaning and disinfection, especially those items that are used by patients, those used during delivery of patient care, and mobile devices that are moved in and out of patient rooms frequently (e.g., daily).

Textiles and laundry

Handle used textiles and fabrics with minimum agitation to avoid contamination of air, surfaces and persons.

FIGURE 5-8 A standard precautions chart. Note when certain PPE is to be used in different situations. Reprinted with permission from Brevis Corporation (www.brevis.com).

Droplet precaution (Figure 5-9), in addition to standard precautions, may need to be followed when caring for patients with a respiratory illness. Health care personnel should avoid direct patient contact when they have a respiratory illness. A less desirable option would be for the infected health care worker to wear a mask while providing direct patient care. Strict adherence to proper hand hygiene techniques should be reinforced.

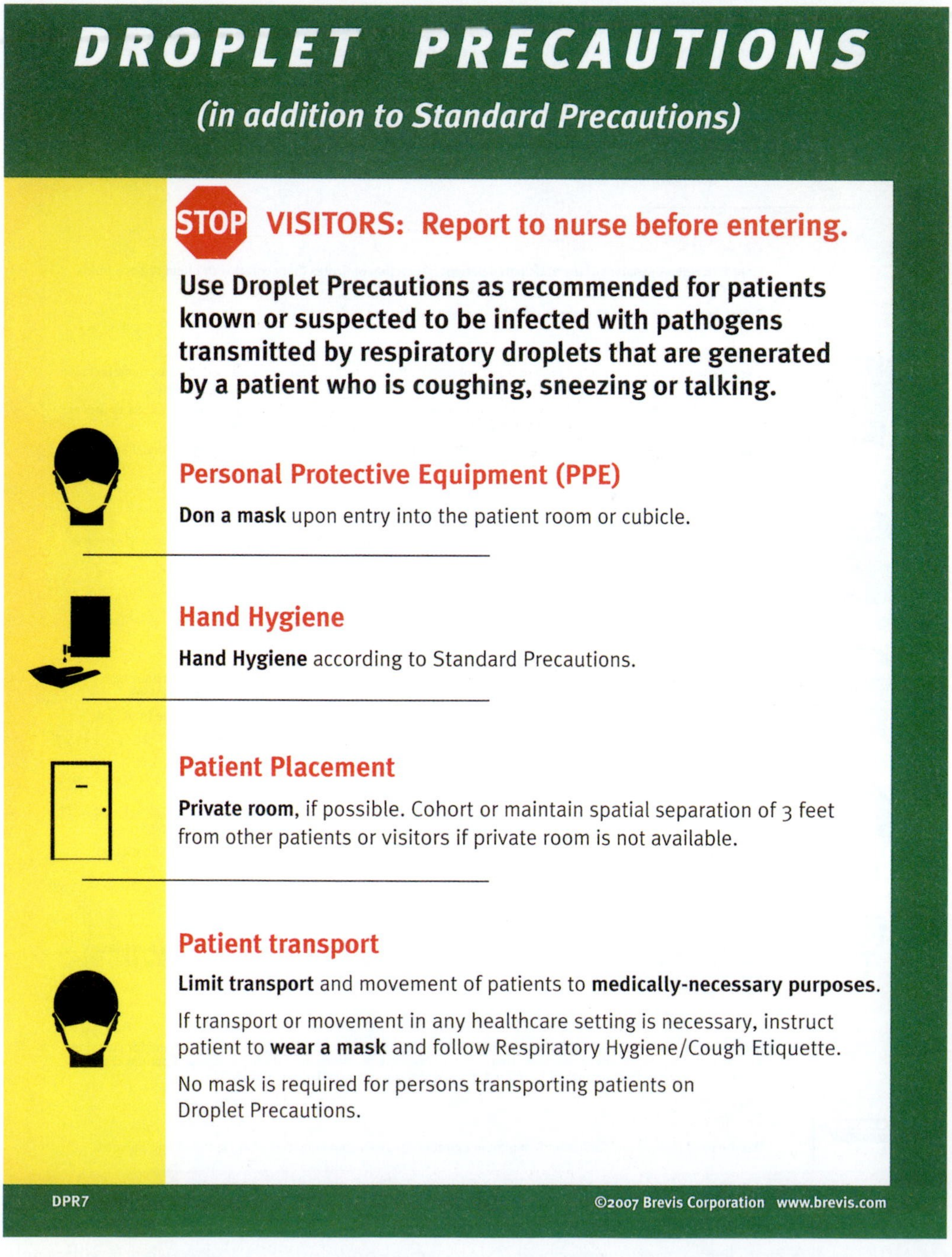

DROPLET PRECAUTIONS
(in addition to Standard Precautions)

STOP **VISITORS: Report to nurse before entering.**

Use Droplet Precautions as recommended for patients known or suspected to be infected with pathogens transmitted by respiratory droplets that are generated by a patient who is coughing, sneezing or talking.

Personal Protective Equipment (PPE)

Don a mask upon entry into the patient room or cubicle.

Hand Hygiene

Hand Hygiene according to Standard Precautions.

Patient Placement

Private room, if possible. Cohort or maintain spatial separation of 3 feet from other patients or visitors if private room is not available.

Patient transport

Limit transport and movement of patients to **medically-necessary purposes**.

If transport or movement in any healthcare setting is necessary, instruct patient to **wear a mask** and follow Respiratory Hygiene/Cough Etiquette.

No mask is required for persons transporting patients on Droplet Precautions.

DPR7   ©2007 Brevis Corporation   www.brevis.com

FIGURE 5-9 Droplet precautions. Reprinted with permission from Brevis Corporation (www.brevis.com).

When the activity of respiratory illnesses is increased in the community (e.g., during influenza outbreaks), prescreening patients for respiratory illnesses prior to their health care visit is useful. It might be possible to schedule a patient at slower times during the day; have him or her don a mask upon entry into the waiting area, or if the reason for the visit is not urgent, reschedule the visit. Placing patients with respiratory illnesses in an empty exam room immediately after registration may be another option if feasible.

Safe Injection Practices

Safe injection practices concern the proper use, handling, and disposal of supplies used for administering injections. Because many of these concerns are beyond the scope of this book, we will mention a few issues applicable to all health care workers. Used syringes and needles should be disposed of at the point of use in a **sharps container** that is puncture-resistant, closable, and leakproof. Single-use, disposable fingerstick devices (e.g., lancets) that are used to obtain blood samples to test for glucose and other tests should be disposed of in a sharps container immediately after use. Figure 5-10 illustrates various types of sharps containers.

sharps container: container in every clinic that is designed for the disposal of sharps; required and regulated by the Occupational Safety and Health Administration (OSHA)

Blood draws (phlebotomy) should be performed in a dedicated area with hand hygiene stations and sharps containers located nearby. Blood tubes should be labeled before the blood is drawn, and tubes containing blood should not be placed on any surface that cannot be properly cleaned.

Safe Handling of Potentially Contaminated Surfaces or Equipment

It is important to have policies and procedures concerning cleaning patient care devices that are reused (e.g., stethoscopes) and rooms used for patient care.

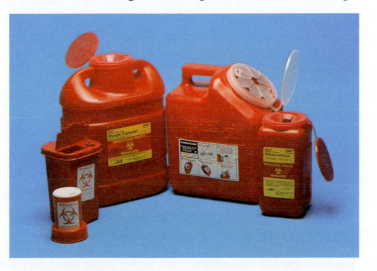

FIGURE 5-10 Various types of sharps containers.
© Cengage Learning®.

Clinical Application

Cleaning Blood and Body Substances

1. Wear gloves and use appropriate personal protective equipment.
2. If the spill contains large amounts of blood or other infectious matter, use absorbent disposable material and dispose of in biohazard waste.
3. Clean area with EPA-registered product that has specific label claims for bloodborne pathogens (e.g., HIV, HCV, etc.). Alternatively a 1:10 dilution of bleach should be used first to clean the infectious material followed by a 1:100 dilution of bleach for subsequent cleaning.

Noncritical devices should be cleaned according to the manufacturer's instructions. Patient care areas should be cleaned at least daily unless there is a blood or other infectious body fluid spill. Those should be cleaned immediately. Rooms should be cleaned first and then disinfected unless a one-step detergent disinfectant is used. Cleaning efforts should be focused on areas that are frequently touched by patients and staff.

Transmission-Based Precautions

Before we begin our discussion of this specialized category of precautions, it is important to remind the reader that these precautions are used in addition to standard precautions. It is important for staff to remain vigilant for any patients with confirmed or suspicion for active infection. These may include patients with fever, respiratory tract symptoms (e.g., cough or runny nose), draining wounds, or skin lesions, to name a few.

Contact Precautions

Contact precautions are instituted when there is a possibility of the transmission of pathogens by body-to-body contact. Use standard precautions plus the following additional precautions. A private room should be used, or a multiple patient room can be used if all patients have the same condition. Equipment should be dedicated to that patient during his or her length of stay. Any equipment removed from the room must be properly disinfected. Perform hand hygiene prior to touching the patient and before wearing gloves. Personal protective equipment used includes:

- Gloves, which should be worn when touching the patient or the patient's immediate environment or belongings.

- Gowns for any direct contact with the patient, environmental surfaces, or any equipment in the room.

Hand hygiene should be performed after glove removal. Soap and water should be used if the hands are visibly soiled or the patient has known or suspected infectious diarrhea (e.g., Norovirus, *Clostridium difficile*). Figure 5-11 illustrates contact precautions.

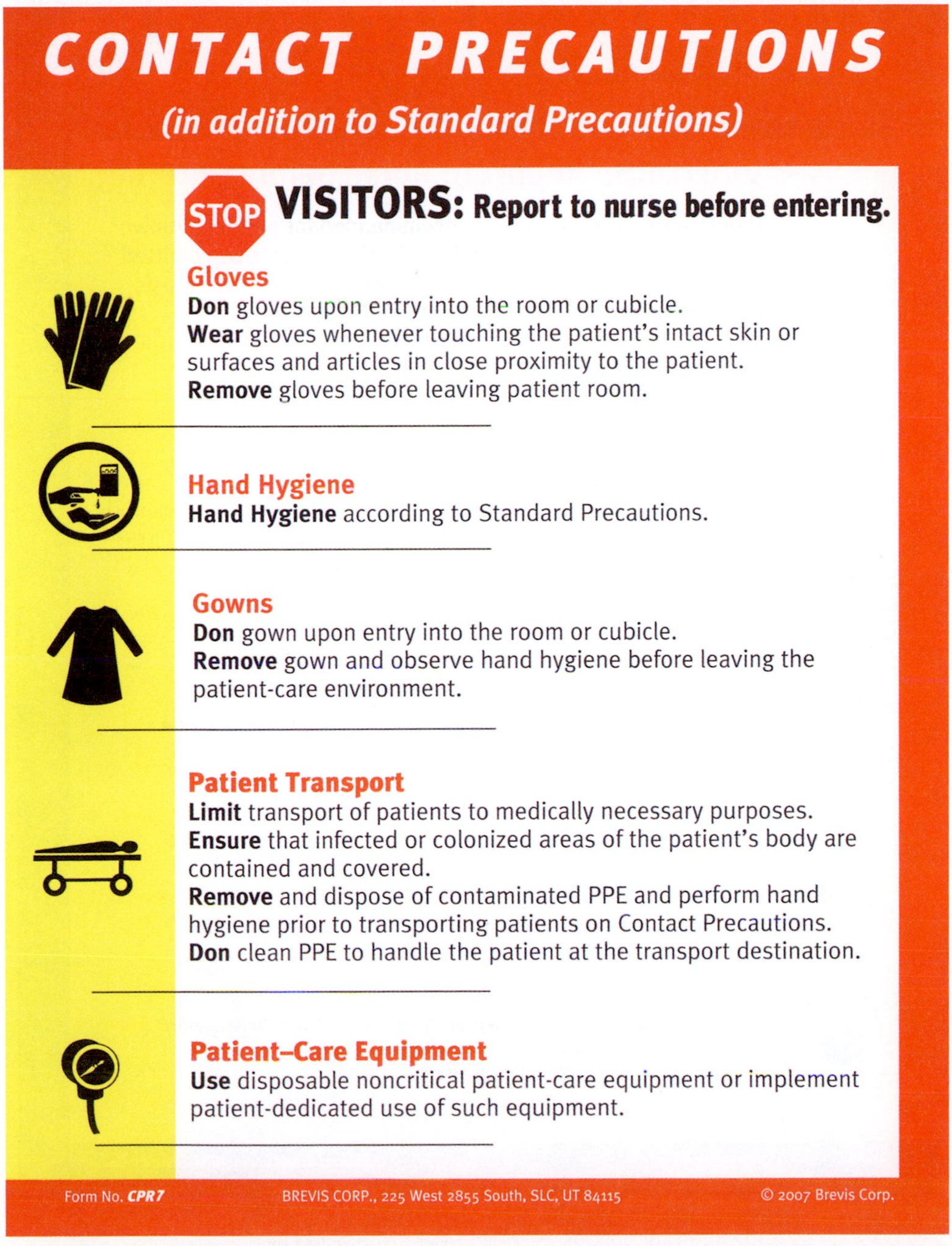

CONTACT PRECAUTIONS
(in addition to Standard Precautions)

STOP **VISITORS: Report to nurse before entering.**

Gloves
Don gloves upon entry into the room or cubicle.
Wear gloves whenever touching the patient's intact skin or surfaces and articles in close proximity to the patient.
Remove gloves before leaving patient room.

Hand Hygiene
Hand Hygiene according to Standard Precautions.

Gowns
Don gown upon entry into the room or cubicle.
Remove gown and observe hand hygiene before leaving the patient-care environment.

Patient Transport
Limit transport of patients to medically necessary purposes.
Ensure that infected or colonized areas of the patient's body are contained and covered.
Remove and dispose of contaminated PPE and perform hand hygiene prior to transporting patients on Contact Precautions.
Don clean PPE to handle the patient at the transport destination.

Patient–Care Equipment
Use disposable noncritical patient-care equipment or implement patient-dedicated use of such equipment.

Form No. *CPR7*   BREVIS CORP., 225 West 2855 South, SLC, UT 84115   © 2007 Brevis Corp.

FIGURE 5-11 Contact precautions. Reprinted with permission from Brevis Corporation (www.brevis.com).

Airborne Precautions

When there is a concern about the possibility for pathogen transmission by droplet spread or by dust particles, initiate standard precautions plus airborne precautions. Patients with confirmed or suspected cases of but not limited to tuberculosis, chickenpox, measles, and herpes zoster are candidates for airborne precautions (Figure 5-12). Place the patient in a negative

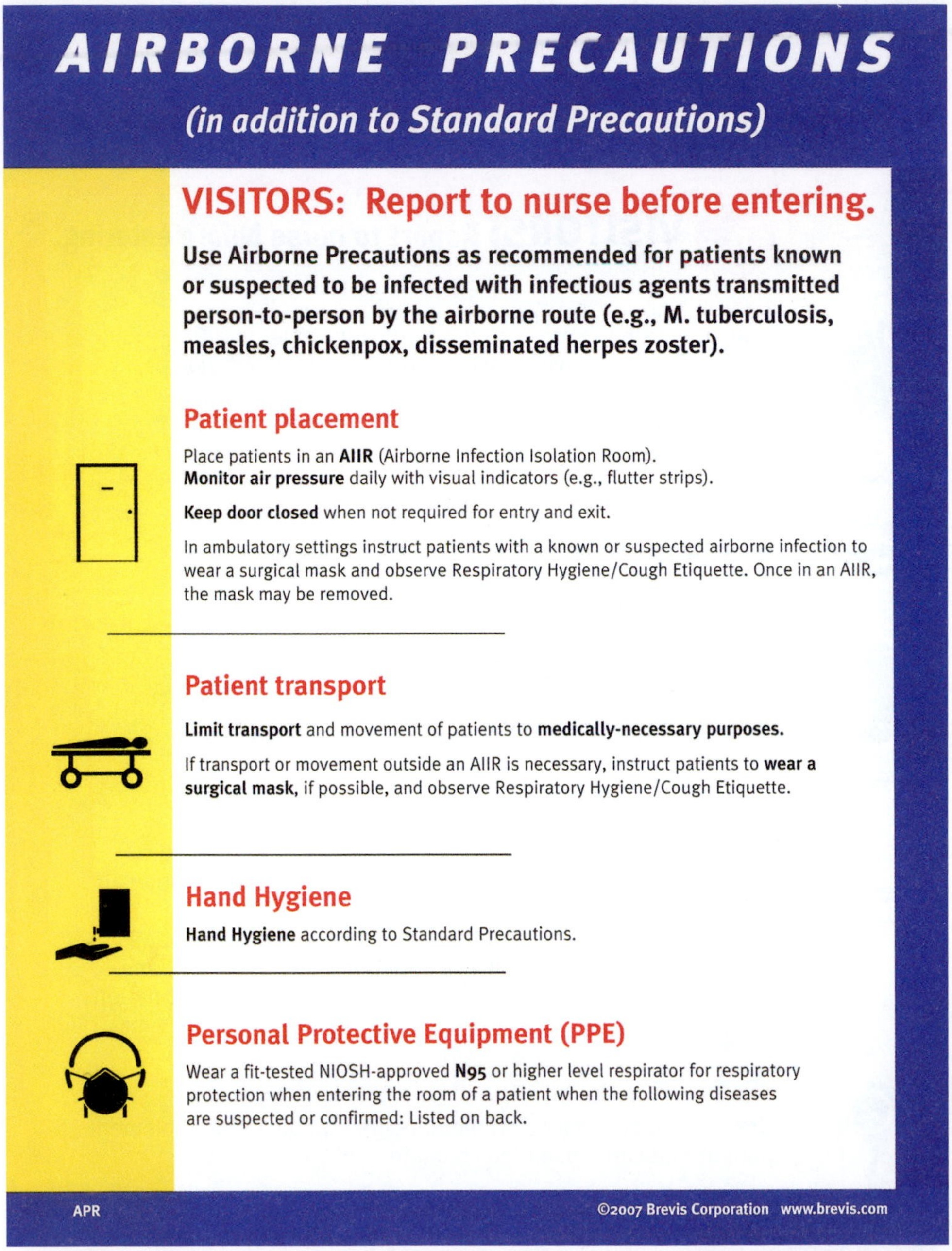

AIRBORNE PRECAUTIONS

(in addition to Standard Precautions)

VISITORS: Report to nurse before entering.

Use Airborne Precautions as recommended for patients known or suspected to be infected with infectious agents transmitted person-to-person by the airborne route (e.g., M. tuberculosis, measles, chickenpox, disseminated herpes zoster).

Patient placement

Place patients in an **AIIR** (Airborne Infection Isolation Room).
Monitor air pressure daily with visual indicators (e.g., flutter strips).

Keep door closed when not required for entry and exit.

In ambulatory settings instruct patients with a known or suspected airborne infection to wear a surgical mask and observe Respiratory Hygiene/Cough Etiquette. Once in an AIIR, the mask may be removed.

Patient transport

Limit transport and movement of patients to **medically-necessary purposes.**

If transport or movement outside an AIIR is necessary, instruct patients to **wear a surgical mask,** if possible, and observe Respiratory Hygiene/Cough Etiquette.

Hand Hygiene

Hand Hygiene according to Standard Precautions.

Personal Protective Equipment (PPE)

Wear a fit-tested NIOSH-approved **N95** or higher level respirator for respiratory protection when entering the room of a patient when the following diseases are suspected or confirmed: Listed on back.

APR

©2007 Brevis Corporation   www.brevis.com

FIGURE 5-12 Airborne precautions. Reprinted with permission from Brevis Corporation (www.brevis.com).

pressure room and keep the door closed. That way no air will escape into the hall or other rooms. If a negative pressure room is unavailable, provide the patient with a face mask and consider transfer to a specialized facility that can manage the patient. The following are requirements for your personal protective equipment:

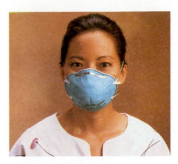

FIGURE 5-13 N-95/HEPA filtered mask. Source: Courtesy of 3M Company, St. Paul, MN.

- Mask: a fit-tested (this means the proper fit of the mask on health care workers who are caring for the patient has been determined ahead of time) N-95 or HEPA (high-efficiency particulate air) filtered mask must be put on before entering the room. If it is a patient with chickenpox or measles and you are immune to those diseases, then the mask is not necessary (Figure 5-13).

- If potential spraying of respiratory secretions is anticipated, gloves, gown, and goggles or face shield should be worn also.

- Do not forget to perform proper hand hygiene before and after touching the patient and after contact with any bodily secretions.

Droplet Precautions

Patients warranting this form of precaution are known to have or are suspected of having a serious illness that is easily spread by large particle droplets such as *Neisseria meningitidis,* respiratory viruses (e.g., influenza, parainfluenza virus, adenovirus), and *Bordetella pertussis* (whooping cough). Use standard precautions and a private room, or multiple patient rooms if all patients exhibit the same condition. The door to the room may be kept open. Use the following personal protective equipment:

- Surgical mask if within 3 feet of the patient.

- If substantial spraying of respiratory fluids is anticipated, gloves, gown, and goggles or face shield should be worn.

- Hand hygiene before and after patient contact and after contact with respiratory secretions or other objects contaminated with respiratory secretions.

Food for Thought
When One Is Not Enough

Not to complicate matters, but occasionally certain microbes require more than one type of isolation. For example, in addition to airborne precautions for herpes zoster, contact precautions should also be used for immunocompromised patients or if herpes zoster has spread throughout the body (this is called disseminated herpes zoster).

Media Connection

For a final summary and review of infection prevention and control, visit the accompanying online resources.

5-3 Stop and Review

1. During _____ outbreaks in the community, prescreening patients for respiratory illnesses prior to their health care visit is useful.

2. Used syringes and needles should be disposed of at the point of use in a(n) _____ that is puncture-resistant, closable, and leakproof.

3. _____ are a form of transmission-based precautions used for patients who are known to have or are suspected of having a serious illness that is easily spread by large particle droplets such as *Neisseria meningitides*, certain respiratory viruses, and *Bordetella pertussis*.

Bloodborne Pathogen Standard: extensive, detailed regulations to be practiced by employers and employees to prevent occupational exposure

Occupational Safety and Health Administration (OSHA) Regulations

The intent of OSHA regulations is to make the work environment safe for employees. Employers must follow these regulations. While there are many regulations mandated by OSHA, the **Bloodborne Pathogen Standard** is something we need to discuss in detail because it plays a large role in protecting us and our patients from acquiring diseases spread by exposure to blood and other body fluids.

The Bloodborne Pathogen Standard became law in 1992 about 11 years after the discovery of HIV in humans. Its principal goal at that time was to prevent occupational-related cases of HIV and hepatitis B infections in health care workers. However, the intent of the standard is to prevent the exposure of health care workers to any infectious microorganism that may be present in blood (hepatitis C virus) or other body fluids. This standard's requirements state what employers must do to protect workers and covers all employees who may be "reasonably anticipated" to come in contact with blood and other infected materials as part of their job duties.

In general, the standard requires employers to:

1. **Establish an exposure control plan.** This is a written plan to eliminate or minimize occupational exposures. The employer must prepare an exposure determination that contains a list of job classifications in which some workers have occupational exposure and a list of job classifications in which all workers have occupational exposure. A comprehensive list of job duties must be compiled that might result in a worker's exposure.

2. **Update the plan annually.** The update should indicate changes in procedures, tasks, and positions that might affect occupational exposure. Employers must document and review the use of safer medical devices that limit worker exposure to bloodborne pathogens. For example, 10 years ago most hospitals used needles to provide most medications given to patients via a vein. Today, needleless medication delivery devices are used throughout health care. Employers must ask employees to assist with identifying, evaluating, and selecting these devices.

3. **Implement the use of standard precautions.** As we discussed previously, this basic level of precautions assumes all blood and body fluids are potentially infectious.

4. **Identify and use engineering controls.** This is a fancy way of saying employers are required to use devices that isolate and/or remove the bloodborne pathogens hazard from the workplace area. Sharps disposal containers, self-sheathing needles, and needleless intravenous systems are some examples of these engineering controls. Figure 5-14 illustrates a shielded blood needle system.

5. **Identify and ensure the use of work practice controls.** These are practice changes that reduce the possibility of worker exposure by mandating appropriate handling of specimens and laundry, cleaning of contaminated surfaces and devices, and handling and disposal of contaminated sharps.

6. **Provide personal protective equipment, such as masks, gloves, gowns, and eye protection.** Employers must not only provide this equipment at no cost to the employee, but they must maintain it in good working order and replace the items as necessary.

7. **Make available hepatitis B vaccinations to all workers with occupational exposure.** After the employee receives the mandatory bloodborne pathogen training, the vaccine must be offered within the first 10 days of employment in a position with occupational exposure.

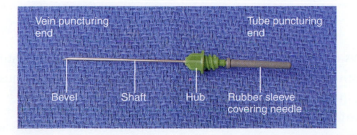

FIGURE 5-14 Shielded blood needle system. © Cengage Learning®.

8. **Make available postexposure evaluation and follow-up to any occupationally exposed worker who experiences an exposure incident.** An exposure incident is defined as a mouth, eye, mucous membrane, or needlestick/sharps injury and exposure to blood or other bodily secretions. The confidential medical evaluation and follow-up must be at no cost to the employee and include:

- Circumstances surrounding the event

- Route or routes of exposure

- Identifying and testing the source individual for HBV, HCV, and HIV if source individual consents or consent not required by law

- Collecting and testing the exposed worker's blood for HCV, HBV, and HIV if the worker consents

- The exposed employee is offered appropriate postexposure prophylaxis if indicated (e.g., hepatitis B immune globulin or HIV postexposure prophylaxis).

9. **Use labels and signs to communicate hazards.** Warning labels must be applied to containers of regulated waste, reusable sharps, refrigerators and freezers storing blood or other potentially infectious material, and contaminated laundry. Red bags or red containers may be used instead of labels (Figure 5-15).

10. **Provide information and training to workers.** Employers must mandate employee training during regular working hours at no cost to the employee. The training must provide information on bloodborne pathogens, ways to control occupational exposure, hepatitis B vaccine, and postexposure follow-up procedures. The training must be offered when an occupational exposure may occur and then annually.

11. **Maintain worker medical training records.** The employer must maintain a sharps injury and bloodborne pathogen exposure log.

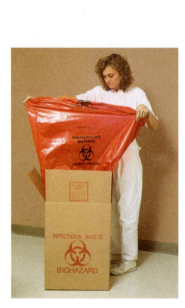

FIGURE 5-15 Red biohazard bag/container.
© Cengage Learning®.

Chapter Summary

- We have discussed numerous ways to protect patients and ourselves from spreading microbes to one another. We began the chapter by addressing ways that microbes may gain access to our bodies through so-called portals of entry.

- It is important to understand that humans as well as animals may carry disease-causing microorganisms without being ill.

- Contact, common vehicle, airborne, and vector are all examples of how diseases may come into contact with our bodies. Collectively these terms are known as routes of transmission.

- If you are sick of us mentioning hand hygiene as the most important way to prevent the spread of disease, then we did our job.

- Resident flora are the relatively harmless microbes that colonize our skin and keep the mostly bad transient flora from taking up residence on our bodies. Transient flora may be picked up from patients during routine patient care and may be removed using proper hand hygiene practices.

- Standard and transmission-based precautions form the foundation of a solid infection control and prevention program.

- When it is necessary to use transmission-based precautions, it is important to remember that they are used on top of or in addition to standard precautions. Standard precautions assume patients may harbor disease-causing microorganisms even if they do not appear ill and practicing proper hand hygiene hopefully prevents you from acquiring these microbes (transient flora) and spreading them to another patient.

- We also reviewed the various types of personal protective equipment and when these items should be used.

- Principles of safe injection practices were discussed along with the safe handling of potentially contaminated surfaces or equipment.

- Finally, we reviewed OSHA regulations with a focus on the Bloodborne Pathogen Standard. This standard details what employers must do to protect workers who may come into contact with blood and other infectious material as part of their job.

Case Study

A 65-year-old female is driven to the hospital emergency room with severe shortness of breath, cough, and fever. She is also complaining of muscle aches stating "it feels like I was hit by a truck." She has a long-standing history of severe lung disease (chronic obstructive pulmonary disease) requiring home oxygen because of a 45-pack-per-year smoking history. It is January, and she declined influenza vaccination when she was seen by her primary care physician in November. She is admitted to the hospital with a diagnosis of severe exacerbation of her chronic lung disease. The next day her attending physician decides to test her for influenza. The test is reported back to the floor as a critical value because the result is positive for influenza Type A. She is started on an antiviral medication for influenza. What type of transmission-based precautions should be used to isolate this patient? What could have been done differently with this case starting with the emergency room?

Chapter Review

1. _____ transient flora
2. _____ vectors
3. _____ standard precautions
4. _____ personal protective equipment
5. _____ alcohol-based hand sanitizers
6. _____ soap and water
7. _____ resident flora
8. _____ Bloodborne Pathogen Standard
9. _____ airborne precautions
10. _____ droplet precautions
11. _____ gloves
12. _____ portals of entry

a. a required way to wash hands that are visibly soiled

b. used on hands when touching a patient in contact precautions

c. flora that normally resides on the surface of our skin

d. precautions for patients with influenza

e. openings in our bodies that allow the entry of microbes

f. flora acquired by direct contact with the patient or the environment

g. organism that carries disease

h. must contain at least 60% alcohol to be effective

i. precaution to isolate patient with tuberculosis

j. specialized clothing worn by health care workers

k. a government law that employers must follow

l. type of precaution that applies to all patients

13. _____ Gloves should always be worn before entering a patient care room.

14. _____ It is not necessary to wash your hands if you are using gloves.

15. _____ Performing proper hand hygiene is the single most important thing you can do to prevent the spread of infection.

16. _____ Sharps containers are used to dispose of soiled linens.

17. _____ Standard precautions are used only in patients with known infections.

18. Name the portals of entry and how they contribute to disease.

19. What is the difference between resident and transient flora?

20. Describe the different types of precautions.

21. What is OSHA's role in protecting health care workers from acquiring infections?

Fill in the blanks.

22. _____ are nonliving objects such as clothing, towels, and medical instruments that may harbor and transmit diseases.

23. Pathogens may find their way inside us and cause infections by using avenues known as the _____.

24. _____ are organisms that carry a disease agent to the host.

25. _____ is specialized clothing worn by the health care worker to protect against acquiring microorganisms.

Additional Activities

1. By reading this chapter you have discovered how important hand hygiene is to prevent the spread of infection. In fact, proper hand hygiene saves lives. Research why compliance with proper hand hygiene is poor. Can you think of some creative solutions to help improve compliance with good hand hygiene?

2. See if your class can obtain some personal protective equipment (e.g., gloves, gowns, and masks). Review when to use this equipment and then practice putting on and removing the gear. Develop a checklist for the proper way to apply and remove the equipment and then critique each other. (Hint: visit the website www.cdc.gov and search personal protective equipment.)

3. Visit your local hospital or have an infection control specialist from a local hospital visit your classroom to discuss infection control and prevention activities. Ask them to discuss their facility's compliance with proper hand hygiene and the various types of patient precautions.

4. Play the "Save a Life Game." Have someone pretend to be a patient with a disease requiring certain types of transmission-based precautions. Divide the rest of the class into teams. Write each team number on the back of a 3 × 5 card. Shuffle the cards and draw a 3 × 5 card to see which team goes first. The team that is picked should attend (e.g., pretend to start an IV, bathe the patient, help him or her to the restroom), to the student patient who requires a certain type of transmission-based precaution. Develop a scoring sheet to include observations for proper hand hygiene and the use and removal of personal protective equipment.

Media Connection

Go to the accompanying online resources and have fun learning as you play games, view animations and videos, and take practice tests to help reinforce key concepts you learned in this chapter.

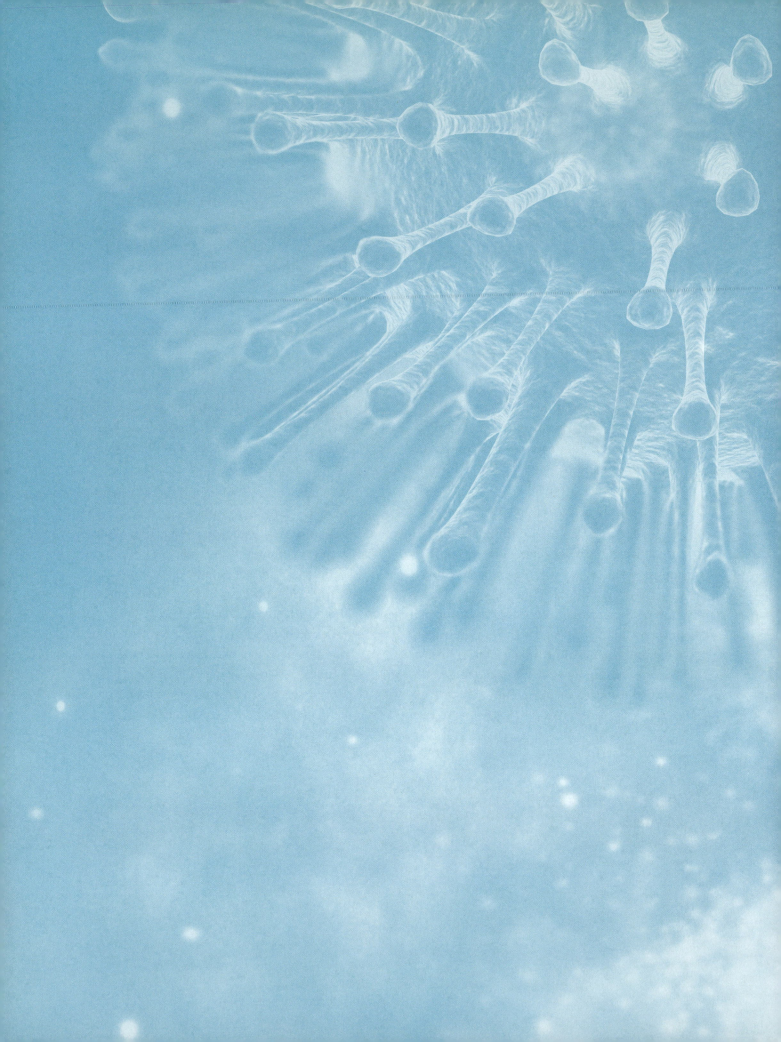

Microbiology-Related Procedures

OBJECTIVES

After studying this chapter, the learner will be able to:

- Contrast infectious and noninfectious waste.

- Describe infectious waste disposal procedures.

- Describe the correct method for applying and removing sterile and nonsterile gloves.

- Distinguish between medical and surgical asepsis.

- Describe guidelines for the maintenance of a sterile field.

- List the general principles of specimen collection to include blood, cerebrospinal fluid (CSF), sputum, and throat, nasal, and wound cultures.

- Describe the procedure for obtaining a urine specimen and stool sample.

- Discuss why appropriate specimen collection is important.

- Given a specific site, discuss the appropriate procedures for obtaining a clinically useful specimen from that body site.

KEY TERMS

asepsis

biological liquid waste

blood cultures

cerebrospinal fluid (CSF) cultures

hand hygiene

infectious waste

medical asepsis

nasal specimens

nonsharp

nonsterile gloves

pathological wastes

resident flora

sharps

sputum cultures

sterile field

sterile gloves

sterile principles

stool specimens

surgical asepsis

throat cultures

transient flora

urine specimen

wound cultures

Introduction

During patient care we may create or come across infectious waste that must be disposed of in the proper manner, so that will be an important topic to discuss in this chapter. Another important goal of this chapter is to outline how samples may be properly obtained from various body sites and properly transported for processing by the microbiology laboratory.

Our discussion of microbiology-related procedures begins with the proper way to dispose of medical waste. Medical waste that may be infectious must be distinguished from noninfectious waste because disposal of infectious waste is costly. We then discuss procedures and considerations for obtaining various cultures. The proper diagnosis of infectious diseases is aided tremendously by obtaining proper culture material from various body sites. Without using the proper techniques to obtain samples for processing in the microbiology laboratory, a diagnosis may be missed or an improper diagnosis made. The old saying *garbage in equals garbage out* applies here. We will also be visiting the proper way to apply and remove sterile dressings, **sterile gloves**, and **nonsterile gloves**.

sterile gloves: clean, germ-free gloves

nonsterile gloves: gloves not put through the process of sterilization

Infectious Waste Disposal

To begin our discussion we first must define what we mean by **infectious waste**. Infectious wastes are solid or liquid wastes that may cause human disease if improperly treated, transported, stored, or disposed of. They may be body fluids themselves or are items that have come in contact with human body fluids and blood. Infectious waste must be handled with gloves and then disposed of by placing this material in the proper biohazard containers. The containers are either purchased by a facility or provided by a licensed contract waste hauler. The infectious waste is properly treated prior to disposal in a sanitary landfill.

Local and state rules and regulations may determine how your infectious waste is handled by a licensed contractor. Your local or state health department office can assist a facility in developing an infectious waste disposal plan and provide names of licensed contractors who can properly dispose of soiled items. Because the disposal of this waste is costly, it is important that all employees are educated about the difference between infectious and noninfectious waste and the proper disposal of each. There are many types of infectious waste, but to simplify things, we will continue our discussion by focusing on waste encountered in health care and dividing infectious waste into two broad categories: **sharps** and **nonsharp** infectious wastes. Table 6-1 contrasts sharp and nonsharp infectious waste, and Figure 6-1 illustrates examples of waste containers.

infectious waste: hazardous waste with infectious characteristics, including contaminated animal waste and human blood and blood products

sharps: any needles, scalpels, or other articles that could cause wounds or punctures to personnel handling them

nonsharp: does not contain pointed edges that can easily penetrate other objects

TABLE 6-1 Types of Infectious Waste

Nonsharp
Biological liquid wastes–blood or any other body fluid
Pathological waste–material obtained during surgery, surgical procedures, or autopsies
Patient care items–bed linens and protective pads, for example, that are visibly soiled with blood and/or body fluids
Sharps
Needles, intravenous tubing with needles attached, scalpel blades, glass or glass ware–any discarded article that may cause punctures or cuts

© 2016 Cengage Learning®.

Food for Thought
Ruined Vacations

In 1988 the federal government passed the Medical Waste Tracking Act. This legislation was in response to syringes and other medical waste washing ashore on beaches on the East Coast of the United States. This act was later repealed in 1991, and states were given the responsibility to regulate and pass laws concerning the tracking and disposal of infectious or medical waste.

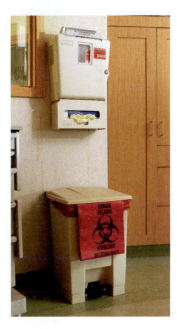

FIGURE 6-1 Sharps disposal (hanging on wall) and infectious waste containers (on floor).
© Cengage Learning®.

biological liquid wastes: a liquid that contains or has been contaminated by a biohazardous agent

pathological waste: waste material consisting of only human or animal remains, anatomical parts and/or tissue, the bags/containers used to collect and transport the waste material, and animal bedding

The proper disposal of infectious waste depends on the type of facility and the state in which the facility is located. Large university medical centers may have the proper equipment to decontaminate infectious waste (e.g., autoclaves), while smaller facilities and medical offices generally will use outside contractors to perform this function. Table 6-2 lists sample infectious waste disposal procedures for facilities without on-site autoclaving.

Applying and Removing Nonsterile Disposable Gloves

Because you previously learned the importance of hand washing, keep in mind that this applies even when gloves are to be worn when caring for patients. Gloves help to prevent the spread of infection and protect both the caregiver and the patient. Before we discuss the proper way to apply gloves, remember that gloves are *not always* worn when caring for a patient. When appropriate, touching patients with bare hands can be comforting and help ease the fear and anxiety of being a patient.

TABLE 6-2 Infectious Waste Disposal Procedures

Procedure for Nonsharp Items

1. Wear gloves and place all infectious waste items immediately in red infectious waste biohazard bags.

2. When the bag is ¾ full, the bag will be sealed and placed in a disposal container for shipment to an outside disposal facility.

3. Liquid infectious waste such as blood and body fluids will be flushed/discarded directly into the sanitary sewer system using copious amounts of water. (Check with your local or state Department of Health.)

4. If liquid infectious wastes are in leakproof containers (e.g., blood transfusion bags), the container should be placed in a red infectious waste biohazard bag for disposal as above.

Procedure for Sharp Items

1. Wear gloves and place disposable sharps directly into leak- and puncture-resistant disposable sharps containers.

2. Sharps containers should be conveniently located anywhere sharps are routinely used.

3. Used disposable needles will be placed directly into sharps containers without recapping.

4. Sharps containers should be sealed and removed when the container is ¾ full.

5. Do not force instruments into the sharps container.

6. Filled containers should be tightly closed and sealed when full to avoid spillage and injury to health care facility personnel.

7. Sharps containers are never placed in a normal waste container after sealing.

© 2016 Cengage Learning®.

The proper procedure for applying and removing disposable nonsterile gloves can be found in Table 6-3. Gloves should always be worn if patient contact is likely to involve exposure to blood, body fluids, or nonintact skin. Don't forget to wash your hands before and after gloving.

Applying and Removing Sterile Gloves

Now we describe the procedure for applying and removing sterile gloves. There are two ways to put sterile gloves on your hands. One technique is called the *open method*. Can you guess the other? If you guessed *closed method*, you are correct. The closed method is used by the scrubbed personnel in the operating room because the possibility of the glove touching the skin is eliminated.

TABLE 6-3 Applying and Removing Nonsterile Gloves

Applying Nonsterile Gloves

1. Wash and dry your hands.

2. Pull a glove out of the box with one hand and slide the glove onto the other hand.

3. With your gloved hand, pull another glove out of the box and slide it onto your bare hand.

4. Interlace fingers and push down between fingers on both hands to ensure proper fit.

Removing Nonsterile Gloves

1. Remove gloves immediately if patient care procedure is finished, the gloves become heavily soiled, the gloves are torn, before touching another part of the body, or before touching any clean surface or object.

2. To remove gloves, firmly grip one glove at the palm and pull it off inside out (Figures 6-2A through D). Hold the removed glove in the palm of the other glove (Figure 6-2E).

3. Slip bare fingers under the gloved hand at the wrist without touching its surface (Figure 6-2F).

4. Push the glove down and off with the first glove tucked inside it. One glove is now inside the other, and both are inside out. Place the gloves in the appropriate waste receptacle according to your facility's policies and procedures.

5. Wash and dry your hands!

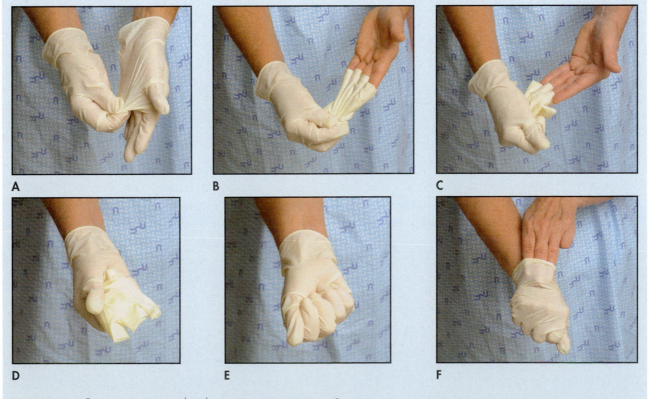

A   B   C   D   E   F

FIGURE 6-2 Removing nonsterile gloves. © Cengage Learning®.

It also may be used by health care providers wearing a sterile gown. For all other procedures, the open method is more frequently used. Practice your technique using nonsterile gloves because sterile gloves are very expensive. Table 6-4 outlines the open gloving technique.

TABLE 6-4 Applying and Removing Sterile Gloves Using the Open Method

Applying Sterile Gloves Using the Open Method

1. Wash your hands.

2. Check the glove package for sterility.

3. Open the outer packages by peeling the upper edges back with your thumbs (Figure 6-3A).

4. Remove the inner package containing the gloves and place it on the inside of the outer package (Figure 6-3B).

5. Open the inner package, handling it only by the corners on the outside (Figure 6-3C).

6. Pick up the cuff of the right-hand glove using your left hand. Avoid touching the area below the cuff (Figure 6-3D).

7. Insert your right hand into the glove (Figure 6-3E). Spread your fingers slightly, sliding them into the fingers. If the glove is not on correctly, do not attempt to straighten it at this time.

8. Insert the gloved fingers of your right hand under the cuff of the left glove (Figure 6-3F).

9. Slide your fingers into the left glove, adjusting the fingers of the gloves for comfort and fit. Because both gloves are sterile, they may touch each other. Avoid touching the cuffs of the gloves.

10. Insert your right hand under the cuff of the left glove and push the cuff up over your wrist (Figure 6-3G). Avoid touching your wrist or the outside of the cuff with your glove.

11. Insert your left hand under the cuff of the right glove and push the cuff up over your wrist. Avoid touching your wrist or the outside of the cuff with your glove.

12. You may now touch sterile items with your sterile gloves (Figure 6-3H). Avoid touching unsterile items.

Removing Sterile Gloves Using the Open Method

1. Grasp the outside of the glove on the nondominant hand, at the cuff. Pull the glove off so that the inside of the glove faces outward (Figure 6-3I). Avoid touching the skin of your wrist with the fingers of the glove.

2. Place the glove into the palm of the gloved hand (Figure 6-3J).

3. Put the fingers of the ungloved hand inside the cuff of the gloved hand. Pull the glove off, inside out. The first glove removed should be inside the second glove (Figure 6-3K).

4. Discard the gloves into a covered container or trash, according to facility policy (Figure 6-3L).

5. Wash your hands.

(Continues)

TABLE 6-4 *(Continued)*

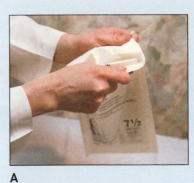

A

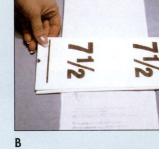

B

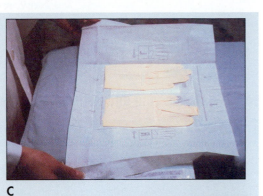

C

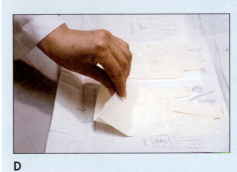

D

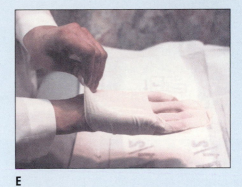

E

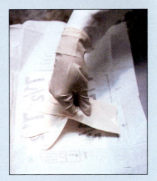

F

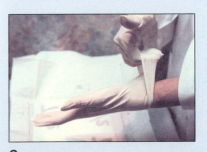

G

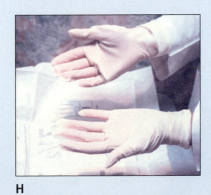

H

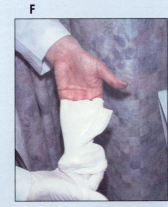

I

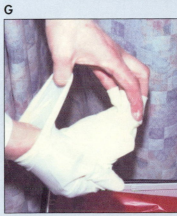

J

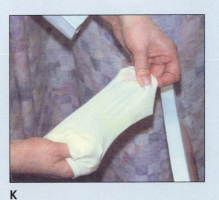

K

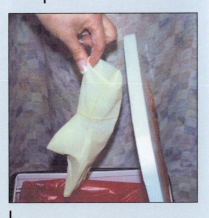

L

FIGURE 6-3 Applying (A-F) and removing (G-L) sterile gloves using the open method procedure.
© Cengage Learning®.

Now review the steps in Table 6-5, which show the closed gloving technique.

TABLE 6-5 Applying and Removing Sterile Gloves Using the Closed Method

Applying Sterile Gloves Using the Closed Method
1. While wearing a sterile gown, use the right hand to pick up the left glove (Figure 6-4A).
2. Place the glove on the upward-turned left hand, palm side down and thumb to thumb with the fingers extending along the forearm and pointing toward the elbow (Figure 6-4B).
3. Hold the glove cuff and sleeve cuff together with the thumb of the left hand (Figure 6-4C).
4. Use the left hand to stretch the cuff of the right glove over the opened end of the sleeve (Figure 6-4D).
5. Work the fingers into the glove as the cuff is pulled onto the wrist.
6. The left glove is done in the same manner (Figure 6-4E).

Removing Sterile Gloves Using the Closed Method
1. Grasp the outside cuff of one glove and pull off, turning inside out (Figure 6-4F). Hold it with the remaining gloved hand.
2. Pull the second glove off without touching the outside of the second glove. Turn the second glove as it is removed. Dispose into receptacle with first glove.
3. Wash your hands.

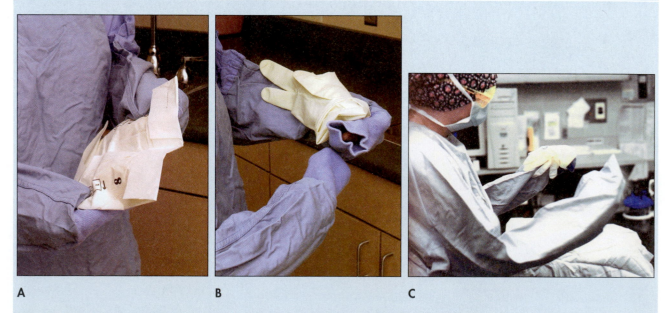

A   B   C

FIGURE 6-4 Applying (A-E) and removing (F) sterile gloves using the closed method. © Cengage Learning®. *(Continues)*

(Continues)

TABLE 6-5 *(Continued)*

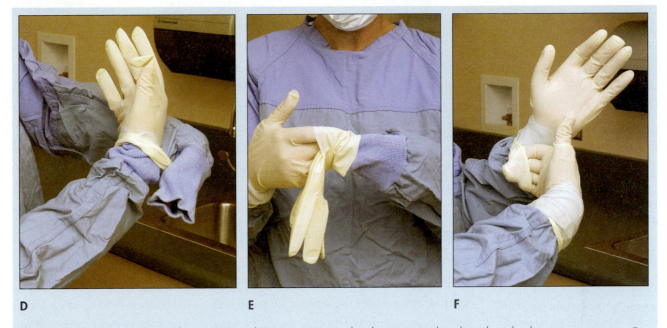

D   E   F

FIGURE 6-4 *(Continued)* Applying (A-E) and (F) removing sterile gloves using the closed method. © *Cengage Learning®*

© 2016 Cengage Learning®.

6-1 Stop and Review

1. _____ are solid or liquid wastes that may cause human disease.

2. _____ are needles, intravenous tubing, or any discarded article that may cause punctures.

3. _____ should always be worn if patient contact is likely to involve exposure to blood and other body fluids.

Media Connection

Go to the accompanying online resources to view methods of donning sterile gloves.

Asepsis

The absence of microorganisms is termed **asepsis**. When patient care is provided using aseptic technique, the chance of spreading microbes that cause health care–associated infections is decreased. The two types of asepsis are *medical* and *surgical*. **Medical asepsis** uses procedures that *reduce* the number, growth, and spread of microbes. **Surgical asepsis** *eliminates* all microbes from an object or area. We have previously discussed many of the common medical aseptic measures such as hand washing and gloving. Other medical asepsis procedures are changing bed linens and cleaning floors and furniture daily. Thank goodness we do not practice medical asepsis at home. How would you like to do those things daily around the house?

asepsis: a condition free from germs, infection, and any form of life

medical asepsis: procedures used to reduce the number of microorganisms and prevent their spread, such as the hand "no touch" dressing technique

surgical asepsis: the exclusion of all microorganisms before they can enter an open surgical wound or contaminate a sterile field during surgery; measures taken include sterilization of all instruments, drapes, and all other inanimate objects that may come in contact with the surgical wound; all personnel coming in contact with the sterile field perform a surgical hand scrub with an antimicrobial agent and put on a surgical gown and gloves

hand hygiene: the removal of visible soil and the removal or killing of transient microorganisms from the hands accomplished by using soap and running water or an alcohol-based hand rub

transient flora: microorganisms that may be present in or on the body under certain conditions and for certain lengths of time; they are easier to remove by mechanical friction than resident flora

The goal of surgical asepsis is the elimination of not only living microbes but their spore forms, if any, as well. The procedures performed to achieve surgical asepsis include surgical hand scrub, sterilization of instruments, dressing in surgical attire (e.g., caps, masks, and eyewear), the handling of sterile equipment and instruments, and establishing and maintaining a sterile field. A sterile field represents a specified surgical area that is free of microorganisms. As you might imagine, surgical asepsis is practiced by health care personnel in the operating room. What you may not know is that it is also practiced when delivering babies and for many diagnostic and therapeutic interventions performed at the patient's bedside. Some examples of these include inserting certain types of intravenous (IV) lines and changing a surgical wound or IV site dressing.

Hand Hygiene for Surgical Asepsis

We previously discussed in detail the importance of hand hygiene and how to perform hand washing correctly. This type of **hand hygiene** is perfect for the day-to-day performance of routine patient duties. The goal is to remove *pathogenic* microorganisms from the hands to prevent patient-to-patient transmission.

Hand cleansing for surgical asepsis is hand hygiene *on steroids*. The goal here is to remove as many microbes, both pathogenic and normal skin flora along with **transient flora** that may contaminate hands after patient or environmental contact prior to wearing sterile gloves and performing surgery or another invasive procedure. Surgical asepsis hand hygiene consists of careful scrubbing of the hands (including nails), wrists, and forearms before applying sterile gloves. Table 6-6 presents a comparison between medical and surgical hand hygiene.

TABLE 6-6 Differences between Medical and Surgical Hand Hygiene

Medical Hand Washing	Surgical Hand Washing
Liquid soap and water adequate for most situations and procedures	Special cleaning solutions may be indicated, may use brush
Approximately 1 minute duration	3 to 6 minutes duration
Wash hands and wrists	Wash hands, wrists, and forearms to the elbows. Always glove for sterility.
Can apply lotion (see note below) for dry hands during frequent washings	Do not apply lotion (see note), especially petroleum based because it may react with latex gloves causing them to deteriorate and increase latex sensitivity of the person using the gloves.

Note: Hand lotions should be chosen based on the type of hand hygiene product used.

Sterile Principles

Sterile principles are guidelines designed to determine the areas and items that are considered sterile and what actions might cause contamination. While this is an obvious need for surgery, it is also required for procedures performed at the bedside. Some surfaces, such as our skin, cannot be sterilized. The size of an object may limit our ability to sterilize it because it won't fit into an autoclave, for example. If a **sterile field** needs to be created in an area where sterility is not possible (e.g., putting an intravenous line into the neck vein of a patient at the bedside), sterile drapes, gowns, and gloves need to be used to create an area that is as sterile as possible. Table 6-7 describes guidelines to protect sterile items and areas from contamination. Figure 6-5 shows practical applications of the knowledge you just learned.

sterile principles: a set of guidelines designed to determine the areas and items that are considered sterile and what actions might cause contamination especially in surgical procedures

sterile field: a specified surgical area that is free of microorganisms

TABLE 6-7 Guidelines for Maintaining a Sterile Field

1. A sterile object may not touch a nonsterile object.

2. Sterile objects should be dry. Moisture can trap microbes on the sterile object.

3. A border of at least 1 inch should be maintained between sterile and nonsterile areas. Sterile items should be placed in the middle of the sterile field away from the borders.

4. Maintain visual contact with the sterile field throughout the procedure. If you cannot see the field, you cannot be sure if anything touched it.

5. Anything below the operator's waist is considered contaminated. Keep all instruments and trays above the waist.

6. Try not to cough, sneeze, or talk over a sterile field. Do not participate in the performance of sterile procedures if you are ill.

7. Do not reach over the sterile area.

8. Do not pass contaminated instruments or other items over the sterile field.

9. When opening sterile packages, the outer wrapper is contaminated. Open the package without touching the inner contents and then drop the contents onto the sterile field.

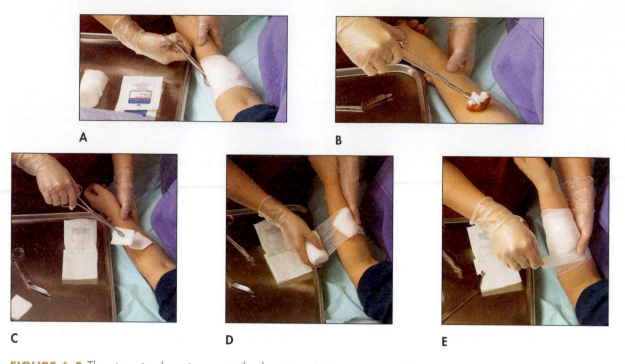

FIGURE 6-5 The steps in changing a sterile dressing. © Cengage Learning®.

Media Connection

Go to the accompanying online resources to view videos on changing sterile dressings and sterile fields.

6-2 Stop and Review

1. _____ and _____ are two types of asepsis.

2. Surgical hand washing should be at least _____ minutes in duration.

3. A border of at least _____ should be maintained between nonsterile and sterile areas.

Specimen Collection

Imagine for a minute that you are an executive baking chef making a dessert for a large party that will be attended by a number of celebrity guests. Unfortunately, you ran out of some important ingredients and did not follow the steps of the recipe that won you awards exactly as you should have. The cake turns out to be a flop, and your career takes a nosedive. Following a *recipe* for the proper way to collect patient specimens is also exceedingly important. The quality of the specimen collected by the health care provider and the results produced by the diagnostic microbiology laboratory are intended to have a positive impact on the care of patients. If you are inattentive to the proper way to collect and transport specimens for processing, a diagnosis may be missed or based on bad information.

General Principles

Specimens should be collected using aseptic techniques from body sites likely to yield microbes that cause disease in humans. Tissue or fluid should be obtained and submitted whenever possible. Specimens such as surface material from skin ulcers and nasal swab specimens from patients with sinusitis are examples of material that is not likely to yield clinically useful information. This is because the normal flora that typically inhabit the surface of those areas may also contaminate the swab. Collection of swab specimens should be limited to throat and urethral cultures. Other reasons swab cultures are inadequate means of specimen collection are because they limit the amount of fluid that can be obtained, interfere with direct Gram staining, and are easy to contaminate. Complete information should be collected and submitted along with the specimen, and both should be transported to the diagnostic microbiology laboratory without delay. Table 6-8 lists examples of information that should be submitted along with the specimen.

Most specimens can be transported in sterile collection containers or in the syringe used for collection. Specimen transport containers are available from different vendors and may assist with the transport of specimens to off-site laboratories. If there will be a delay in the transport or processing of a specimen, most specimens should be refrigerated to maintain the survival of pathogens in their relative numbers and to minimize the growth of contaminants. Blood and **cerebrospinal fluid (CSF) cultures** are exceptions, and they should be kept at room temperature. Figure 6-6 shows examples of specimen containers.

cerebrospinal fluid (CSF) culture: a laboratory test to look for bacteria, fungi, and viruses in the normally sterile fluid that moves in the space surrounding the spinal cord by performing a spinal tap

TABLE 6-8 Guidelines for Specimen Collection

1. Include the date and time the specimen was collected.
2. Indicate the specific site(s) from which specimens were obtained.
3. List any antibiotics, if any, the patient was receiving at the time of specimen collection.
4. Indicate the collection method used for obtaining the specimen (e.g., sterile syringe).
5. If the patient is suspected of having an infection that may be hazardous to laboratory workers, that should be indicated (e.g., *Mycobacterium tuberculosis*).

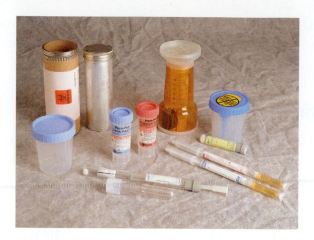

FIGURE 6-6 Labeled examples of specimen containers. © Cengage Learning®.

Blood Cultures

blood culture: a microbiological culture of blood employed to detect infections that are spreading through the bloodstream

resident flora: species of microorganisms that are always present on or in the body and are not easily removed by mechanical friction

The blood in our body is normally sterile; thus, when microorganisms invade the bloodstream and cause disease, it is usually very serious. Proper collection and processing of **blood cultures** is extremely important. Only about 8%–9% of blood cultures yield microbes judged to be the cause of disease, and it is very important to properly collect the specimens avoiding contamination with normal **resident flora**. This is especially true because normal skin flora can at times cause serious disease such as a heart valve infection that would cause the blood culture to be positive for organisms normally found on our skin. The best way to prevent contamination includes proper preparation of the skin prior to the venipuncture and avoiding drawing blood from existing intravenous lines. Reportedly, even with good collection techniques about 1%–3% of blood cultures are found to be contaminated with outside sources such as normal flora.

The technique to obtain a blood culture is as follows. The tourniquet should be applied and the vein palpated prior to disinfecting the site. Next, the site should be disinfected with 70% isopropyl alcohol (rubbing alcohol) followed by an application of chlorhexidine or 1%–2% tincture of iodine. Allow the disinfectant to dry for 1–2 minutes before attempting the blood collection. Povidone-iodine solutions such as Betadine should not be used as a disinfectant because they result in higher rates of contamination than iodine or chlorhexidine. If palpation of the skin is necessary, a sterile glove should be worn to do this. The blood should be collected directly into blood culture bottles that contain growth medium. This is done by removing the caps on the media bottles, swabbing the septum of the bottle with 70% isopropyl alcohol, and then collecting at least 10 mL into each blood culture bottle. One blood culture bottle is to recover aerobic organisms, and the other bottle will recover anaerobic microbes. Generally two sets of blood cultures are obtained with 20 mL for each collection (10 mL collected for the aerobic bottle and 10 mL collected for the anaerobic bottle $\times$ two different sites). For infants and small children the volume of blood collected is usually 1–5 mL.

Once the blood is collected, it should be transported to the laboratory immediately. If this is not possible, the blood may be kept at room temperature or stored temporarily in an incubator at 35°C. The bottles should *never* be refrigerated.

Cerebrospinal Fluid (CSF) Cultures

Physicians or other licensed independent practitioners (e.g., nurse practitioner) perform a lumbar puncture to obtain CSF for Gram stain, culture, and susceptibility. Because other health personnel may be asked to assist with this procedure, we will detail it here. Because CSF, like blood, is normally sterile, it is important to avoid contamination of the specimen. The skin of the back at the lumbar spine (L3–L5 level) should be cleaned first with isopropyl alcohol and then disinfected with chlorhexidine. After proper disinfection of the skin, a sterile drape should be used with an opening over the previously disinfected area. A spinal needle is inserted, and a total of 8–15 mL of fluid is withdrawn.

CSF specimens should be transported immediately to the laboratory and should not be refrigerated prior to transport. CSF can be drawn to diagnose different diseases but is most often obtained to diagnose meningitis. Because meningitis is a life-threatening disease, delays in specimen transport should never occur.

Sputum Cultures

Obtaining **sputum cultures** (lung secretions) from patients who have symptoms of respiratory tract infections such as pneumonia is common. Unlike blood and CSF, sputum is not sterile, and many bacterial species are normal colonizers of this area of the body. Therefore they may or may not be the cause of the lung infection in a given patient. Careful specimen collection and screening of the specimen for quality by the laboratory is necessary if clinically useful information is to be obtained.

At least one-third of patients with pneumonia may not be able to produce sputum suitable for culture. Some recommendations to enhance the quality of sputum specimens obtained from patients may be found in Table 6-9.

Media Connection

Go to the accompanying online resources to view a video on the proper way to collect blood cultures.

Media Connection

Go to the accompanying online resources to view a video on lumbar puncture.

Media Connection

Go to the accompanying online resources to view a video on obtaining a sputum sample.

sputum culture: a test to find and identify the microorganism causing an infection of the lower respiratory tract by obtaining a sample of sputum (mucus coughed up from the lungs) from the mouth

TABLE 6-9 Obtaining a Sputum Specimen

1. Try to obtain the specimen before antibiotics are given to the patient.
2. Ask the patient to rinse his or her mouth if possible prior to providing a specimen.
3. Ideally no food should have been consumed 1 to 2 hours prior to obtaining the sample.
4. Hand the sterile specimen cup to the patient and instruct him or her to remove the lid and expel secretions while attempting a deep cough. Emphasize that secretions *must* be obtained from the lungs and not saliva, or spit, from the mouth to be valid.
5. Seal the specimen cup and immediately transport the specimen to the laboratory. If the specimen cannot be transported immediately, it should be refrigerated.
6. After the laboratory receives the specimen, laboratory employees will Gram stain the specimen to screen for contamination by saliva. Laboratories may reject specimens if contaminated by saliva.
7. Specimens submitted for detection of *Mycobacterium tuberculosis* or *Legionella* sp. are not screened because recovery of these pathogens is not necessarily affected by the quality of the specimen.

© 2016 Cengage Learning®.

wound culture: a laboratory test in which microorganisms from a wound are grown in a special growth medium to find and identify the microorganism causing an infection in a wound or an abscess

urine specimen: clean-catch, midstream urine specimen for routine urinalysis and culture

stool specimen: a test to identify bacteria in patients with a suspected infection of the digestive tract by taking a sample of the patient's feces and placing it in a special medium where the bacteria is then grown

Wound Cultures

Wound culture is a general term used to describe material obtained from both superficial and deep wounds. It is important to distinguish between surface and deep or surgical wound specimens when submitting material to the diagnostic microbiology laboratory because it is not appropriate to culture superficial wounds for anaerobic bacteria. Because colonization of wounds with bacteria is common, it is challenging to sort out which organisms may be colonizing the wound from those causing true infection.

Common culture techniques for wounds listed in order of their clinical utility include obtaining swabs, needle aspiration, and deep tissue culture. If needle aspiration or fluid/material from a deep tissue culture may be obtained, this is always preferred over swab material. Table 6-10 presents some tips on collecting wound cultures.

TABLE 6-10 Obtaining a Wound Culture Specimen

1. If the lesion is open, the surface flora should be removed (e.g., irrigation or debridement) prior to obtaining culture material.

2. Material from burn wounds should be obtained only after extensive debridement and cleaning because it will always be colonized by flora.

3. Specimens of wounds should be obtained from the leading margin (edge) of the wound.

4. Culture material from an unruptured abscess should be obtained by needle aspiration after decontamination of the overlying skin.

5. For an open lesion or abscess, irrigate the wound to remove as much superficial flora as possible, then firmly sample the margin of the lesion with a swab (Figure 6-7).

6. Label the specimen describing the body site location from which the specimen was obtained.

7. Submit material for the appropriate cultures:

   a. Aerobic cultures—superficial lesions, open wounds, lacerations, and open abscesses

   b. Anaerobic cultures—surgical aspirates, biopsy tissue, closed abscess aspirates

8. Refrigerate the specimen if it cannot be transported immediately.

9. The laboratory should perform a Gram stain of the material. The presence of squamous epithelial cells indicates surface contamination, and consideration should be given for obtaining a more suitable specimen.

© 2016 Cengage Learning®.

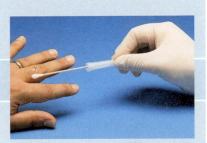

FIGURE 6-7 Obtaining a wound culture. © Cengage Learning®.

Urine Specimens

Urine specimens may be important to collect to assist in the diagnosis of urinary tract infections (Figure 6-8). In collecting these specimens, it is important to avoid contamination, especially from bacteria that may be found in the distal urethra. Suprapubic aspiration and straight catheter technique are two procedures that may avoid contamination but are invasive and are rarely used. Most urine specimens are obtained from adult patients using a clean-catch midstream technique. This technique is simple and inexpensive and is neither invasive nor uncomfortable for the patient. Table 6-11 outlines this procedure.

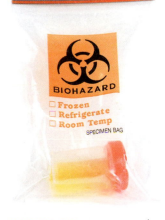

FIGURE 6-8 Urine sample in biohazard bag. ©iStock.com/leezsnow.

Stool Specimens

Stool specimens may be obtained to aid in the diagnosis of bowel (enteric) infections. Specimens may be evaluated for the presence of intestinal microbes such as *Giardia lamblia*, *Salmonella*, *Shigella*, or *Clostridium*

TABLE 6-11 Obtaining a Clean-Catch Midstream Urine Specimen

Female Patient
1. Stand in a squatting position over the toilet.
2. Open three prepackaged towelettes.
3. Separate the folds of the skin around the urinary opening.
4. Using a towelette wipe first the left side from front to back. Repeat this using a towelette for the right side and then another down the center.
5. Void the first portion of urine into the toilet. Stop the flow, then void the next portion of urine in the sterile container. Do not touch the inside of the sterile container with any body part including the hands. Void the remainder of the urine into the toilet.
6. Cover the specimen with the lid provided.
7. Wipe away any excess urine from the outside of the container.
8. Wash hands.
9. Deliver immediately to the lab or refrigerate the specimen.

Male Patient
1. Wash hands.
2. Cleanse the end of the penis with a towelette by starting at the urethral opening and working away from it. Retract the skin in males who are not circumscribed prior to performing this procedure. Repeat this cleansing procedure twice using new towelettes.
3. Void the first portion of urine in the toilet. Stop the urine flow and resume voiding urine into the sterile collection container. Do not touch the inside of the container with any body part. Finish voiding urine into the toilet.
4. Cap the specimen with the lid provided and touch only the outside of either the lid or container.
5. Wash hands.
6. Deliver immediately to the lab or refrigerate the specimen.

© 2016 Cengage Learning®.

difficile to name a few. Optimal test results are obtained when testing is performed on fresh specimens. Unfortunately this is often impractical, especially in outpatient settings, so a variety of commercially available containers with transport medium (e.g., 10% neutral-buffered formalin)

TABLE 6-12 Obtaining a Stool Specimen

1. Instruct the patient to defecate into a clean bedpan or container and discard any tissue into the toilet.

2. Make sure the patient is instructed to collect only stool. The specimen must not be contaminated with urine because the substances in urine may kill microbes.

3. A tongue depressor may be used to transfer approximately 2 or 3 tablespoonfuls of stool to the specimen transport container.

4. The specimen should be transported to the laboratory immediately. If receipt of the specimen by the lab cannot occur within 2 hours, it should be refrigerated.

© 2016 Cengage Learning®.

are available. If a specimen cannot be transported immediately, it should be refrigerated. Table 6-12 details the proper procedure to collect a stool sample.

Throat Culture

Most sore throats (pharyngitis) are caused by viruses. However, *Streptococcus pyogenes* remains an important bacterial cause particularly in children. Because it is not possible to reliably distinguish infection with this organism from infection with common viruses, **throat cultures** remain an important method of diagnosis. Table 6-13 outlines the steps for obtaining a throat culture.

Nasal Specimens

Nasal specimens are generally considered the specimen of choice for the diagnosis of respiratory viruses. They are not useful in the diagnosis of sinus infections because the nasal cavity is often inhabited by bacteria even in a person without a sinus infection. Nasal swabs are usually obtained from one nostril at a depth of 2 to 3 centimeters using a sterile cotton swab. After the specimen is obtained, it is then inserted into a container of viral transport medium. The specimens should be immediately transported to the microbiology laboratory for processing. Viruses such as influenza, respiratory syncytial virus, parainfluenzae, enterovirus, and rhinoviruses may be detected using either automated methods that detect viral material or less commonly by culture.

throat culture: a technique for identifying disease bacteria in material taken from the throat; most throat cultures are done to rule out infections caused by beta-hemolytic streptococci, which cause strep throat

nasal specimen: a specimen obtained using a cotton swab on a stick, passed up the nostril to obtain a sample of exudate and epithelial debris for microbiological or cellular examination; not recommended unless testing for viruses

Media Connection

Go to the accompanying online resources to view a video on throat culture technique.

TABLE 6-13 Obtaining a Throat Culture

1. Position the patient so that the patient's mouth is at eye level.
2. Ask the patient to tilt his or her head back and open the mouth.
3. Don gloves. Obtain a sterile swab and remove it from its wrapper. Place the tongue depressor on the patient's tongue and ask him or her to say, "Ah-h-h" (Figure 6-9A).
4. Swab both tonsils and the back of the mouth by sweeping the cotton tip from side to side. Do not allow the cotton tip to touch the tongue, sides of the mouth, or uvula.
5. Remove the cotton tip without touching any other parts of the mouth and place the swab in its container (Figure 6-9B).
6. If a dual swab system is used, one swab is used to detect the antigen (rapid Strep test) while the second swab is sent to the laboratory for culture if the direct test is negative.
7. Label the swab prior to sending to the lab (Figure 6-9C).

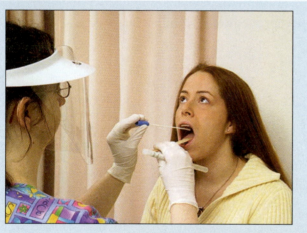

A

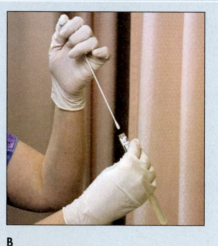

B

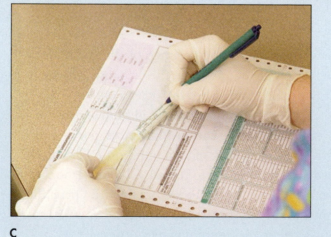

C

FIGURE 6-9 Obtaining a throat culture. © Cengage Learning®.

6-3
Stop and Review

1. Collection of _____ specimens should be limited to throat and urethral cultures.
2. _____ should not be used as a disinfectant prior to collecting blood cultures since contamination rates are higher.
3. _____ specimens are considered the specimen of choice for the diagnosis of respiratory viruses.

Chapter Summary

- Is it not great to take the theories you learned in previous chapters and put them into practical application? That is what this chapter was all about.

- We discussed the proper way to dispose of medical waste, which you learned could be contaminated with bloodborne pathogens.

- The disposal of sharps is different than disposal of regular medical waste, not only because we need to protect ourselves, but also because laundry workers and waste haulers do not want to be injured by a needlestick.

- We discussed applying and removing both sterile and nonsterile gloves in detail. Do not

forget to wash your hands before and after glove removal!

- We addressed the meaning of sterility and asepsis by building on our knowledge of how microorganisms cause disease.

- The proper diagnosis of infectious diseases is aided tremendously by obtaining proper culture material from various body sites. Finally, we discussed the proper techniques to obtain a wide variety of samples for processing in the microbiology laboratory so a proper diagnosis may be obtained.

- This chapter built on your previously acquired knowledge of medical microbiology by showing you how this knowledge can be put into practice.

Case Study

Mr. Jones is a 69-year-old male who underwent an umbilical hernia repair operation 1 week ago. He was doing well until a day or so ago when he noticed the incision site on his abdomen was getting red and draining a small amount of fluid that he described as thick and yellowish in color. After discussing this problem with Mr. Jones on the phone, you schedule him to be seen by his surgeon. The surgeon asks you to obtain a culture of the material draining from the incision to be sent to the local microbiology laboratory. How should the specimen be obtained to provide the most useful information?

Chapter Review

Match the cellular component with its function.

1. _____ transient flora

2. _____ stool specimens

3. _____ blood cultures

4. _____ surgical asepsis

5. _____ wound culture

6. _____ cerebrospinal fluid cultures

7. _____ resident flora

8. _____ medical asepsis

9. _____ sharps

10. _____ nasal specimens

11. _____ infectious waste

12. _____ open method

a. 1%–3% are found to be contaminated

b. procedures reduce the number and growth of microorganisms

c. flora that normally resides on the surface of our skin

d. goal is to eliminate all microbes

e. needles and scalpels

f. a way of putting on gloves

g. transport to lab immediately or refrigerate

h. only useful to diagnose respiratory viral infections

i. needle aspiration is preferred over a swab specimen

j. medical waste contaminated with blood or other potentially infectious body fluids

k. flora that may contaminate our hands after patient or environmental contact

l. type of caution that applies to all patients

Identify if each statement is true or false.

13. _____ If a person reaches over a sterile field, the field is still sterile.

14. _____ The border edge of a sterile field is considered part of the sterile field.

15. _____ Performing proper hand hygiene is the single most important thing you can do to prevent the spread of infection.

16. _____ Medical and surgical asepsis are considered to be the same.

17. _____ Proper specimen collection is essential to assist in obtaining a medical diagnosis.

Discuss the answers to the following questions with your instructor.

18. Why is it necessary to properly obtain specimens from various body sites?

19. What is the difference between medical asepsis and surgical asepsis?

20. Many health care workers assume that wearing gloves means they do not have to wash their hands. How would you explain why hand washing is necessary even if gloves are worn?

21. What two types of testing can be performed on throat cultures to diagnose Strep throat?

22. If specimens are not properly stored or transported to the laboratory, what types of problems may occur?

Additional Activities

1. By reading this chapter you have discovered how important hand hygiene is to prevent the spread of infection. In fact, proper hand hygiene saves lives. Research why compliance with proper hand hygiene is poor. Can you think of some creative solutions to help improve compliance with good hand hygiene?

2. Create a sterile field and add items to the field using proper techniques.

3. Visit your local hospital's operating room to observe surgical aseptic procedures. Observe the surgeons, surgical technicians, and scrub nurses washing their hands and donning gloves and gowns.

4. Divide the class into groups and distribute cards with a specific specimen to be obtained. Let each group draw a specimen card and then practice obtaining that specimen from someone else in the group or explain the steps in the proper technique.

5. Have a contest in class to see who can properly apply gloves using each of the different methods (open versus closed method). Use checklists to score each contestant.

Media Connection

Go to the accompanying online resources and have fun learning as you play games, view animations and videos, and take practice tests to help reinforce key concepts you learned in this chapter.

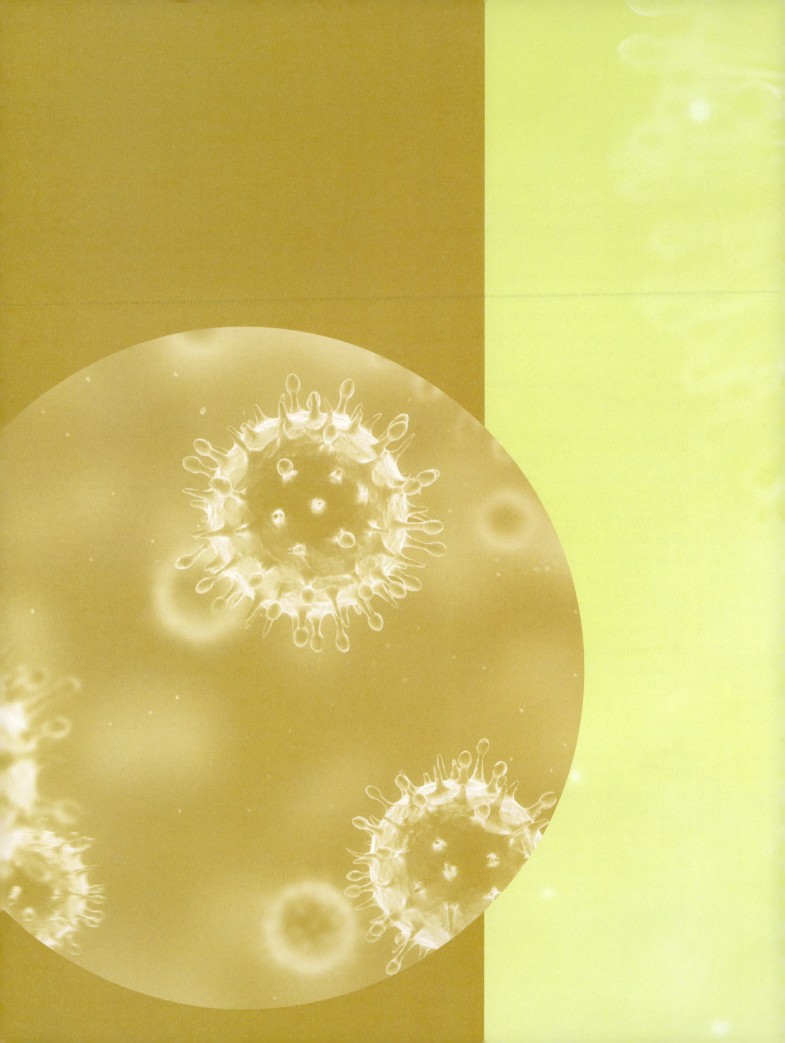

The Infectious Diseases: A Systems Approach

Now that you are familiar with the background and science of microbiology and how to prevent the spread of infections, it is time to learn about infectious diseases using a systems approach. In the next several chapters, we discuss immunizations, antimicrobials, monitoring therapy, and the types of infections commonly encountered by health care practitioners. The first chapter of this section provides a background on disease terminology, immunizations, monitoring therapy, and the drugs we use to treat infections. We call these medications antimicrobials rather than antibiotics because we discuss medications used to treat bacteria (antibiotics), fungi (antifungals), and viruses (antivirals). After you are finished studying immunizations and antimicrobials, you will use this new knowledge to better understand the following two chapters, which discuss the treatment of infections. The infections will be categorized by body systems. For example, we talk about infections occurring in the head and neck and from there move on to discuss cardiovascular infections, and so on. With each body location or system, we will first mention the type of symptoms the patient may exhibit. From there we discuss the type of microorganisms commonly encountered. Finally, we discuss antimicrobial treatments, if any exist. For some infections, no drug treatments are available, and we must depend on a competent immune system to do the job of eradicating the infection.

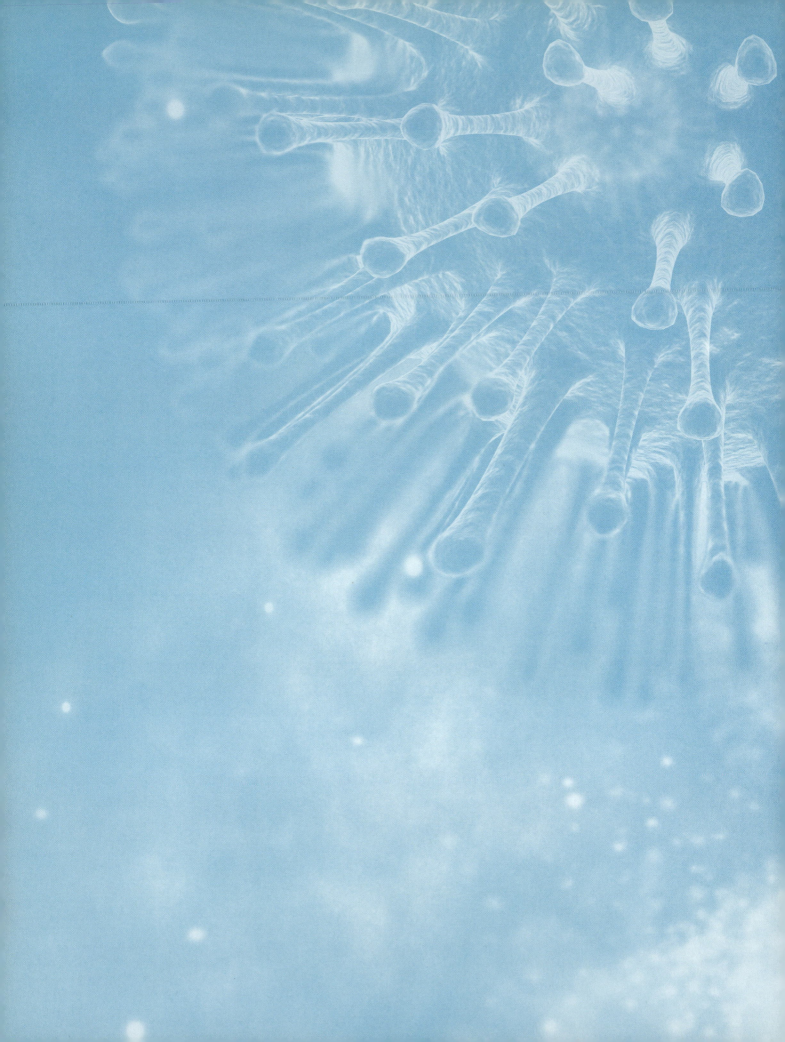

Immunizations and Antimicrobials

OBJECTIVES

After studying this chapter, the learner will be able to:

- Define basic disease terminology and concepts.

- Contrast the difference between active and passive immunity.

- Describe why drugs that induce passive immunity in a patient are important to assist in the treatment of patients with certain infectious diseases.

- Discuss how patients with infectious diseases are monitored both clinically and from a laboratory perspective.

- List the various mechanisms of antimicrobial resistance.

- Discuss the importance of appropriate prescribing and consumption of antimicrobials.

- Compare and contrast the different ways of classifying antibiotics.

- Given a particular antibiotic, provide the classification or grouping to which it belongs, potential therapeutic uses, and toxicity.

- Discuss the various types of antivirals, their potential clinical uses, and toxicity.

- Compare and contrast antifungal drugs according to their spectrum of activity, route of administration, and toxic effects.

KEY TERMS

active immunity

aminoglycosides
[a ME noh GLY koh sides]

antifungal drugs

antitubercular drugs
[AN tee too BER kyu ler]

antiviral drugs

bactericidal
[back TEER ih SIGH dul]

bacteriostatic
[back teer ee oh STAT ik]

beta-lactams

broad-spectrum drugs

carbapenem
[kahr buh PEN um]

cephalosporins
[SEF uh loh SPORE ins]

chief complaint or concern (CC)

(Continues)

KEY TERMS (Continued)

clindamycin
[KLIN duh MY sin]

daptomycin [DAP toe MY sin]

diagnose

echinocandins
[ee KYE noh KAN dins]

endemic

epidemic

epidemiology

etiology

exacerbation

folate inhibitor

glycopeptide
[GLY koh PEP tide]

immunity

immunoglobulins
[IM you noh GLOB you lins]

macrolides

metronidazole
[MET roh NYE duh zole]

monobactam
[MAHN oh back tam]

morbidity

mortality

multidrug-resistant (MDR) TB

narrow-spectrum drugs

oxazolidinones
[ock SAY zoh LYE di nohns]

pandemic

passive immunity

penicillins

prognosis

quinolones [KWIN oh lohns]

quinupristin-dalfopristin
[kwin YOU pris tin
dal FOE pris tin]

relapses

remission

resistance

**respiratory syncytial virus
(RSV)** [sin SISH ul]

signs

superinfection

symptoms

syndrome

tetracyclines
[TET ruh SIGH kleens]

vital signs

Introduction

The goal of this chapter is to familiarize the reader with disease terminology and concepts, immunizations, and antimicrobials. We begin with a discussion of general disease terminology and concepts. Next we cover immunizations and discuss the difference between active and passive immunity. Before launching into the specific antimicrobial drugs, we discuss the increasing public health problem of resistance and then follow up with ways of classifying antibiotics. Then we begin our discussion of antimicrobials, organizing each section when possible by grouping the medicines into a therapeutic class. We do the same for **antiviral drugs** and **antifungal drugs**. This chapter serves as a building block for the next chapters as we explore infectious diseases using a systems approach.

We have used this "building block" approach throughout the book, and we hope that it has facilitated your learning. Finally, we need to emphasize

antiviral drug: drug that can destroy viruses and help treat illnesses caused by them

antifungal drug: destructive to fungi, or suppressing their reproduction or growth; effective against fungal infections

the importance of using antimicrobials appropriately in an attempt to slow the development of resistance to these miracle drugs. Society as a whole and readers of this book in particular have a responsibility to use antimicrobials wisely. With your newly acquired knowledge, we hope you will do what you can to make that happen.

General Disease Terminology

The word *disease* literally means not (*dis*) at ease and is a condition in which the body fails to function normally. Disease can come from several causes, but certainly infections rank high on the list of causes or etiologies for disease. A brief discussion of some of the unique language of disease, especially as it relates to infectious diseases, is needed to lay the foundation for future discussions.

Signs and Symptoms of Disease

Think back to a time when you were sick. You may have had a fever, cough, nausea, dizziness, joint aches, or a generalized weakness. These are examples of **signs** and **symptoms** of disease. Although the terms *signs* and *symptoms* are often used interchangeably, each has its own specific definition. Signs are more definitive, *objective* (measurable), obvious indicators of an illness that can actually be measured and expressed as numbers. Fever is a good example of a common sign in many infectious diseases. **Vital signs** are common, measurable indicators that help us assess the health of our patients. Vital signs are the signs vital to life and include pulse (heart rate), blood pressure, body temperature, and respiratory rate. The vital sign standard values can change according to the patient's age and sex and are often affected in the infectious disease process.

Symptoms, on the other hand, are more *subjective*, based on the individual's perception, and are therefore more difficult to measure consistently. Although pain is now being considered the fifth vital sign, it is still a subjective evaluation very much like a symptom. For example, tolerance to pain varies among individuals, so an equal amount of pain (as in a needlestick) applied to a number of people could be perceived as a light, moderate, or intense level of pain, depending on each individual's perception. Symptoms are hard to measure. They are, however, still very important in the diagnosis of disease. Sometimes a disease exhibits a set group of signs and symptoms that may occur at about the same time. This specific grouping of signs and symptoms is known as a **syndrome**. The flu syndrome, for example, can include fever, muscle aches, tachycardia, difficulty breathing, and generalized weakness and malaise.

Discovering as many signs and symptoms as possible can help to **diagnose** a disease. A diagnosis is an identification of a disease determined

sign: any objective evidence or manifestation of an illness or disordered function of the body

symptom: any change in the body or its functions as perceived by the patient

vital signs: medical assessment during a physical examination in which the temperature, pulse, and respirations (TPR), as well as the blood pressure, are measured

syndrome: a set of symptoms and signs associated with, and characteristic of, one particular disease

diagnose: determine the cause of the patient's symptoms and signs

Learning Hint
Using Medical Terminology

The word *gnosis* is Greek for knowledge. *Dia* means through or complete, and therefore *diagnosis* literally means "know through or completely." *Pro* is a prefix meaning before or in front of, and *prognosis* literally means the foreknowledge or predicting of the outcome of a disease.

chief complaint or concern (CC): the main sign or symptom that caused an individual to seek health care

etiology: the specific cause of the disease

prognosis: the predicted outcome of a disease

remission: a lessening of severity or disappearance of symptoms

relapse: a recurrence of a disease or symptoms after an apparent recovery

exacerbation: a worsening or flare-up of a disease process

mortality: condition of being dead or the number of deaths in a given population

morbidity: state of being diseased

epidemiology: the study of the origin, distribution, and determinants of diseases

endemic: a condition or disease related to a specific population or region of the world

epidemic: an outbreak of a disease that suddenly affects a large group of people in a geographical region or a defined population group

pandemic: disease or condition that affects many people worldwide

immunity: the protection against infectious disease conferred either by the immune response generated by immunization or previous infection or by other nonimmunological factors

by studying the patient's signs, symptoms, history, and results of diagnostic tests. The diagnostic procedure is done by first obtaining a patient history and determining the patient's **chief complaint or concern (CC)**. Although the individual may have many medical problems, the chief complaint is what brought him or her *now* to seek medical help. Obtaining a complete medical history can help in determining the **etiology**, or cause, of the disease. The **prognosis** is the prediction of the outcome of a disease.

It is also helpful to determine if the chief complaint was gradual or of a sudden onset. Quite often, symptoms gradually develop from a disease process that may have been there for some time. These often are *chronic conditions* as opposed to *acute conditions* that exhibit a rapid onset of signs and symptoms. The signs and symptoms of a chronic disease may disappear at times, and this period is known as **remission** of the disease. **Relapses** are recurrences of the signs and symptoms of disease. If the signs and symptoms acutely *flare up*, this is known as an **exacerbation** of the disease. **Mortality** is the measure of the number of deaths attributed to a specific disease in a given population over a period of time. **Morbidity** is the measure of the disabilities and extent of problems caused by an illness. For example, although polio has a low mortality rate (few deaths associated with the disease), it does have a high morbidity rate because of the paralysis, limb deformities, and difficulty breathing later in life.

Epidemiology is the science that studies the patterns, causes, spread, and effects of disease conditions in defined populations. The Centers for Disease Control and Prevention (CDC) uses epidemiology to track disease worldwide. If a disease is continually present within a specific population or region, it is called **endemic**. If the disease occurs suddenly in large numbers over a specific region, it is called an **epidemic**. If the disease spreads countrywide or worldwide, it is called a **pandemic**. The CDC is the infectious disease surveillance agency that helps prevent and control the spread of diseases throughout our population.

Immunizations

Immunity is inherited, acquired, or induced resistance to infection by a specific pathogen. Once foreign invaders are recognized, our bodies produce an immune response that tries to eliminate the intruder. The immune response, among other things, consists of producing antibodies against the foreign invaders (microbes). These antibodies are specific for certain microbes or closely related microbes. There are basically two broad types of immunity that a person can acquire: *active* and *passive*.

Passive immunity involves injecting already formed antibodies called **immunoglobulins** into a patient who has an infection or to prevent an infection. This immunity is short-lived because the immunoglobulins are not produced or made by the patient. Once they are used up, the immunity is gone. For this reason, passive immunity is generally only used in patients who have not been immunized against the disease or are immunocompromised and would not be able to produce antibodies on their own. Table 7-1 presents some examples of products that can be used to passively immunize a patient.

The other type of immunity, which is long-lasting, is active immunity. **Active immunity** can be produced artificially by vaccination or naturally by becoming ill with a particular disease. Because our goal is to prevent disease, the best way to acquire active immunity is through vaccination (Figure 7-1). The goal of active immunity is to have our bodies produce our own antibodies against invading microorganisms. Vaccines contain antigens that are used to fool our body into making antibodies to fight a particular disease. This

passive immunity: immunity acquired by the introduction of preformed antibodies into an unprotected individual

immunoglobulin [IM you noh GLOB you lins]: protein of animal origin with known antibody activity, synthesized by lymphocytes and plasma cells and found in serum and in other body fluids and tissues; abbreviated Ig; there are five distinct classes based on structural and antigenic properties: IgA, IgD, IgE, IgG, and IgM

active immunity: a type of immunity that can be produced artificially by vaccination or naturally by becoming ill with a particular disease

TABLE 7-1 Agents for Passive Immunization

Generic Name	Brand Name	Use(s)
Antithymocyte globulin	Atgam	Aplastic anemia, organ transplant rejection
Botulism immune globulin	BabyBIG	Infant botulism
Cytomegalovirus immune globulin	CytoGam	Prevention of CMV disease
Hepatitis B immune globulin	HepaGam B	Passive immunity after acute exposure to hepatitis B
Immune globulin	Gammagard	Treatment of immunodeficiency
Rabies immune globulin (human)	Imogam	Used to provide passive immunity after a rabies exposure
Tetanus immune globulin	Hypertet	Prophylaxis against tetanus following injury if immune status is uncertain
Varicella-zoster immune globulin	VariZIG	Passive immunization of pregnant women exposed to varicella

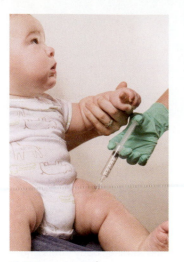

Learning Hint

Keeping Up-to-Date on Vaccines

Information regarding vaccines and immunizations changes from time to time, and requirements may vary by state, territory, or country. Therefore, the most up-to-date information regarding vaccines, immunization recommendations, and requirements can be obtained by contacting the Centers for Disease Control and Prevention (CDC) and the National Immunization Program at http://www.cdc.gov/vaccines. The best source of up-to-date vaccine information is the CDC Website, Advisory Committee on Immunization Practices (ACIP).

FIGURE 7-1 Infant receiving vaccination. Source: CDC/ Amanda Mills

type of immunity is long-lasting because cells are produced that may rapidly produce antibodies any time the invader reappears.

Because the vaccine does not cause disease, we achieve our goal without making the patient sick. For example, if we caught the flu (influenza) we would become very ill. To help us get well, our bodies would eventually make antibodies against the influenza type that was causing our illness. To prevent us from getting influenza, we use vaccination. We must be vaccinated yearly against influenza because the virus is constantly changing, so our bodies may not recognize the invading flu strain if we have not been immunized against it previously. Another reason vaccines must be given again is because the immunity does not last a lifetime, as discussed in Section I.

Monitoring Antimicrobial Therapy

When we treat patients with antimicrobials, we want to ask ourselves two basic questions. First, is the disease we are treating getting better, staying the same, or getting worse? The second question we need to ask is, Is the treatment causing side effects that may be worse than the disease?

To answer our first question we usually use a combination of bedside (clinical) and laboratory monitoring. For example, if patients have pneumonia, they usually have a fever, cough with yellowish phlegm, shortness of breath, a high white blood cell count, and a shadow (infiltrate) on their chest x-ray. If we choose the right antibiotic, hopefully we will see these clinical and laboratory findings improving as treatment progresses (Figure 7-2). In the subsequent chapters we will discuss in a bit more detail the clinical findings of different infectious diseases that should improve with the proper treatment.

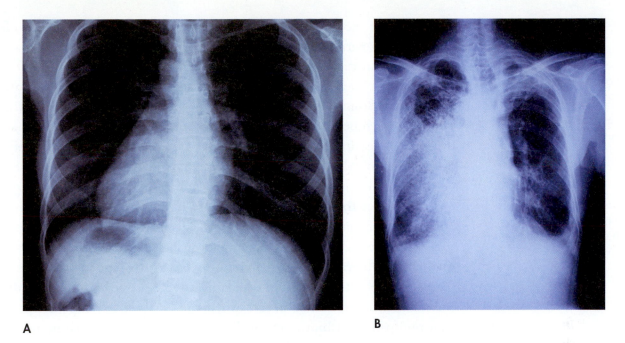

FIGURE 7-2 A. Normal chest x-ray. © leungchopan/Shutterstock.com. **B.** Chest x-ray showing pneumonia in the right middle and lower lobe. © joloei/www.Shutterstock.com. Note: keep in mind right and left are always referenced to the patient.

To answer our second question, we also use a combination of clinical and laboratory monitoring. If we are using vancomycin to treat an MRSA infection, we will monitor the patient during the drug infusion for red itchy skin, especially in the upper body (red man syndrome). We may order a platelet and white blood cell count because, in rare cases, vancomycin may cause these to decrease. Sometimes our monitoring reveals serious toxicity that would lead us to stop the medication and substitute another. As you read about antimicrobials, you will note some of the possible side effects that may occur and what to monitor.

Some antimicrobials such as aminoglycosides and vancomycin can be monitored using drug levels measured in a patient's blood to see if they are at levels needed to achieve the desired effect (therapeutic effect). These levels may be used to adjust drug doses in an attempt to prevent side effects or to increase the chance of a cure.

Microbial Resistance Mechanisms

The development of so-called *superbacteria* has been facilitated by the widespread misuse of antibacterial agents to treat viral infections (e.g., common colds and influenza), the use of antibiotics to prevent disease in

broad-spectrum drug: drug that acts on a wide range of disease-causing bacteria

narrow-spectrum drug: drug that is effective against specific families of bacteria

resistance: a lack of response of a pathogen to treatment such as antibiotic therapy

animals, and the continued use of broad-spectrum agents to treat infections when a narrow-spectrum agent would do. Use of antibiotics that are effective against a wide range of microorganisms (**broad-spectrum drugs**) can result in overkill if a drug effective against fewer microorganisms (a **narrow-spectrum drug**) would do. Even with appropriate use of antimicrobials, microbes are very capable of becoming resistant to certain antimicrobials, leaving physicians with limited treatment options. Viruses and fungi are also able to evolve into *superpathogens* when they are exposed to antifungals and antivirals.

Resistance to antimicrobials develops in many ways. As one example, an antibiotic may actually be destroyed by bacterial enzymes. Bacteria that produce the enzyme β-lactamase can inactivate cephalosporins and penicillins. Alteration in protein binding is another type of resistance that prevents the antibiotic from attaching to the altered protein. Another mechanism of resistance occurs when the bacteria develop pumps that can pump the antibiotic out of the organism (bacteria become resistant to macrolides this way), thus preventing it from destroying the bacteria.

Resistance also develops when patients take antibiotics whether or not they are clinically indicated. Appropriate use of antibiotics will also eventually result in resistance, but this problem is magnified when we take antibiotics for the wrong reasons. A rather common occurrence is for patients with acute bronchitis to be seen by a health care provider and given an antibiotic prescription even though the majority of these cases are caused by viruses. Educating patients to understand what infections require antibiotics (e.g., bacterial pneumonia and cellulitis) and which do not (e.g., acute bronchitis and colds) is an important role for every health care provider. For more information on the CDC's efforts to educate the population, check out the CDC's Get Smart campaign at http://www.cdc.gov/getsmart/

Food for Thought
Patient and Family Education

Every health care provider should assist with educational efforts to decrease the inappropriate use of antimicrobials. Few new antibiotics are being introduced for use in part because it is difficult for companies to profit from drugs that clinicians are told not to use until resistance becomes a problem. Figure 7-3 shows a simplified model of how antibiotic resistance develops and how it spreads.

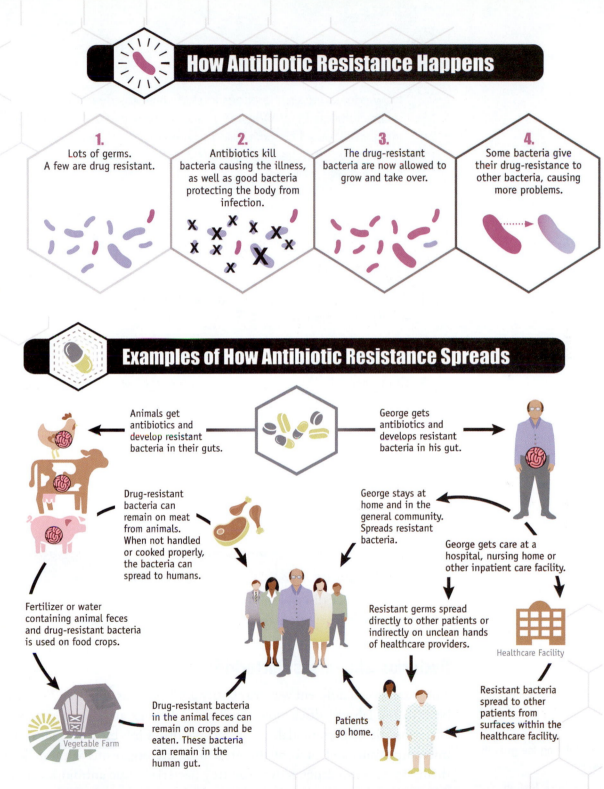

FIGURE 7-3 A. Simplified model of antibiotic resistance. **B.** Examples of the spread of antibiotic resistance. It is important to note that simply using antibiotics causes resistance, and therefore prudent use is critical.
Source: CDC/Melissa Brower

Food for Thought

Do Your Part

How can you assist the efforts to stop unnecessary use of antimicrobials? Hint: When was the last time you or your family member received an antibiotic prescription? After reading this chapter, was the prescription necessary? If it was, did the person finish the prescription?

7-1
Stop and Review

1. _____ is the number of measured deaths attributed to a specific disease.

2. _____ is the measure of disability and problems caused by a disease.

3. The science that studies patterns, causes, and spread of disease is _____.

4. Resistance in bacteria develops when patients take _____ unnecessarily.

5. Antibiotics that are effective against a wide range of bacteria are termed _____.

Antibacterial Drug Classification

Before we begin our discussion of antibacterial drug classes, a few important general properties that apply to all antibiotics will be discussed.

Bacteriostatic versus Bactericidal

bacteriostatic [back teer ee oh STAT ik]: inhibiting the growth of bacteria

bactericidal [back TEER ih SIGH dul]: capable of killing bacteria

There are several different ways to classify antibacterials. The first way relates back to the lab test discussion. Antibacterial drugs are classified as either bacteriostatic or bactericidal. **Bacteriostatic** drugs inhibit the replication of microorganisms and prevent the growth of the organisms without killing them. **Bactericidal** drugs actively destroy bacteria. Some antibiotics are bacteriostatic at low concentrations, but at higher concentrations, may be bactericidal. See Table 7-2 for some common bacteriostatic and bactericidal drugs. In theory, it would seem you should always use an antibiotic that is bactericidal. However, both -cidal and -static antibiotics may result in a cure of the infection.

TABLE 7-2 Bactericidal versus Bacteriostatic Antibiotics

Bactericidal	Bacteriostatic
Beta-lactams	Tetracyclines
Vancomycin	Macrolides
Fluoroquinolones	Trimethoprim-sulfamethoxazole
Daptomycin	Linezolid*
Metronidazole	Clindamycin*

*May exhibit both properties depending on the type of bacteria.
© 2016 Cengage Learning®.

Spectrum of Activity: Broad versus Narrow

Antibacterials can also be classified according to their spectrum of activity. Broad-spectrum antibiotics are effective against a wider range of bacteria than are narrow-spectrum antibiotics. Broad-spectrum antibiotics may be used initially to treat infections in patients who are very ill because they are less likely to miss the microbial cause. Once the organism is known, a narrow-spectrum drug may then be substituted. See Table 7-3 for examples of this classification system.

Based on Mechanism of Action

Just as there are many ways of classifying bacteria (aerobic/anaerobic, gram-positive/gram-negative), there are also multiple ways to classify

TABLE 7-3 Broad- and Narrow-Spectrum Antibiotics

Classification	Spectrum of Activity
Broad	
Carbapenems	Gram-positive cocci and bacilli, gram-negative bacilli including Pseudomonas, anaerobes
Ceftaroline	Gram-positive cocci including MRSA, gram-negative
Narrow	
Penicillin G	*Streptococci*
Nafcillin	Methicillin-susceptible *Staphylococcus aureus*

© 2016 Cengage Learning®.

antibacterial agents. Antimicrobials may be classified based on their mechanism of action. This method is commonly used to classify HIV medications. HIV disease is treated with at least three active drugs, and the classification scheme based on mechanism of action allows the clinician flexibility to pick and choose different agents from each class. Besides HIV disease, drugs are rarely selected clinically according to their mechanism of action.

Antibacterial Agents

The first broad class of antimicrobials we will discuss are medications that are used to fight bacteria. Antibacterial agents are grouped according to their chemical structure.

Beta-Lactams

beta-lactams: any of a class of antibiotics that is structurally and pharmacologically related to the penicillins and cephalosporins

Beta-lactams are chemically related drugs and include penicillins, cephalosporins, monobactams (Azactam), carbacephems (Loracarbef), and carbapenems (Imipenem and Meropenem). All beta-lactam antimicrobials act by inhibiting materials needed for bacterial cell wall synthesis. Bactericidal activity requires sensitive bacteria to be actively dividing. Their action prevents the repair of the bacteria's cell wall, causing cell death. These enzymes are generally referred to as penicillin-binding proteins (PBPs) and are located just under the cell wall.

Penicillins

penicillin: any group of antibiotics biosynthesized by several species of molds

The **penicillins** can be further subdivided into natural penicillins, penicillinase-resistant semisynthetic penicillins, aminopenicillins, extended-spectrum penicillins, and penicillins combined with beta-lactamase inhibitors. By changing the basic penicillin structure, researchers have developed many penicillin derivatives. Combining a penicillin with a beta-lactamase inhibitor may prevent the beta-lactam drug from being inactivated by enzyme-producing bacteria. Extended-spectrum penicillins are more active than natural penicillins against gram-negative bacteria because of their ability to enter the larger cell membrane.

Diarrhea is a main side effect of penicillins and most antibiotic classes. Otherwise, penicillins have very little toxicity; however, 15% to 20% of people are allergic to this drug. The allergy can vary from an itchy, red, mild rash to wheezing and anaphylaxis. Table 7-4 lists commonly used penicillins.

TABLE 7-4 Commonly Used Penicillins

Type	Generic Name	Brand Name
Natural penicillins	Penicillin G	
	Penicillin V	Veetids
Aminopenicillins	Ampicillin	Omnipen
	Amoxicillin	Amoxil
Penicillinase-resistant penicillins	Dicloxacillin	Dynapen
	Nafcillin	Unipen
Extended-spectrum penicillins	Piperacillin	Pipracil
Beta-lactam with beta-lactamase inhibitor	Amoxicillin–clavulanate	Augmentin
	Ampicillin-sulbactam	Unasyn
	Piperacillin-tazobactam	Zosyn

Clinical Application
Pencillins and Prophylaxis

Penicillins are frequently used for prophylaxis to decrease the risk of infection in patients with conditions such as mechanical heart valves that may predispose them to infection. For example, some patients with a history of rheumatic heart disease take amoxicillin before a dental appointment to prevent a cardiac infection. That infection could occur as a result of bacteria being spread through the blood from the mouth, with dental manipulation, to a vulnerable site such as the heart.

Cephalosporins

Cephalosporins have a mechanism of action that is similar to penicillins. They differ from penicillins in their antibacterial spectrum, resistance to beta-lactamase, and duration of action. One of the advantages of some cephalosporins over most penicillins is that they have a longer duration of action, which allows for infrequent outpatient parenteral dosing for chronic infections. This may keep some patients out of the hospital allowing them to be treated as outpatients.

cephalosporin [SEF uh loh SPORE ins]: a subtype of beta-lactam antibiotics that kill bacteria or prevent their growth; used to treat infections in different parts of the body, such as the ears, nose, throat, lungs, sinuses, and skin

The cephalosporins are generally divided into five generations. Each generation tends to be a little broader in their spectrum of activity. First-generation cephalosporins are usually more active against gram-positive than gram-negative organisms and may be chosen for community-acquired infections. Second-generation cephalosporins are used for otitis media in pediatrics and for respiratory and urinary tract infections in hospitalized patients. Third-generation cephalosporins are used in community and health care–associated infections because of their enhanced gram negative activity. Because they survive in the body for longer periods of time, they are useful to treat patients outside the hospital—they require less frequent dosing (e.g., once daily instead of three or four times daily). Fourth-generation cephalosporins are used to treat health care–associated infections such as pneumonia, urinary tract infections, and skin infections. The fifth-generation ceftaroline is the first cephalosporin to have activity against methicillin-resistant *Staphylococcus aureus* as well as keeping the broad spectrum of activity for gram-negative pathogens that are seen in the later cephalosporin generations. However, it loses the activity against *Pseudomonas aeruginosa* that is found in its third- and fourth-generation relatives. Adverse effects from cephalosporins are similar to those seen with penicillins, and they are less toxic than many antibiotics. See Table 7-5 for some commonly used cephalosporins.

TABLE 7-5 Commonly Used Cephalosporins

Generation	Generic Name	Brand Name	Route of Administration
First	Cephalexin	Keflex	PO
	Cefazolin	Ancef	IM, IV
Second	Cefaclor	Ceclor	PO
	Cefoxitin	Mefoxin	IM, IV
	Cefotetan	N/A	IM, IV
	Cefuroxime	Ceftin, Zinacef	PO, IM, IV
Third	Ceftriaxone	Rocephin	IM, IV
	Ceftazidime	Fortaz	IM, IV
	Cefixime	Suprax	PO
Fourth	Cefepime	Maxipime	IM, IV
Fifth	Ceftaroline	Teflaro	IV

Clinical Application
Allergic Reactions

Many patients who say they are allergic to penicillin are able to safely receive a different beta-lactam antibiotic such as a cephalosporin. The reason is partly related to confusion over what is a true serious allergy (e.g., hives, difficulty breathing, drop in blood pressure, and anaphylaxis) versus what is an adverse reaction or side effect (e.g., nausea and diarrhea). The other reason is related to the structural dissimilarity among the beta-lactam antibiotic classes.

Monobactams

Aztreonam (Azactam) is the only antimicrobial in this drug class. Aztreonam is only available parenterally and has a wide spectrum of activity against gram-negative organisms but little to none against gram-positive or anaerobic microorganisms. An advantage of this drug is that it is safe to use in patients who report serious allergies to other beta-lactams. Side effects may include injection site reactions, nausea, vomiting, and diarrhea.

Learning Hint
What Is in a Name?

As indicated in the class name, **monobactams** have one (mono-) beta-lactam ring.

monobactam [MAHN oh back tam]: a class of synthetic antibiotics with a cyclic beta-lactam nucleus; may be useful in patients with severe beta-lactam allergies

Carbapenems

Four **carbapenems** are currently available for use in the United States: imipenem-cilastatin (Primaxin), meropenem (Merrem), ertapenem (Invanz), and doripenem (Doribax). There are some differences within this group with respect to spectrum of activity and side effects. Ertapenem is not active against *Pseudomonas*, and imipenem-cilastatin may cause seizures in patients with kidney failure. They have pharmacological activity that is similar to other β-lactam antibiotics, and they are broad-spectrum and active against many organisms that are resistant to other classes of antibiotics. For this reason, they are usually reserved for serious infections. Side effects include nausea, which may be related to the infusion rate, seizures, dizziness, and confusion.

Now that we have finished our discussion of beta-lactam antibiotics, we can move on to other classes.

carbapenem [kahr buh PEN um]: a subtype of beta-lactam antibiotics, including imipenem and meropenem, which are effective against a wide range of bacteria

7-2
Stop and Review

1. What are some of the ways antibiotics may be classified?

2. What is meant by a broad-spectrum antibiotic? When might using a broad-spectrum antibiotic be important?

3. As you move from a first-generation cephalosporin to a third-, fourth-, or fifth-generation, how has the spectrum of activity changed?

Match the following:

4. Carbapenems   _____ ampicillin

5. Monobactams   _____ aztreonam

6. Cephalosporin   _____ doripenem

7. Penicillin   _____ ceftazidime

Quinolones

quinolone [KWIN oh lohns]: a class of broad-spectrum antibacterial drugs

Quinolones block two enzymes responsible for DNA growth, which causes breakage of the DNA, resulting in bactericidal activity. Human cells do not have this enzyme, so the drug is specific for microorganisms. This drug class has been available for years starting with nalidixic acid (no longer available), which was used for urinary tract infections caused by gram-negative pathogens. Fluoroquinolones have a much broader spectrum of activity, which makes them useful to treat infections caused by both gram-positive and gram-negative microbes.

The newer agents have a fluorine atom chemically attached to the quinolone structure and are called fluoroquinolones. This chemical change allows the antibiotic to penetrate the bacteria better than plain quinolones can. Fluoroquinolones are used primarily for lower respiratory tract infections.

There are many drug interactions with quinolones. These drugs should not be taken with antacids or minerals because they may interfere with quinolone absorption. Quinolones may increase theophylline (a medication occasionally used to help breathing in patients with asthma) levels resulting in toxic effects such as increased heart rate, nausea, and seizures. Quinolones, like many antibiotics, may cause enhanced sensitivity to sunlight (photosensitivity), so patients should use sunscreen when taking them. Prolonged use of quinolones may cause **superinfection**, which is the appearance of a new infection with a different strain or species of microorganism during antibiotic treatment. Usually the organism responsible for the superinfection is resistant to the antibiotic being given and may be more difficult to treat. Superinfections may appear several days after antibiotic initiation and require treatment with a different antibiotic or antifungal and discontinuation of the

superinfection: infection occurring after or on top of an earlier infection, especially following treatment with broad-spectrum antibiotics

current antibiotic. Superinfection can also occur with other anti-infective agents. Other quinolone side effects include nausea, dizziness, and an unpleasant taste. Common fluoroquinolones include:

- ciprofloxacin (Cipro)

- levofloxacin (Levaquin)

- moxifloxacin (Avelox)

- gatifloxacin (Tequin)

Clinical Application

Quinolones and Tendon Injury

Quinolones have been linked to tendon inflammation and rupture. This may occur even after the medication has been discontinued. Strenuous physical activity may be a risk factor for this rare side effect. If signs of tendon pain or inflammation occur, the prescriber should be notified immediately and the medication may need to be discontinued.

Aminoglycosides

Aminoglycosides are used in many serious infections for gram-negative coverage. They are often initially used with other antibiotics in very ill patients to ensure broad coverage against potentially drug-resistant organisms. They are bactericidal and dosed on the basis of weight, renal function, and serum blood levels. Because they may cause hearing loss and kidney failure, they are not used for infections that could be treated with other less toxic antibiotics. Sometimes they are used for short-term coverage in intensive-care patients on breathing machines for additive *Pseudomonas* coverage. Aminoglycosides may increase muscle weakness because of a potential blockage of signals at the neuromuscular junction. Sometimes they are given as aerosol treatments by inhaling them directly into the lungs. This method of administration would lower the concentration of the drug in the blood, thereby possibly preventing the serious side effects of hearing loss or kidney failure. Examples of aminoglycosides include:

aminoglycosides [a ME noh GLY koh sides]: a group of antibiotics used to treat certain bacterial infections primarily aerobic, gram-negative bacteria

- amikacin (Amikin)

- gentamicin (Garamycin)

- tobramycin (Nebcin)

Glycopeptides

glycopeptide [GLY koh PEP tide]: any of a class of peptides that contain carbohydrates, including those that contain amino sugars

Vancomycin (Vancocin) is a bactericidal **glycopeptide** antibiotic. It binds to a portion of the cell walls of reproducing microorganisms and prevents cell wall development. The cell dies because the cell wall cannot grow. Vancomycin is indicated for infections caused by gram-positive cocci. It is frequently reserved for methicillin-resistant *Staphylococcus aureus* (MRSA) or *Staphylococcus epidermidis*. Hospitals closely monitor their vancomycin sensitivity patterns because there are few alternatives should resistance become prevalent. Vancomycin can cause side effects with intravenous administration such as low blood pressure and, rarely, kidney failure and hearing loss. Rapid infusion can cause a histamine release and flushed skin, or what is called red man syndrome (seriously). Vancomycin may be monitored by serum drug levels, which can be helpful in adjusting doses, especially for serious infections because of MRSA (Figure 7-4).

Telavancin (Vibativ) is a relatively new glycopeptide antibiotic that inhibits cell wall synthesis and causes a disruption in cell membrane permeability. This antibiotic is a welcome addition because of its activity against *Staphylococcus aureus* isolates that are resistant to not only methicillin but to vancomycin as well. It has a long duration of action so it may be given once daily. Adverse effects include nausea, insomnia, and taste disturbance. This antibiotic should only be considered in patients with documented resistance or clinical failure to other antibiotics.

Macrolides

macrolide: a class of antibiotics discovered in *Streptomyces*, characterized by molecules made up of large-ring lactones

Macrolides inhibit bacterial protein synthesis and, as their name implies, have a large or "macro" ring as their basic structure. They are commonly

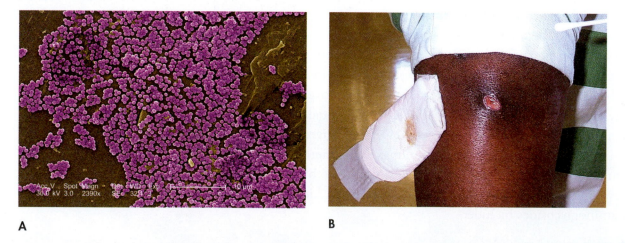

A   **B**

FIGURE 7-4 A. Colorized scanning electron micrograph (SEM) of MRSA. Source: CDC/Jeff Hageman, M.H.S. Photo credit: Janice Haney Carr. **B.** Cutaneous abscess of knee caused by MRSA. Source: CDC/Bruno Coignard, M.D.; Jeff Hageman, M.H.S.

used to treat pulmonary infections because of their spectrum of activity, which includes many common respiratory organisms such as *Streptococcus pneumoniae,* Legionella, Chlamydophila, and *Moraxella catarrhalis.* In addition, they are used for skin soft tissue infections. Erythromycin was the first macrolide available in this class and may be bactericidal or bacteriostatic, depending on the organism's susceptibility and the drug concentration. Erythromycin may cause stomach distress and diarrhea and has been largely replaced by the newer macrolides clarithromycin and azithromycin, which are better absorbed in the stomach and cause less gastrointestinal upset. Because macrolides have been commonly prescribed for respiratory infections, resistance to this class of antibiotics has been increasing. The newest member of this class, telithromycin, is reserved for more serious infections because it may cause injury to the liver. Common macrolides include:

- erythromycin (E-Mycin)

- clarithromycin (Biaxin)

- azithromycin (Zithromax)

- telithromycin (Ketek)

Tetracyclines

The **tetracyclines** have been available for approximately 50 years and have a relatively broad spectrum of activity, including activity against gram-positive and gram-negative aerobic and anaerobic bacteria as well as Mycoplasma, some mycobacteria, Chlamydia, and spirochetes. They are produced by soil organisms and are bacteriostatic. Uses include treatment for acne, Rocky Mountain spotted fever, Lyme disease, and as part of a combination treatment regimen for peptic ulcer disease caused by *Helicobacter pylori.*

tetracycline [TET ruh SIGH kleens]: a class of broad-spectrum bacteriostatic antibiotics

Tetracycline cannot be taken with antacids, minerals, or dairy products because they will bind with each other and not be absorbed. Pregnant women and children under the age of 9 years should not take tetracycline because permanent tooth discoloration could result. Tigecycline (Tygacil) is a new parenteral derivative of minocycline. Common tetracyclines include:

- doxycycline (Vibramycin)

- minocycline (Minocin)

- tigecycline (Tygacil)

Clinical Application

Saving Medication Can Be Dangerous

Many people save antibiotics left over from a previous infection for another time. Most drugs simply lose effectiveness when they become out of date; tetracycline, however, can cause kidney failure if it is used after its expiration date.

7-3
Stop and Review

1. Would you rather be treated with a bacteriostatic or a bactericidal antibiotic? Why?

2. What is the mechanism of action of beta-lactams compared with fluoroquinolones? Macrolides?

Match the following:

3. Tetracyclines _____ clarithromycin

4. Macrolides _____ vancomycin

5. Glycopeptides _____ tobramycin

6. Aminoglycosides _____ minocycline

Folate Inhibitors

folate inhibitor: agent that inhibits folic acid synthesis

Sulfonamides are classic examples of **folate inhibitors** and are considered bacteriostatic. They block a step in the synthesis of folic acid resulting in the inhibition of the susceptible microorganisms. The most common side effects are rash, drug fever, and low blood cell counts. Their main use is in the treatment of urinary tract infections. Sulfonamides are frequently used in combination with trimethoprim, another folate inhibitor, to treat urinary tract infections, infectious diarrhea, and for *Pneumocystis jiroveci* pneumonia in AIDS patients which is discussed more in Chapter 9. Common sulfonamides include:

• sulfamethoxazole/trimethoprim (Bactrim, Septra)

• sulfadiazine

Oxazolidinones

oxazolidinones [ock SAY zoh LYE di nohns]: heterocyclic organic compound containing both nitrogen and oxygen in a 5-membered ring; antibiotic used against gram-positive pathogens

Linezolid (Zyvox) is the only **oxazolidinone** available at present in the United States. The oxazolidinones are antibiotics with a novel mechanism

> ### Clinical Application
> #### Importance of Hydration
> Patients taking sulfonamide antibiotics should drink plenty of fluids daily to prevent the drug from depositing as crystals in the urine or kidneys.

of action of inhibiting bacterial protein synthesis. Linezolid is bacteriostatic against enterococci and staphylococci and bactericidal against streptococci. It is available orally and as an IV for treatment of vancomycin-resistant *Enterococcus faecium* infections, community-acquired pneumonia, health care–associated pneumonia (MRSA), and skin and soft tissue infections. Complete blood counts should be monitored weekly in patients on linezolid because bone marrow suppression (anemia, leukopenia, pancytopenia, and thrombocytopenia) has been reported, especially in patients on prolonged therapy.

Quinupristin-Dalfopristin

Quinupristin-dalfopristin (Synercid) is an intravenous product composed of two drugs from the chemical class called streptogramins. Both drugs work together to inhibit bacterial protein synthesis and are bacteriostatic against gram-positive bacteria. They may be bactericidal against staphylococci, including the methicillin-resistant strains, and have been used to treat MRSA infections that have failed to respond to vancomycin. Muscle aches, joint pains, and infusion site reactions are commonly reported side effects. They may have a role in infections associated with vancomycin-resistant *Enterococcus*.

quinupristin-dalfopristin [kwin YOU pris tin dal FOE pris tin]: a combination of two antibiotics used to treat infections by staphylococci and by vancomycin-resistant *Enterococcus faecium*

Daptomycin

Daptomycin (Cubicin) is a lipopeptide bactericidal antibiotic that works by interfering with the electrical activity of the cell membrane. It is active against gram-positive organisms such as MRSA and VRE. It is useful to treat MRSA bloodstream infections, especially after the occurrence of vancomycin failure or side effects. It cannot be used to treat pneumonias because its activity is inhibited by pulmonary surfactant. This drug may cause diarrhea, vomiting, leg and arm pain, and a release of muscle enzymes into the bloodstream. Rarely, this rise of muscle enzymes may be severe and result in kidney failure, so close clinical monitoring for these conditions is warranted.

daptomycin [DAP toe MY sin]: a miscellaneous anti-infective used to treat complicated skin and skin structure infections caused by *Staphylococcus aureus*, *S. agalactiae*, *S. dysgalactiae*, and *Enterococcus faecalis*

Clindamycin

clindamycin [KLIN duh MY sin]: a semisynthetic derivative of lincomycin used systemically, topically, and vaginally as an antibacterial, primarily against gram-positive bacteria

Clindamycin is available in oral, topical, and intravenous formulations. Its spectrum of activity includes gram-positive cocci and anaerobes with the exception of bacteroides because most species are resistant. As you will see in upcoming chapters, it is used in the treatment of aspiration pneumonia, skin soft tissue infections, osteomyelitis, serious infections of the female pelvis caused by susceptible bacteria, and for *Pneumocystis jiroveci* pneumonia associated with HIV. Clindamycin may work to treat community acquired MRSA infections depending on local susceptibility patterns. Side effects of clindamycin that frequently occur can include nausea, vomiting, diarrhea, and *Clostridium difficile* colitis (drug should be stopped if this condition occurs).

Metronidazole

metronidazole [MET roh NYE duh zole]: an antiprotozoal and antibacterial effective against obligate anaerobes; used as the base or the hydrochloride salt and also used as a topical treatment for rosacea

Metronidazole (Flagyl) is a synthetic drug with an anaerobic spectrum of activity (e.g., *Clostridium difficile*). It inhibits bacterial protein synthesis, resulting in cell death. It is part of a cocktail of drugs used to treat peptic ulcer disease caused by *Helicobacter pylori*. Side effects include a metallic taste, diarrhea, nausea, and intolerance to alcohol. Patients on metronidazole should not drink alcohol for up to 3 days after discontinuing the drug to prevent adverse effects of nausea and flushing that may result from the combination.

Antituberculosis Agents

antitubercular drug [AN tee too BER kyu ler]: any agent or group of drugs used to treat tuberculosis; at least two drugs, and usually three, are required in various combinations in pulmonary tuberculosis therapy

multidrug-resistant (MDR) TB: a lack of expected therapeutic response in tuberculosis patients to several disease-specific pharmaceutical agents, especially antibiotics

Tuberculosis (TB) is a disease that is usually confined to the lungs, but it can also affect the kidney, spine, and brain (Figure 7-5). The disease is spread through the air from one person to another by inhaling the bacteria that cause TB when a person who is infected coughs, sneezes, or speaks. TB can be symptomatic or asymptomatic (latent TB), but it is a chronic disease requiring months of treatment with the appropriate antibiotics. Even though the person with latent TB is not ill and cannot spread the disease, treatment is recommended for these individuals to prevent them from developing disease later in life or if they become ill. TB is treated with a combination of **antitubercular drugs** for 6 to 9 months.

Multidrug-resistant (MDR) TB can occur because of suboptimal treatment of tuberculosis. At diagnosis, most TB is susceptible to the chosen drugs, but because of the long duration of treatment needed, inappropriate drug doses, and noncompliance with drugs, MDR TB often develops. This is a major public health problem because there are currently few new drugs for TB in clinical research trials.

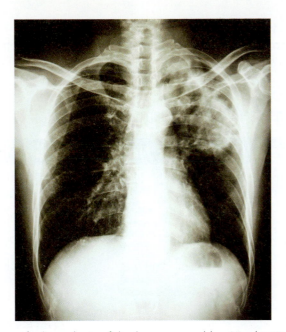

FIGURE 7-5 X-ray of tuberculosis of the lungs caused by *Myobacterium tuberculosis*. TB is transmitted by aerosol droplet when coughing and sneezing.
© Puwadol Jaturawutthichai/www.Shutterstock.com.

 Clinical Application

Red Tears and Sweat

Rifampin, used to treat TB, can cause urine, feces, saliva or sputum, sweat, and tears to be colored red-orange. Patients should be warned to expect this and should be cautioned about staining soft contact lenses. If you see someone with orange perspiration you may not be imagining it. It could be someone taking rifampin.

TB treatment consists of a combination of drugs categorized as first-line drugs. Second-line drugs are reserved for MDR TB or drug intolerance. Second-line drugs are secondary because they are either more toxic or have limited clinical experience in TB treatment. Table 7-6 presents a list of drugs used to treat TB.

Isoniazid can cause liver injury, which is enhanced when alcohol is used concurrently, so patients should avoid alcohol. Patients frequently complain of a numbness or tingling sensation in their hands and feet with isoniazid or ethionamide. Pyridoxine (vitamin B_6) supplementation may be recommended to try to prevent this adverse reaction. Ethambutol may cause visual problems such as color blindness and decreased visual acuity, so routine eye exams and prescriber notification of changes in vision are important information to provide patients. Bedaquiline is a relatively new drug approved for treatment of MDR TB and is used with at least three other drugs that have activity against the MDR TB isolate.

TABLE 7-6 Drugs Used to Treat Tuberculosis

Type of Drug	Generic Name	Brand Name
Primary	isoniazid	INH
	rifampin	Rimactane
	pyrazinamide	Tebrazid
	ethambutol	Myambutol
	rifabutin	Mycobutin
Secondary	streptomycin	Streptomycin
	cycloserine	Seromycin
	ethionamide	Trecator
	bedaquiline	Sirturo

© 2016 Cengage Learning®.

Food for Thought
Life-Span Considerations

Young and old patients alike should keep up-to-date lists of true medication allergies. If a patient states that he or she is allergic to a particular antibiotic, for example, asking a few additional questions may help clarify the reaction as an adverse effect or intolerability rather than a true allergy. Hives, hypotension, and difficulty breathing should be taken seriously. Patient reports of nausea, vomiting, and diarrhea are adverse reactions and not true allergies.

Antivirals

Viruses are the most common infectious agents in humans. A virus can only replicate in a living host cell because it lacks the necessary structures and energy stores to replicate on its own. This makes it difficult to kill the virus without harming the host cell. Because this is a different situation than with bacteria, different drugs are needed to treat viruses than bacteria. Viruses contain DNA and RNA molecules, so they are classified by whether they contain RNA or DNA. RNA viruses cause diseases such as influenza, polio, HIV, rabies, and encephalitis. DNA viruses cause adenovirus respiratory disease, papilloma warts, herpes simplex, and Epstein-Barr mononucleosis (Figure 7-6).

Prevention of viral infections by vaccination, rather than treatment when they occur, has been an effective strategy for many viral infections such as influenza, measles, mumps, polio, and rubella. Only recently have more antiviral drugs become available for diseases such as HIV and hepatitis C. Viral infections may be classified by their severity, length of time present,

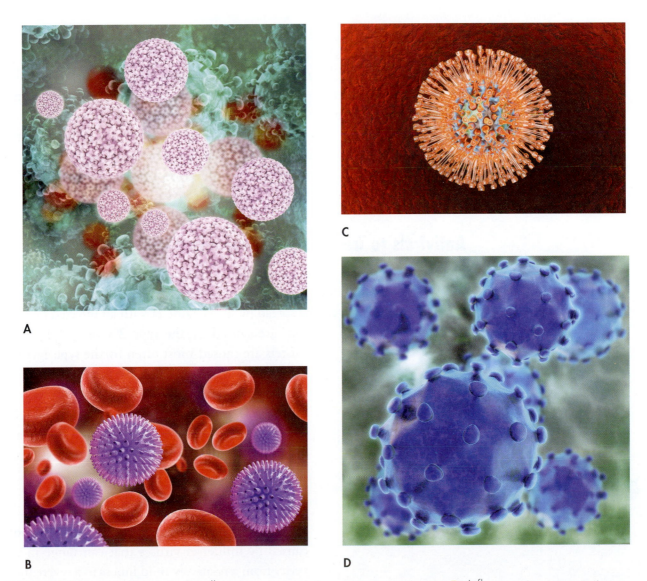

A

B

C

D

FIGURE 7-6 Various viruses. **A.** Papillomavirus or wart virus. © iStockphoto/xrender. **B.** Influenza virus type; notice the spikes on the virus that can attach to host cells. © dream designs/www.Shutterstock.com. **C.** Herpes simplex viruses. © Spectral-Design/www.Shutterstock.com. **D.** Hepatitis C virus. © iStockphoto/xrender.

Clinical Application
Killing the Virus but Not the Host

After the initial infection with HIV (which resembles many acute viral illnesses causing fever, rash, sore throat, and swollen lymph nodes), the virus takes up residence in CD4 lymphocytes during which time it can be in the cell, latent and undetectable, and surface long after the initial transmission. The role of antivirals is to search for and destroy the virus in its host cell while not interfering with the normal function of that host cell.

and body parts affected. Infections such as the common cold and influenza can be acute and resolve quickly, or they can be slow and have a progressive course, as with HIV. Viral infections can be local and affect just the lungs, for example, or generalized and spread throughout the bloodstream. Some viruses can be dormant and then, under certain conditions, reproduce again. This is called *latency* and implies that a disease may surface years after transmission or after the initial breakout. An example of this would be a person who had chickenpox as a child and then develops shingles as he or she ages. Both diseases are caused by the herpes zoster virus.

Antivirals to Treat Herpes Virus Infections

Herpes simplex virus (HSV) is a DNA virus that can cause the skin blisters most people know as fever blisters or cold sores (Figure 7-7). It can also cause genital herpes, which can be spread by sexual contact with an infected person. Most genital HSV infections are caused by the type 2 virus, while fever blisters are caused most often by the type 1 virus. The main drugs to treat herpes are acyclovir (Zovirax), famciclovir (Famvir), and valacyclovir (Valtrex). These drugs interfere with viral DNA synthesis and inhibit viral replication. They are also used to treat shingles caused by herpes zoster.

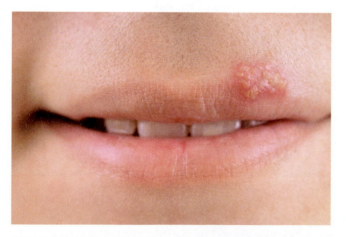

FIGURE 7-7 Example of herpes infection. © Levent Konuk/ www.Shutterstock.com.

Antivirals to Treat Influenza Virus

Influenza or *the flu* is a common viral infection caused by influenza viruses that can range in severity from a relatively mild illness to a severe lung infection and death. There are three types of influenza (A, B, and C). Serious illness because of influenza is caused by either type A or B, while type

C may cause a mild respiratory illness but does not cause pandemics. Certain patients are at higher risk for complications from influenza, including the elderly, diabetics, and patients with heart, kidney, and lung problems. Influenza agents include amantadine (Symmetrel), rimantadine (Flumadine), zanamivir (Relenza), and oseltamivir (Tamiflu). Amantadine and rimantadine have been available for years. They are effective against influenza A virus, but their use may be limited, especially in elderly adults, by their side effects involving the brain, such as confusion, hallucinations, and agitation.

Zanamivir and oseltamivir have been marketed as drugs to cut the duration of mild flu by at least 1 day and maybe 3 days, but they may decrease the risk of death in patients who require hospitalization. These two drugs are called neuraminidase inhibitors. They are indicated for treatment of both influenza A and influenza B. Zanamivir is available as an inhaled medication delivered by a breath-activated *diskhaler*. It has been associated with adverse respiratory effects such as cough and nasal congestion, especially in patients with asthma or lung disease from smoking. These agents are most effective in treating or preventing influenza if started within 30 hours of symptoms or exposure, respectively.

Antivirals to Treat Respiratory Syncytial Virus

Respiratory syncytial virus (RSV) is a pathogen that causes inflammation of lung tissues and pneumonia and is a major cause of lung disease in children. Ribavirin is an antiviral with inhibitory activity against both RNA and DNA

respiratory syncytial virus (RSV)
[sin SISH ul]: virus that causes infection of the lungs and breathing passages

viruses (e.g., RSV, influenzas A and B, and herpes simplex). Although its mechanism of action is not fully known, it may inhibit nucleic acid formation in viral particles. Severe cases of RSV are treated with inhaled ribavirin (Virazole). Ribavirin is administered through a device that generates small particles capable of penetrating the small airways of the lung when inhaled. It is administered for 12 to 18 hours daily for 3 to 7 days. Because ribavirin can escape into the air around the patient, visitors and staff may be exposed to the drug; because of its potential to cause birth defects, this is a concern. It should not be mixed with any other aerosol medications.

7-4
Stop and Review

1. Why are viruses more difficult to eradicate from the human body?
2. How are viruses classified?

Match the following drug and disease.
3. Herpes simplex   _____ metronidazole
4. Tuberculosis   _____ oseltamivir
5. Influenza   _____ acyclovir
6. *Clostridium difficle* _____ rifampin

Antivirals to Treat Hepatitis C Virus

New breakthroughs in antiviral treatment for hepatitis C virus (HCV) infection deserve special mention in this chapter because HCV is the most common bloodborne infection in the United States. It is estimated that 3.2 million people are chronically infected with HCV. There are six unique genotypes of HCV (1–6), and they respond to treatment differently. Therefore, it is important to obtain the viral HCV genotype that an infected patient carries because it is predictive of response to treatment and how long the infection must be treated. HCV, like HIV, is treated with a combination of drugs. Unlike HIV infection, HCV is a potentially curable viral infection.

Telaprevir and boceprevir are two new antivirals approved for use in patients with chronic hepatitis C infection. They are both classified as first-generation protease inhibitors, and they inhibit viral replication. Unfortunately, each of these agents requires the patient to consume multiple pills two to three times daily. Anemia is a common adverse effect for both of these new medications, while rashes, some of which may be serious, are more common with telaprevir.

The introduction of a second-generation protease inhibitor was a significant improvement over its first-generation relatives. Simeprevir offers improved dosing schedules, a lower number of pills that must be taken by the patient for each dose, and less severe adverse reactions. Photosensitivity (patients should use sunscreen and limit sun exposure) and rash were the most commonly reported adverse effects. Sofosbuvir is a recently approved nucleoside polymerase inhibitor that is used in combination with other drug therapies to treat different genotypes of hepatitis C. It is taken once daily and has a very favorable adverse effect profile with fatigue, nausea, headache, and vomiting being the most common.

Peginterferon and ribavirin have been mainstays of treatment for years but are associated with numerous side effects such as fatigue, depression, flu-like illness, and bone marrow suppression. Peginterferon is given as a subcutaneous injection once weekly. Peginterferon works to inhibit viral reproduction through a variety of complicated pathways. Ribavirin inhibits viral protein synthesis, which results in a slowing of viral replication. Table 7-7 lists common antivirals used to treat HSV, hepatitis, influenza, and RSV.

TABLE 7-7 Common Antivirals

Disease	Generic Name	Brand Name
Herpes (HSV)	acyclovir	Zovirax
	famciclovir	Famvir
	valacyclovir	Valtrex
Influenza	zanamivir (inhaled)	Relenza
	oseltamivir	Tamiflu
	amantadine	Symmetrel
	rimantadine	Flumadine
RSV	ribavirin	Virazole
Hepatitis C	ribavirin	Copegus, Rebetol
	peginterferon alfa-2a	Pegasys
	boceprevir	Victrelis
	telaprevir	Incivek
	simeprevir	Olysio
	sofosbuvir	Sovaldi

Clinical Application

From Annoying to Life Threatening

Fungal infections may range from annoying cosmetic problems such as toenail infections to life-threatening infections such as invasive aspergillosis in a bone marrow transplant recipient.

Antivirals to Treat Human Immunodeficiency Virus (HIV) Infection

Human immunodeficiency virus (HIV) infection that is left untreated progresses eventually in most infected individuals to AIDS, which is a fatal disease caused by the retrovirus HIV. Treatment of HIV includes several different drugs to suppress the virus. These drugs are termed *antiretrovirals*. The virus is difficult to treat because it infects cells of our immune system. There are several drug classes used to treat HIV infection with names that are difficult to pronounce and remember. Medication classes include nucleoside reverse transcriptase inhibitors (NRTIs), non-nucleoside reverse transcriptase inhibitors (NNRTIs), protease inhibitors (PIs), integrase strand transfer inhibitor, fusion inhibitor, and CCR5 antagonists (Table 7-8). In addition, several HIV vaccines are undergoing clinical testing. As mentioned before, the HIV virus infects CD4 cells taking over the cellular machinery and eventually resulting in the death of these important immune-fighting cells. This destruction of the infected patient's immune system causes the patient to be susceptible to a wide range of pathogens that do not cause disease when immunity is normal. These can include widespread herpes simplex virus infections, cytomegalovirus (CMV), Kaposi sarcoma, and commonly *Pneumocystis jiroveci,* which can lead to severe pneumonia in AIDS patients. In 1981 the CDC reported a cluster of unusual pneumonias occurring in homosexual men in the San Francisco Bay area. These pneumonias were caused by *Pneumocystis jiroveci.* The men were susceptible to infections with this organism because their immune systems were severely weakened by HIV infection.

Antifungal Agents

Fungi are one-cell or multicellular organisms consisting of two basic forms that may cause disease in humans: yeasts and molds. Fungi reproduce by spores, have a rigid cell wall, and contain no chlorophyll. Fungi have

TABLE 7-8 Common Antiretrovirals*

Type of Antiretroviral	Generic Name	Brand Name
Nucleoside reverse transcriptase inhibitors (NRTIs)	abacavir	Ziagen
	didanosine (ddI)	Videx
	lamivudine (3TC)	Epivir
	zidovudine (AZT)	Retrovir
	tenofovir	Truvada
Non-nucleoside reverse transcriptase inhibitors (NNRTIs)	efavirenz	Sustiva
	nevirapine	Viramune
	etravirine	Intelence
Protease inhibitors	indinavir	Crixivan
	ritonavir	Norvir
	atazanavir	Reyataz

*For a more complete listing, visit www.aidsinfo.gov.

© 2016 Cengage Learning®.

ergosterol in their cell walls instead of cholesterol, which is found in human cells. Some antifungals work by preventing the production of ergosterol, which is a building block for the cell membranes. Serious fungal infections are most likely to develop in patients with impaired immune systems, but if you have ever had athlete's foot, you had a fungal infection. In addition, taking antibiotics for bacterial infections may knock out our normal bacterial flora and allow fungi to take over because they would not be killed by the antibiotic. This is another good reason to make sure we use antibiotics appropriately.

Some examples of fungal infections include ringworm, athlete's foot, and jock itch, all of which can be treated with topical antifungal creams. More serious fungal infections include histoplasmosis within the lung and *Candida albicans* (thrush) in the mouth. These can progress to whole body infections. Figure 7-8 illustrates oral candidiasis (thrush) and some other fungal diseases.

Nystatin (Mycostatin) is an antifungal medication that is available as an oral suspension and topical cream; it is used to treat *Candida albicans* and skin fungal infections. Another class of antifungal drugs is the

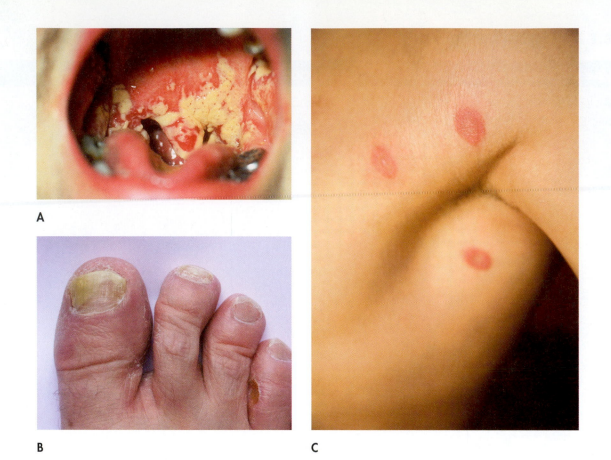

FIGURE 7-8 Photos of fungal diseases. **A.** Oral thrush (*candida albicans*). Source: CDC. **B.** Athlete's foot (tinea pedis). © David Reilly/www.Shutterstock.com. **C.** Fungal infection (ringworm/tinea corporis). © iStockphoto/alejandrophotography.

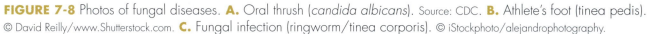

echinocandins [ee KYE noh KAN dins]: antifungal drugs that inhibit the synthesis of glucan in the cell wall

azoles. This class includes miconazole (Monistat), which is used as a topical treatment for superficial or vaginal yeast infections, and fluconazole (Diflucan) or voriconazole (VFEND), which can be administered IV or orally for whole body fungal infections. The next class of whole body antifungal agents are the **echinocandins**, including caspofungin (Cancidas), anidulafungin (Eraxis), and micafungin (Mycamine). The echinocandins are generally reserved for *Candida* species that are resistant to fluconazole.

Amphotericin B deoxycholate (Fungizone) was used intravenously for decades as the standard drug treatment for serious *Candida* infections. When amphotericin B is given intravenously, it requires close clinical monitoring because of common side effects. Toxicity from amphotericin B may include electrolyte abnormalities and injury to the kidneys. Taking the parent compound and manufacturing it with lipid has reduced the toxic effects on the kidneys, but these products are significantly more expensive. Table 7-9 lists some common antifungal agents.

TABLE 7-9 Common Antifungals

Generic Name	Brand Name	Route
Nystatin	Mycostatin	Topical for skin candidiasis or oral thrush
Miconazole	Monistat	Topical preparations for cutaneous yeast or vaginitis infections
Amphotericin B	Fungizone	IV
Liposomal amphotericin B	Ambisome	IV
Fluconazole	Diflucan	PO and IV
Voriconazole	VFEND	PO and IV
Ketoconazole	Nizoral	Local scalp shampoo or PO
Caspofungin	Cancidas	IV
Anidulafungin	Eraxis	IV
Micafungin	Mycamine	IV

© 2016 Cengage Learning®.

Chapter Summary

- The goal of this chapter was to familiarize the reader with disease terminology and concepts, immunizations, and a representative sampling of antimicrobials.

- We began with a discussion of immunizations because, after all, it is better to prevent infections than it is to treat them.

- Before launching into the specific antimicrobials, we began by discussing ways antibiotics may be classified.

- Then we began our discussion of antimicrobials by discussing antibiotics, organizing each section when possible by grouping the medicines into a therapeutic class based on chemical structures.

- Next, antivirals and antifungals were discussed.

- This chapter will serve as an important foundation as the reader moves on to learn about infectious diseases using a systems approach.

- We need to again emphasize the importance of using antimicrobials appropriately in an attempt to slow the development of resistance to these miracle drugs. In the next two chapters, we will use the knowledge gained from this chapter as we discuss common infections and their treatment.

Case Study

Mrs. Smith is a 34-year-old, otherwise healthy woman who developed a temperature of 104°F with teeth chattering chills and shortness of breath. She was transported to the emergency room by ambulance. Upon arrival, the emergency room physician decided to place her on a breathing machine, administer several liters of intravenous fluids, and use strong medicines to raise her falling blood pressure. Antibiotics were started right after blood cultures were obtained. Do you think the emergency room physician started broad- or narrow-spectrum antibiotics and why?

Chapter Review

Match the term with its description.

1. _____ immunoglobulins
2. _____ clindamycin
3. _____ doripenem
4. _____ bacteriostatic
5. _____ vancomycin
6. _____ superinfection
7. _____ tigecycline
8. _____ tobramycin
9. _____ caspofungin
10. _____ ceftriaxone

a. carbapenem
b. infection resulting from antibiotic use
c. tetracycline
d. echinocandin
e. cephalosporin
f. agent used for passive immunity
g. glycopeptide
h. may have activity against MRSA
i. aminoglycoside
j. inhibits but does not kill bacteria

Define the following.

11. Active immunity _____

12. Passive immunity _____

13. Bacteriostatic _____

Fill in the blanks.

14. _____ may be treated with boceprevir.

15. Passive immunity may be given to a patient infected with rabies by giving _____ .

16. _____ antibiotics result in the death of the microorganism.

17. The most common bloodborne viral pathogen is _____.

18. Vaccines are used to provide patients with _____ against pathogenic microbes.

Additional Activities

1. Research the appropriate immunizations for an infant, teenager, and adult using www.cdc.gov/vaccines. What are some of the diseases that are reemerging as infectious disease threats because of a lack of vaccination or decreasing immunity? List the pros and cons of vaccinations.

2. Research the use of antibiotics to support the production of food in this country. What evidence exists to support this use as a mechanism of increasing antibiotic resistance?

3. Develop a vaccination report card for yourself. Are you up-to-date? Discuss ways to track your vaccinations. (Hint: Consider Web-based tools.)

4. Research new antibiotics under development. (Hint: Visit www.clinicaltrials.gov and search the Web site using various terms such as antibiotics, antivirals, etc.) List your findings and how these findings may affect the treatment of infectious diseases in the future.

Media Connection

Go to the accompanying online resources and have fun learning as you play games, view animations and videos, and take practice tests to help reinforce key concepts you learned in this chapter.

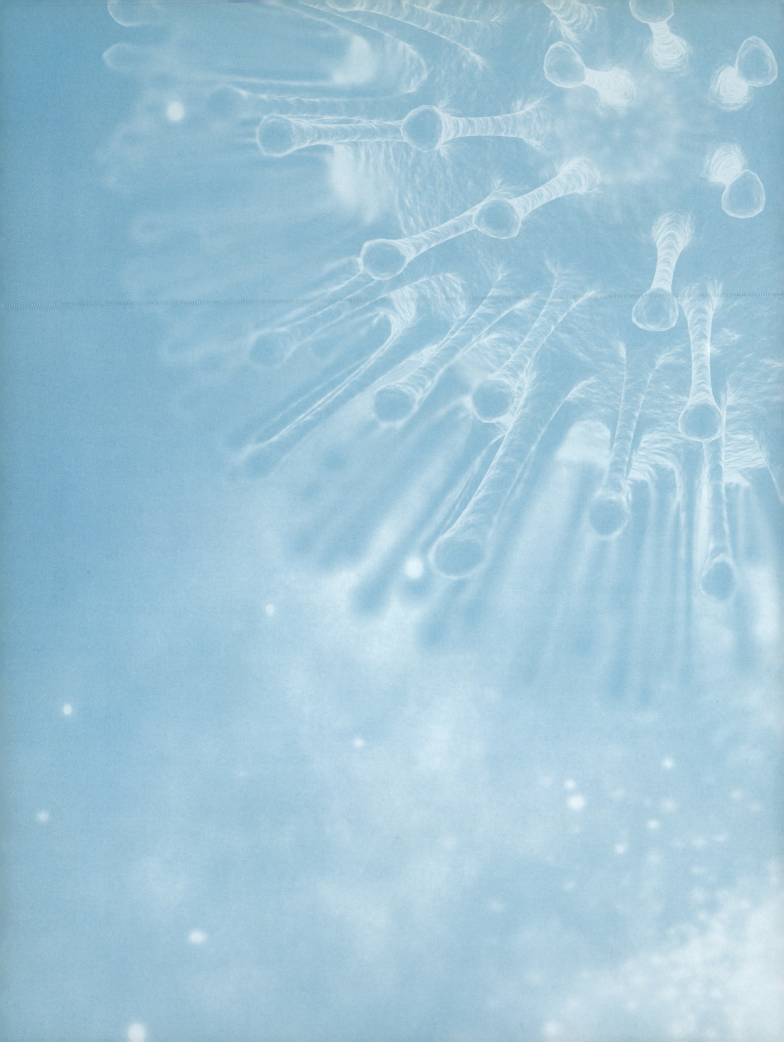

CHAPTER 8

Microbiological Diseases: Nonrespiratory Infectious Diseases

OBJECTIVES

After studying this chapter, the learner will be able to:

- Describe the symptoms, the types of organisms, and treatment for infectious diseases of the head and neck to include meningitis, encephalitis, otitis media, and parotitis.

- Given a particular infection, list the possible antimicrobial treatments for a patient with that infection.

- List the viral causes of encephalitis.

- Discuss when a clinician should initially avoid antimicrobials for a child with acute otitis media.

- Describe the symptoms, the types of organisms, and treatment for infectious diseases of the eye to include conjunctivitis and keratitis.

- Discuss differences in the clinical presentation of viral versus bacterial conjunctivitis.

- Describe the symptoms, the types of organisms, and treatment for infectious diseases of the cardiovascular system to include endocarditis and catheter-related bloodstream infections (CRBSIs).

- Describe the symptoms, the types of organisms, and treatment for infectious diseases of the skin and soft tissue.

- Compare and contrast erysipelas with cellulitis.

- Describe the symptoms, the types of organisms, and treatment for intra-abdominal infectious diseases to include appendicitis, acute cholecystitis, diverticulitis, *Clostridium difficile* colitis, and infectious diarrhea.

- Discuss measures to prevent or limit the spread of *Clostridium difficile*.

- List high-risk foods associated with infectious diarrhea.

- List common sexually transmitted infectious diseases and their treatment.

- Describe the symptoms, the types of organisms, and treatment for urinary tract infections.

- Discuss bone and joint infections to include osteomyelitis and septic arthritis.

KEY TERMS

acute cholecystitis
  [KOH luh sis TYE tis]

appendicitis

catheter-related bloodstream infections (CRBSIs)

cellulitis

Chlamydia [klah MID ee ah]

Clostridium difficile
  [klos TRID ee um
  dif us SEEL]

conjunctivitis

cystitis

diverticulitis
  [DYE ver tick you LYE tis]

encephalitis [EN sef ah LYE tis]

endocarditis
  [EN doh kar DYE tis]

erysipelas [ER i SIP eh les]

genitourinary tract infections

gonorrhea

herpes simplex viruses

infectious diarrhea

keratitis [KER ah TYE tis]

meningitis [MEN in JIGH tis]

necrotizing fasciitis
  [NECK roh TIZE ing
  FAS ee EYE tis]

necrotizing skin and soft tissue infections

osteomyelitis
  [OSS tee oh MY eh LYE tis]

otitis media

parotitis [PAH roh TYE tis]

pyelonephritis
  [PYE eh loh neh FRY tis]

septic arthritis

sexually transmitted diseases (STDs)

Introduction

Chapter 7 laid the foundation of antimicrobial therapy. In Chapters 8 and 9, we use a systems approach to discuss and learn about specific infectious diseases and their treatment. For each body system, we describe the common complaints a patient with the disease may have, laboratory results focusing on material we have previously discussed, and finally, briefly discuss initial treatment. Because this is quite a bit of material to cover, we have divided the topics into two chapters to facilitate learning. We start with the head and work our way down through the various parts of the body that may succumb to an infection. In this chapter we bypass the respiratory system infectious diseases. In Chapter 9, we focus on the respiratory system because it is prone to a host of infections.

Infectious Diseases of the Head and Neck

In this section we will discuss infections of the brain, ears, parotid gland, and eyes.

Meningitis

Meningitis is by definition an inflammation of the meninges—membranes surrounding brain tissue. It may affect people who are otherwise healthy as well as patients who are hospitalized. Patients who are hospitalized usually develop meningitis related to either surgery they have had on the brain (e.g., evacuation of a blood clot after a stroke or a ventriculoperitoneal shunt to drain excess fluid from the brain) or from a traumatic brain injury requiring some form of brain-monitoring equipment (e.g., a catheter inserted into a ventricle inside the brain to monitor brain pressure called a ventriculostomy).

Patients with bacterial meningitis are usually very sick, often seeking medical attention within a day of becoming ill. Not only is meningitis responsible for a large number of deaths worldwide, but survivors may often have disabilities such as hearing loss or some other abnormal neurological finding. Common symptoms of bacterial meningitis include:

- fever

- neck stiffness (nuchal rigidity)

- decline in mental status

- headache

Blood cultures and a lumbar puncture for cerebrospinal fluid (CSF) should be obtained as soon as possible. A Gram stain and culture of the CSF is useful to differentiate bacterial from viral meningitis. Antibiotics should be administered as soon as the diagnosis of bacterial meningitis is suspected. The common pathogens and their antimicrobial treatment may be found in Tables 8-1 and 8-2.

Meningitis caused by *Neisseria meningitides* may be spread to other persons via respiratory droplets. Individuals who have prolonged close contact or direct exposure to respiratory fluids are most at risk. Prophylaxis with

meningitis [MEN in JIGH tis]: a serious inflammation of the meninges, the thin, membranous covering of the brain and the spinal cord, most commonly caused by infection (by bacteria, viruses, or fungi), although it can also be caused by bleeding into the meninges, cancer, diseases of the immune system, and an inflammatory response to certain types of chemotherapy or other chemical agents

TABLE 8-1 Common Causes of Community-Acquired Bacterial Meningitis

Common Organisms	Gram Stain Result	Initial Treatment
Streptococcus pneumoniae	Gm + diplococci	Vancomycin + ceftriaxone ± ampicillin in patients >50 years of age
Neisseria meningiditis	Gm − diplococci	
Group B *Streptococcus*	Gm + cocci	
Haemophilus influenzae	Gm − coccobacilli	
Listeria monocytogenes	Gm + bacillus	

© 2016 Cengage Learning®.

TABLE 8-2 Common Causes of Health Care–Associated Meningitis

Common Organisms	Gram Stain Results	Initial Treatment
Enterobacteriaceae (e.g., *E. coli, K. pneumoniae, P. mirabilis,* etc.)	Gm – bacilli	Vancomycin + cefepime or ceftazidime
Pseudomonas aeruginosa	Gm – bacilli	*or*
Staphylococcus aureus	Gm + cocci	Vancomycin + meropenem

© 2016 Cengage Learning®.

either rifampin or ciprofloxacin is indicated for persons exposed to a patient who has meningitis because of this organism. A vaccine to prevent meningococcal meningitis is available and is indicated for immunocompromised adults, adults with increased risk of exposure, and college students.

Encephalitis

Viruses may also cause **encephalitis**. Encephalitis is inflammation of the brain tissue, specifically the white and gray matter. With meningitis, the patient may feel tired and have a headache. Patients with encephalitis on the other hand have those symptoms and abnormal brain function such as memory deficits, seizures, paralysis, and abnormal movements. A wide variety of viruses may infect the brain. Table 8-3 lists viruses that may cause infections in the brain.

A lumbar puncture is usually performed to obtain CSF for testing. When a clinician suspects a viral cause for the brain infection, specialized testing may need to be performed. However, the cause often remains unknown. Herpes simplex virus (HSV) is an important viral cause that should be tested for using a polymerase chain reaction (PCR) test. This test detects HSV DNA, and therapy with acyclovir should begin even before the test results are known because this virus can cause death if not treated.

encephalitis [EN sef ah LYE tis]: an inflammation of the brain, usually caused by a direct viral infection or a hypersensitivity reaction to a virus or foreign substance

Media Connection

To view an introduction to infection control, pathogens, and learning how to control disease, visit the accompanying online resources.

TABLE 8-3 Viral Causes of Meningitis or Encephalitis

Virus	Distinguishing Characteristic
Cocksackie, echovirus	Belongs to a group called enteroviruses
West Nile, St. Louis encephalitis, Eastern equine encephalitis	Spread by mosquitoes
Mumps, measles	Peak incidence is in winter or spring
Herpes simplex virus (HSV)	Fatal if not treated

© 2016 Cengage Learning®.

8-1
Stop and Review

1. Contrast meningitis and encephalitis in terms of disease process, etiology, and treatment.
2. _____ is a treatable form of viral encephalitis.
3. Rifampin or ciprofloxacin could be used to treat meningitis in people exposed to the _____ organism.
4. _____ virus causes an encephalitis that is spread by the bite of a mosquito.

Otitis Media

Otitis media, or inflammation of the middle ear, is one of the most common causes of sickness in infants and children. Typical symptoms include irritability, ear tugging, lack of energy and appetite, fever, and vomiting. These usually occur in a child who has had cold symptoms of runny nose, nasal stuffiness, or cough.

Diagnosis of acute otitis media is actually very difficult. Infants are not able to describe their symptoms, and viewing the tympanic membrane is often difficult and not always useful. Because the infection is behind the tympanic membrane, it is also not possible to culture the middle ear fluid without puncturing the membrane. Delay in appropriate treatment can lead to hearing loss, and therefore antibiotics are often given without a clear diagnosis. This has led to a divergence of opinion on when to start antibiotic therapy. Many clinicians are concerned that unnecessary antibiotic treatment of otitis media has led to the emergence of multidrug-resistant bacteria. Figure 8-1 illustrates otitis media, and Table 8-4 lists risk factors for otitis media.

Treating the symptoms and observation are good for all children (and parents as well) in the treatment of acute otitis media; however, the question of when to give antibiotics is a difficult one to answer. The use of *Haemophilus influenzae* type B vaccine has been very effective at decreasing middle ear infections caused by this organism and gives us proof that prevention is important in this disease. Measures should be taken to avoid exposure to allergens, irritants, and other sick children and adults.

Table 8-5 lists the typical causes and how often they are the culprit. Protection of the middle

Media Connection

To view a video on otitis media, visit the accompanying online resources.

otitis media: an infection of the middle ear space, behind the eardrum (tympanic membrane) characterized by pain, dizziness, and partial loss of hearing

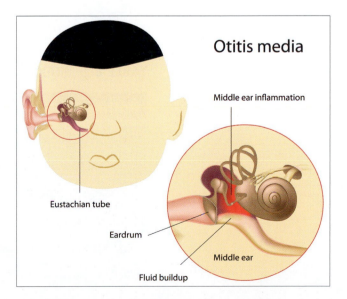

FIGURE 8-1 Schematic drawing of otitis media.
© Alila Medical Media/Shutterstock.com.

ear from microbial or viral invasion depends on the length of the eustachian tube, the pressure difference between the middle ear and the nose and throat, and the angle of the eustachian tube opening. Infants are most likely to get otitis media because their eustachian tubes are shorter and wider and are at a flatter angle relative to their nose and throat than in older children or adults. Acute otitis media generally occurs when an infant develops a viral respiratory tract infection, which results in edema and congestion of the entire respiratory tract. Middle ear secretions cannot be drained into the nose and throat because of blockage of the eustachian tube. These accumulated secretions become an excellent environment for the growth of bacteria.

TABLE 8-4 Factors That Increase the Risk of Otitis Media in Children

Male gender
Sibling in the home
Early age at onset of acute otitis media
Bottle feeding
Group day care
Exposure to tobacco smoke
Nationality—Native American and Alaskan and Canadian Eskimo
Use of pacifier

© 2016 Cengage Learning®.

TABLE 8-5 Microbial Causes of Acute Otitis Media

Pathogen	Percentage of Cases*
Streptococcus pneumoniae	approximately 40%
Haemophilus influenzae	approximately 20%
Moraxella catarrhalis	approximately 20%
Streptococcus pyogenes	approximately 3%
Staphylococcus aureus	approximately 2%
Viral	approximately 40%

*These percentages are estimates compiled by data from the CDC.

© 2016 Cengage Learning®.

Clinical Application
Tubes in the Ears

Do you know someone who has had "tubes" put in his or her ears? A frequent nonpharmacological treatment for recurrent otitis media is myringotomy and insertion of tympanostomy tubes. This procedure reduces the recurrence of otitis media by approximately 50%. The insertion of tympanostomy tubes interrupts the cycle of recurrent infections and helps prevent hearing loss by allowing the fluid to drain from behind the tympanal membrane.

The first decision in the management of acute otitis media is whether to treat the patient with antibiotics. Children and adults with acute otitis media should receive therapy for associated symptoms; antihistamines and decongestants may be used for relief of symptoms of respiratory tract congestion. Topical steroids may help reduce the symptoms and recurrence.

The medications we just discussed provide relief of symptoms, but they do not resolve the fluid that has accumulated behind the eardrum called effusions. Effusions are important because they can result in hearing loss and impaired speech. Effusions may also be a barrier to antibiotic penetration. Whether antibiotics are used for acute otitis may depend on whether the patient has an effusion.

Analgesics and antipyretics such as acetaminophen or nonsteroidal anti-inflammatory agents (ibuprofen, naproxen, etc.), and aspirin, are helpful in relieving the fever and ear pain that is often present with otitis media. Aspirin is not used in children because of its association with Reye syndrome. A significant percentage of children recover from their acute episode of otitis media with symptomatic treatment only. Clinically, there is no way to know which patients need antibiotics and which will recover on their own. The American Academy of Family Physicians and the American Academy of Pediatrics published guidelines in 2004 suggesting that children older than 6 months with less severe illness should be observed first (so called "watchful waiting") before treating with antibiotics.

Most cases of acute otitis media are treated without knowing the bacteria causing the infection. If treatment fails, it is likely that the infection was caused by a virus or a resistant type of bacteria. The development of resistance is rapidly becoming an all-too-common problem, and all health care providers must carefully evaluate the antibiotics to be used.

The three most common bacterial pathogens in acute otitis media are *Streptococcus pneumoniae*, *Haemophilus influenzae*, and *Moraxella catarrhalis*.

Resistant strains of these bacteria have emerged, which complicates therapy choices. There is no one preferred antimicrobial for all children or adults with acute otitis media. Amoxicillin is usually used first in young children who are not allergic to penicillins. Older children are more likely to harbor resistant organisms because of their prior treatment with antibiotics. First-line therapies in children over 3 years of age and adults include:

- high-dose amoxicillin
- cefuroxime axetil (Ceftin)
- amoxicillin–clavulanate (Augmentin)
- cefpodoxime proxetil (Vantin)
- cefdinir (Omnicef)

These agents have good coverage against resistant pneumococcal infections.

Parotitis

The parotid gland is located on each side of the face between the earlobe and the back teeth. When the parotid gland becomes infected, that area of the face appears red, swollen, and firm. Patients usually complain of severe pain, difficulty swallowing, and high fever and chills, and they appear quite ill.

Usually these infections are polymicrobial with *Staphylococcus aureus* (including methicillin-resistant strains) and anaerobes leading the pack as the most common causes. For patients who develop **parotitis** in the hospital, gram-negative microbes such as *Escherichia coli*, *Klebsiella pneumoniae*, and others are found more commonly.

Initial antibiotic therapy for patients who develop this infection outside the hospital consists of regimens containing vancomycin plus either metronidazole or clindamycin. For hospitalized patients, empiric therapy with vancomycin plus piperacillin-tazobactam or meropenem should be considered to cover MRSA as well as gram-negative aerobic organisms and anaerobes.

parotitis [PAH roh TYE tis]: inflammation or infection of one or both parotid salivary glands

✋ 8-2
Stop and Review

1. What are some of the issues related to antibiotic usage in otitis media?
2. Describe the treatment for parotitis.

Infections of the Eye

In this section we will discuss infections that occur in parts of the eye including the sclera and cornea.

Conjunctivitis

Have you ever been told you have *pink eye?* That is a lay term for **conjunctivitis**, which in plain language means an inflammation of the white part, or sclera, of the eye (see Figure 8-2A). Acute conjunctivitis may also be caused by noninfectious causes such as allergies, but we will focus our discussion on infectious causes. Patients with bacterial conjunctivitis usually complain of discharge and redness in the eye. The discharge may be heavy enough to cause the affected eye to be stuck shut in the morning. The discharge of patients with a bacterial cause for their conjunctivitis is usually thick and purulent as opposed to the thin watery discharge from an allergic cause.

Bacterial causes of conjunctivitis include *Staphylococcus aureus, Streptococcus pneumoniae, Haemophilus influenzae,* and *Moraxella catarrhalis. Neisseria gonorrhoeae* can cause a serious form of conjunctivitis that is rapidly progressive and can result in blindness if untreated.

Viruses may also cause conjunctivitis, and they are usually found in patients with an upper respiratory tract infection that precedes the eye infection. Adenoviruses are the usual culprit. Both viral and bacterial causes of conjunctivitis are contagious, and patients and their contacts should perform frequent hand hygiene.

Viral, and even in most cases bacterial, conjunctivitis, with the exception of *Neisseria* sp., is self-limited. Treating bacterial conjunctivitis with

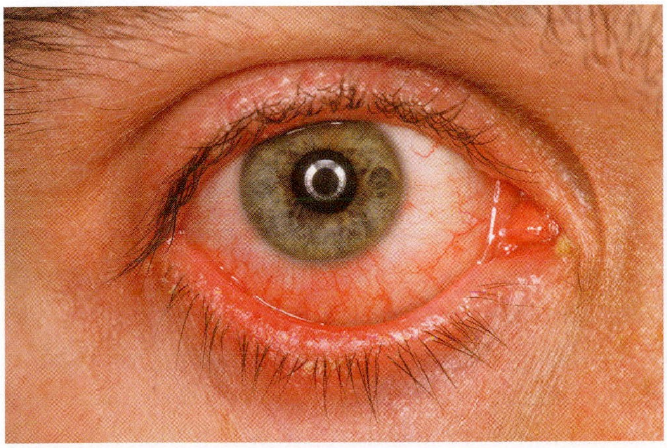

conjunctivitis: an inflammation or redness of the lining of the white part of the eye and the underside of the eyelid (conjunctiva) that can be caused by infection, allergic reaction, or physical agents such as infrared or ultraviolet light

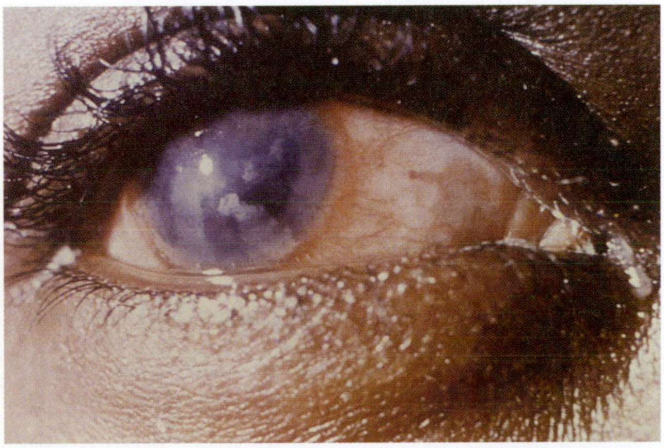

FIGURE 8-2 Infections of the eye. **A.** Conjunctivitis, or pink eye. © Pavel L Photo and Video/Shutterstock.com. **B.** Bacterial keratitis where cornea is inflamed due to bacterial infection. Source: CDC/Robert Sumpter

topical antibiotics may shorten the course and prevent spreading the infection to other individuals. For bacterial causes, polymyxin/trimethoprim eyedrops, sulfacetamide eyedrops, and erythromycin eye ointment are good inexpensive choices. There are no specific antiviral medications available for viral causes. However, topical antihistamine/decongestant eyedrops may be used for symptomatic relief.

Keratitis

keratitis [KER ah TYE tis]: an inflammation of the cornea, the transparent membrane that covers the iris (colored part) and pupil of the eye

Inflammation of the cornea is the hallmark of **keratitis** (Figure 8-2B). It can be caused by almost any type of microbe including viruses, bacteria, parasites, and fungi. Patients typically complain of having trouble keeping their eyelid open and of a foreign body sensation in the affected eye. Patients should be referred to an ophthalmologist as soon as the diagnosis is suspected because they are at risk of losing their sight.

Cultures should be obtained to determine the cause before antibiotics are started. The eyedrops used to treat bacterial keratitis are not commercially available and must usually be compounded by a pharmacist. Viral causes are usually either herpes simplex or adenoviruses and are generally self-limited. Infrequently, antivirals may be used; acyclovir may be used to treat herpes simplex viral keratitis.

Cardiovascular Infections

Cardiovascular infections include infections of the heart valves and as well as infections of the blood stream caused by catheters inserted into large veins for patient treatment or monitoring purposes.

Endocarditis

endocarditis [EN doh kar DYE tis]: inflammation of the endocardium, when microorganisms from the bloodstream can become lodged on the heart valves or heart lining

Endocarditis is a serious infection occurring on one or more heart valves. This infection may be found in patients who have had a valve replacement with either a mechanical valve or pig valve (also called bioprosthetic valve). It may also be found in patients who still have their own valves. Patients who have had pacemakers or defibrillators placed to treat abnormal heart rhythms and patients requiring central venous catheters for hemodialysis or medication therapy may also develop this type of infection. Intravenous drug users may inadvertently introduce bacteria into their bloodstream, which then infect the heart valves on the right side of the heart (tricuspid and pulmonic valves).

Symptoms of endocarditis may be nonspecific such as difficulty breathing, fever, and swelling in the legs and feet. It may also cause a stroke or kidney

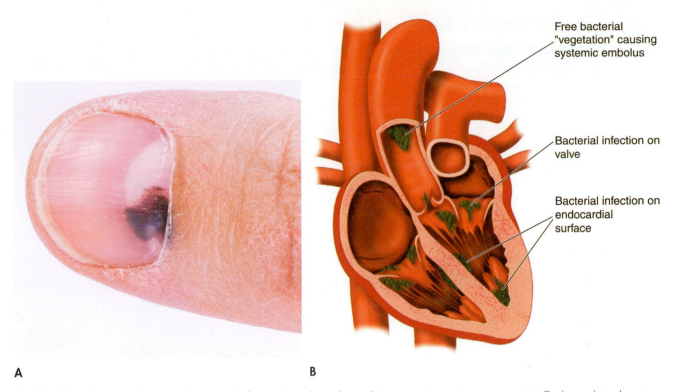

Free bacterial "vegetation" causing systemic embolus

Bacterial infection on valve

Bacterial infection on endocardial surface

A   B

FIGURE 8-3 A. Petechiae on fingernail of patient with endocarditis. ©iStock.com/claudiodivizia. **B.** Endocarditis showing vegetative growth. © Blamb/Shutterstock.com.

damage if pieces of the infection break off and travel to other organs in the body. Patients with endocarditis may have petechiae as well as certain lesions on their skin, eyes, or fingernails (Figure 8-3). A special test called an echocardiogram is useful to look for bacteria growing on the heart valves called vegetations.

Endocarditis is a serious infection that may result in death if not properly treated. Some patients may need their heart valve replaced either because it is severely damaged from the infection or because it is difficult to eradicate the organism without the operation. Table 8-6 lists some common microbial causes of endocarditis and their treatments. Treatment for 2 to 6 weeks with intravenous antimicrobials is usually required depending on the organism and the valve location and type (native vs. prosthetic valve).

Catheter-Related Bloodstream Infections (CRBSIs)

Patients who need medications or fluids intravenously when the oral route is either not possible or feasible require the placement of a catheter in a vein. Some patients on dialysis (e.g., hemodialysis) require the dialysis treatment to be administered using an intravenous catheter. Patients with cancer often have specialized catheters implanted or "tunneled" under their skin to provide access to their bloodstream for the administration of chemotherapy medications. In general, there are two types of catheters based on their

TABLE 8-6 Microbial Causes of Endocarditis and Treatment

Microorganism	Risk Factors	Treatment
Viridans streptococci and *Streptococcus bovis*	Poor dentition	Penicillin G or ceftriaxone ± gentamicin
Streptococcus pneumoniae	Alcoholism	Penicillin G or vancomycin
Enterococci	Prosthetic valves	Penicillin G or ampicillin ± gentamicin
Staphylococcus aureus (methicillin susceptible)	Injection drug users, hemodialysis	Nafcillin
Methicillin-resistant *Staphylococcus aureus* or coagulase-negative staphylococci	Injection drug users, hemodialysis	Vancomycin or daptomycin
Haemophilus aphrophilus, Actinobacillus actinomycetemcomitans, Cardiobacterium hominis, Eikenella corrodens, Kingella kingae*	No specific risk factors identified	Ceftriaxone or ampicillin-sulbactam
Candida sp.	Prosthetic valves, injection drug users, catheters	Flucytosine + liposomal amphotericin

*This group is known collectively by the acronym HACEK.

© 2016 Cengage Learning®.

catheter-related bloodstream infections (CRBSIs): bloodstream infections related to the invasive introduction of a peripheral or central catheter

location in the body. The two types of catheters are known as *central* and *peripheral intravenous catheters*. Catheters inserted into peripheral veins (e.g., veins in the arm or hand) or arteries rarely become infected. However, catheters inserted into the subclavian (vein in the upper chest on both the left and right sides), internal jugular (vein in the neck on both sides), or femoral veins (vein in the groin on both sides) may become infected and cause the bacteria to enter the bloodstream resulting in a seriously ill patient. These infections are called **catheter-related bloodstream infections (CRBSIs)**.

Patients with a CRBSI may have redness of the skin and pus draining from the IV catheter site. Fever, low blood pressure, or a change in mentation may also signal the health care worker that a patient's catheter may be infected. It is important to consider the catheter as a potential source anytime a patient with a central catheter is suspected of having an infection. Blood cultures are obtained both from the catheter and from a peripheral vein to assist in the diagnosis. After blood cultures are obtained, antimicrobials may be started, and usually both gram-positive and gram-negative organisms are covered until an organism is identified. Once a CRBSI is confirmed, it is often necessary to remove the catheter to assist in treating this infection. The types of organisms and their respective antimicrobial treatment can be found in Table 8-7.

TABLE 8-7 CRBSI Organisms and Antimicrobial Treatment

Microorganism	Treatment
Staphylococcus aureus	Nafcillin
Methicillin-resistant *Staphylococcus aureus* (MRSA)	Vancomycin or daptomycin
Coagulase-negative staphylococci	Vancomycin
Enterococcus sp.	Ampicillin or vancomycin
Gram-negative rods (*E. coli, Klebsiella* sp., *Enterobacter* sp., *Pseudomonas aeruginosa*)	Piperacillin-tazobactam or imipenem or cefepime
Candida sp.	Caspofungin or fluconazole

© 2016 Cengage Learning®.

8-3 Stop and Review

1. _____ is an infection of the sclera of the eye that may be caused by bacteria or viruses.
2. The acronym CRBSI stands for _____.
3. Splinter hemorrhages occurring in the nail beds may be a sign of _____.

Infectious Diseases of the Skin and Soft Tissues

In this section we discuss infections occurring in the largest organ of the body: the skin and soft tissue underneath the skin.

Cellulitis and Erysipelas

Cellulitis and **erysipelas** are similar in that they are both infections of the skin. Erysipelas is an infection of the upper dermis and lymphatics of the skin, while cellulitis is an infection of the lower dermis and fat tissue. Erysipelas is a disease found most often in children, and it causes the tissue to swell above the level of the skin forming a red-raised area. Cellulitis infections are more often found in adults and cause the skin to turn red but remain flat to the body. It is more difficult to distinguish the border of the infection from normal skin in cellulitis compared with erysipelas. Fever and chills are more likely to be found in patients with erysipelas, which generally has a fairly abrupt onset. Cellulitis tends to develop slowly over

cellulitis: inflammation of skin and subcutaneous tissues

erysipelas [ER i SIP eh les]: an infection of the skin that is marked by a bright red, swollen, sharply defined rash on the face, scalp, arms, legs, or trunk

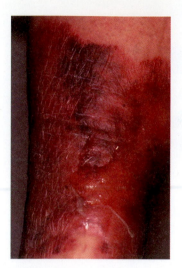

FIGURE 8-4 Cellulitis of the leg. © Biophoto Associates/Science Source/Getty Images.

a few days and at times may have an associated discharge of fluid from the area (Figure 8-4).

The diagnosis of both diseases is usually made clinically by careful examination of the area. It is important for the clinician to exclude the possibility of a necrotizing soft tissue infection because it generally requires emergency surgical treatment and may result in death or permanent disability even if appropriately treated. Cultures are usually not helpful in the treatment of simple cellulitis and erysipelas because they rarely yield an organism. If the infection was caused by an exposure such as a dog or cat bite, then the likely pathogen and treatment will be different. The causative microbes and treatments are found in Table 8-8.

Risk factors for developing cellulitis may include breaks in the skin from athlete's foot infection and/or chronic swelling of the extremity from lymphedema or venous insufficiency. Treatment of these conditions may prevent recurrent cellulitis and should be implemented along with antibiotic therapy. The Infectious Diseases Society of America 2014 Guidelines

TABLE 8-8 Causative Microbes and Treatments for Erysipelas and Cellulitis

Disease	Likely Pathogens	Treatment
Erysipelas	Beta-hemolytic streptococci	Very ill—Ceftriaxone, cefazolin Mild illness—Amoxicillin, cephalexin
Cellulitis	*Staphylococcus aureus* (methicillin susceptible or resistant), beta-hemolytic streptococci (Groups A, B, C, F, G)	Purulence, mild infection—Clindamycin, TMP-SMX,* doxycycline Purulence, serious infection—Vancomycin, clindamycin, or linezolid Nonpurulent—Oral clindamycin, cephalexin, or dicloxacillin
Cellulitis (dog bite)**	*Capnocytophaga canimorsus*	Prophylaxis—Amoxicillin-clavulanate Treatment—Piperacillin/tazobactam
Cellulitis (cat bite)	*Pasteurella multocida*	Same as for dog bite
Cellulitis (water exposure)	*Aeromonas hydrophila, Vibrio vulnificus*	doxycycline plus ciprofloxacin or ceftazidime

*Trimethoprim-sulfamethoxazole (TMP-SMX)

**Found in diabetics, may rapidly result in death

suggest basing empiric therapy of cellulitis depending on the presence or absence of purulence:

- If the cellulitis has purulent drainage or exudates then treatment should include coverage for methicillin-resistant *Staphylococcus aureus* (MRSA).

- For patients with mild infections, oral clindamycin, trimethoprim-sulfamethoxazole, or doxycycline are good options because they should have activity against community strains of MRSA.

- Serious infections should be treated with IV vancomycin, clindamycin, or linezolid. Oral clindamycin, cephalexin, or dicloxacillin would be good choices for patients without purulence.

Treatment of erysipelas for children with mild infections may include options such as amoxicillin, cephalexin, or erythromycin. For more seriously ill patients, therapy should begin with intravenous agents such as ceftriaxone or cefazolin which may be changed to oral agents as the child improves.

Necrotizing Skin and Soft Tissue Infections

Necrotizing skin and soft tissue infections are very serious infections involving rapid destruction of skin and other soft tissues (fascia) with highly virulent anaerobic and/or aerobic bacteria. These infections require early recognition by health care practitioners because, without antibiotics and surgery, the likelihood of death is high. You can find these infections categorized in different ways, but to keep it simple, we will be discussing these serious infections as a group. Patients with these infections often look ill and complain of severe pain in the area of the infection. Most will have fever and a rapid heart rate. As the infection proceeds, low blood pressure, confusion, and reduced urine output alert the health care team to the severity of illness. The involved skin may appear swollen with fluid-filled blisters, and the patient may complain of severe pain when the affected area is touched.

necrotizing skin and soft tissue infections: usually rare but very severe type of bacterial infection that can destroy the muscles, skin, and underlying tissue

Food for Thought
Early Discovery Credited

Fournier's gangrene is a serious necrotizing skin and soft tissue infection that occurs in the perineal area. It may involve the scrotum and penis in males. The name comes from a French physician, Jean-Alfred Fournier, after he described five cases of this serious infection in 1883.

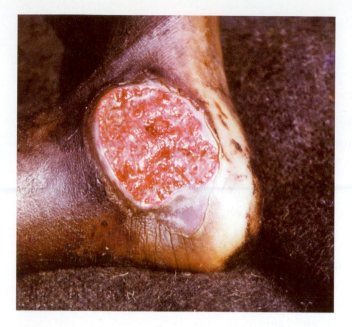

FIGURE 8-5 Necrotizing fasciitis tissue infection.
Source: CDC/Mae Lennon, Tulane Medical School; Clement Benjamin

necrotizing fasciitis [NECK roh TIZE ing FAS ee EYE tis]: bacterial infections that can destroy the deep layers of skin; also known as flesh eating disease

Microorganisms that are commonly found with these infections include both aerobes and anaerobes. Group A streptococcus can cause these infections in both healthy individuals and in patients who have chronic diseases such as diabetes. *Clostridium perfringens* is an anaerobic organism that may be found in patients who have had surgery or trauma. **Necrotizing fasciitis** is an infection of the subcutaneous tissue that may be caused either by group A streptococcus alone or by a mixture of both aerobic and anaerobic bacteria (Figure 8-5).

The treatment of these serious infections requires a combination of surgical debridement (removal of dead or damaged tissue) of the infected tissue and antibiotics. Initial antibiotic therapy should be directed against both aerobic and anaerobic organisms. Treatment with piperacillin/tazobactam or imipenem/cilastatin plus vancomycin would provide broad-spectrum coverage until culture results from both the wound and blood become available. If group A streptococcus is recovered or known to be the causative agent, therapy with both clindamycin and penicillin is recommended.

Intra-Abdominal Infections

Intra-abdominal infections include appendicitis, cholecystitis, diverticulitis, *Clostridium difficile* colitis, and infectious diarrhea. With the possible exception of infectious diarrhea, patients who become ill with these infections almost always have abdominal pain of varying severity.

Appendicitis

appendicitis: inflammation and infection of the appendix

The appendix is a wormlike structure that extends from the cecum of the GI tract. Acute **appendicitis** is a common problem that occurs in patients usually in their 20s or 30s. Individuals with an acute appendicitis attack usually complain of abdominal pain that starts around the belly button and radiates to the right lower side of the abdomen. The disease process usually starts as an inflammation of the wall of the appendix with subsequent abscess formation or rupture causing peritonitis. Nausea, vomiting, and loss of appetite are also common features of this disease process.

As you continue reading about intra-abdominal infections, you will find that many of these require surgery in addition to antibiotics. As a matter of fact, surgery is a more definitive treatment because antibiotics alone are not curative except in rare circumstances. In the case of appendicitis, the usual surgical approach is to perform an appendectomy either laparoscopically or by laparotomy. Because the appendix is located between the large and small bowel, the antimicrobial coverage is directed at both gram-negative rods (e.g., *E. coli*) and anaerobes (*Bacteroides* sp.).

If the appendix is intact, a single dose of an antibiotic given within 60 minutes of the surgical incision is adequate. If the appendix has ruptured, therapy is begun immediately and usually continued for a 5–7 day period. Piperacillin-tazobactam or ceftriaxone plus metronidazole would provide the necessary spectrum of activity required for these infections. Culture material should be obtained during surgery, and the empiric regimen should be adjusted based on the culture and susceptibility results.

Acute Cholecystitis

Gallbladder infections can either be caused by a stone that obstructs the flow of bile in the common bile duct or can occur in critically ill patients without evidence of stones (called acalculous cholecystitis). Patients with this infectious problem usually are ill-appearing and complain of fever and abdominal pain on the right upper side of the abdomen that may radiate to the back or right shoulder. Nausea, vomiting, and lack of appetite are common complaints along with the onset of pain 1 hour after eating a fatty meal. An ultrasound of the gallbladder is usually obtained to aid in the diagnosis.

The symptoms of **acute cholecystitis** are due primarily to inflammation of the gallbladder, but infection occurs in at least one-quarter of patients with this condition. The most frequently encountered bacteria include *Escherichia coli,* Enterococcus, Klebsiella, and Enterobacter.

As mentioned, some form of surgery is usually required for most intra-abdominal infections. In addition to a surgical procedure, empiric antibiotic therapy for acute cholecystitis is similar to that used for appendicitis and would include either ceftriaxone plus metronidazole, piperacillin-tazobactam, or a carbapenem (e.g., ertapenem). Once culture results become available, antibiotic therapy should be directed at the pathogen(s) isolated. The duration of therapy depends on the severity of illness, which could range from 24 hours after surgical intervention up to 5–7 days for patients who are very ill on presentation or have numerous other underlying illnesses.

acute cholecystitis [KOH luh sis TYE tis]: inflammation of the gallbladder

Diverticulitis

diverticulitis [DYE ver tick you
LYE tis]: inflammation of the
diverticulum in the intestinal
tract causing possible pain,
anorexia, and fever

Diverticulitis is an inflammatory condition occurring in the colon. Diverticula are weakened areas of the colonic mucosa that form fingerlike projections into the colon (Figure 8-6). These herniations of the colon can become inflamed and rupture spilling the contents of the colon into the abdominal cavity. These ruptures can either wall themselves off and cause few additional problems, or they can cause disease ranging from a localized abscess to diffuse peritonitis and death if not quickly treated surgically. A CT scan of the abdomen is usually obtained to aid in management decisions. Pain in the lower left side of the abdomen that has usually been present for several days is the most common complaint from patients. Most patients have been experiencing similar episodes of this pain for days prior to seeking medical attention. Nausea, vomiting, constipation, and diarrhea are also nonspecific symptoms associated with this disease.

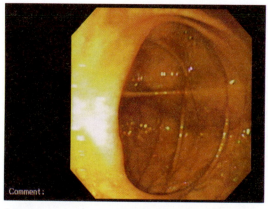

A1

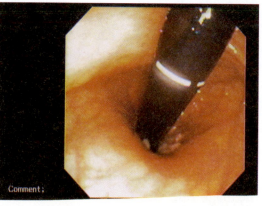

A2

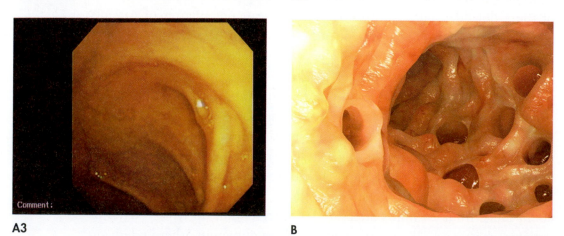

A3

B

FIGURE 8-6 A1-A3. Endoscopic views of healthy colon. ©iStock.como/leezsnow. **B.** Endoscopic view of colon with diverticula (small pouches) in the lining of the colon. © Juan Gaertner/Shutterstock.com.

The usual microbes involved in diverticular infections are those found in the colon. *E. coli* and *Bacteroides fragilis* are the most likely culprits, and empiric therapy is directed at these bacteria. Mild infections (uncomplicated) may be treated in the outpatient setting for 10–14 days. Moderate to severe infections (complicated) require hospitalization and possibly surgical intervention along with antibiotics.

Trimethoprim-sulfamethoxazole plus either metronidazole or clindamycin orally could be used for patients with mild infections treated outside the hospital. Intravenous antibiotic therapy with piperacillin-tazobactam or ceftriaxone plus metronidazole are options for empiric therapy of hospitalized patients. As the disease process resolves and the patients resume oral intake, a 10–14 day course of antibiotics may be completed with an oral regimen similar to the one mentioned for patients with mild disease. Once culture results become available, antibiotic therapy may be directed at the pathogens identified. Anaerobic coverage should be maintained even if anaerobes are not identified by cultures because they are always involved in colonic infections. Some type of surgical procedure is usually required with the exception of patients who have mild disease that resolves with antibiotic therapy.

Clostridium difficile Colitis

This organism can cause disease ranging from a mild form associated with diarrhea and abdominal pain to a very severe, life-threatening infection that may result in death (Figure 8-7). It is one of the most common health care–associated infections (HAIs) so it deserves special attention in our book. The prior consumption of antibiotics alters our normal gastrointestinal tract flora allowing this organism to move in and take up residence.

Watery diarrhea that is frequent, abdominal pain with cramping, mild increase in temperature, and elevation in the white blood cell count are commonly found in patients with this disease. Patients may also present with a very severe colitis with little if any diarrhea (termed toxic megacolon). These patients are very ill with bloated abdomens, very high white blood cell counts, and low blood pressure. In very ill patients

Clinical Application
The Medical History Is Important

Most patients with *Clostridium difficile* colitis have a prior history of consuming antibiotics either when the disease starts or in the past 10 weeks prior to the onset of disease.

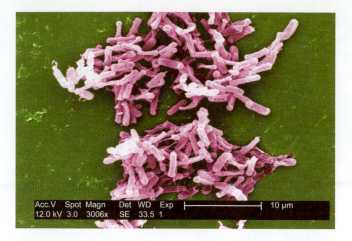

FIGURE 8-7 Micrograph of *Clostridium difficile* bacterial cells. C-diff is one of the most common health care–associated infections (HAIs). Source: CDC/Lois S. Wiggs. Photo credit: Janice Carr.

Clostridium difficile [klos TRID ee um dif us SEEL]: gram-positive anaerobe bacteria that causes watery diarreha, fever, appetite loss, and abdominal pain; sometimes accompanied by pseudomembraneous colitis

without diarrhea, it may be necessary to examine the colon looking for pseudomembranes to confirm the diagnosis.

The diagnosis of **Clostridium difficile** infection is made based on patient symptoms, a history of antibiotic use, and laboratory testing. Anaerobic organisms such as *C. difficile* are difficult to grow so cultures are usually not obtained. However, because the organism produces disease by secreting toxins, testing usually is performed to detect toxin presence in the stool. Because toxins A and B are secreted by the *C. difficile* organism, many laboratories test for the presence of toxins A and B using an enzyme immunoassay (EIA). Because of the high false negative rate (the disease may be present but the test is negative) of the EIA test, it is rapidly being replaced by a polymerase chain reaction test. These tests detect the genes responsible for producing the toxins thereby improving the ability of the test to detect infected patients.

In previous chapters we have spent a considerable amount of time talking about infection prevention. This disease represents the perfect opportunity to show you how we tie the various book chapters together. This organism is shed in the stool and forms spores that can exist on environmental surfaces everywhere for months. The organism is spread to individuals by the fecal–oral route of transmission. Spores are picked up from contaminated surfaces and then are ingested when hands touch our mouths. Patients with this disease are placed in contact precautions (review Chapter 5) isolation. Health care workers should use soap and water to wash hands because the spores resist the action of alcohol-based hand rubs and must be removed from the hands by good hand washing technique (review Chapter 5). Finally, the spores are very resistant to environmental cleaning, and 1:10 dilutions of bleach (sodium hypochlorite) are much more effective at killing the spore form of the organism than quaternary ammonium compounds (review Chapter 4). If an outbreak occurs, antibiotic restriction targeting the antibiotic(s) that were implicated in the outbreak may be important in curtailing further spread of the organism.

If patients develop this disease while on an antibiotic, the antibiotic should be stopped as soon as possible because continued use may prevent the cure of this infection. Patients who have mild infection may be treated with either oral metronidazole or oral vancomycin. It is important to emphasize that intravenous vancomycin should not be used because it is not secreted into the colon. Severe disease may be treated with both oral vancomycin and intravenous metronidazole. In contrast to vancomycin, metronidazole obtains high concentrations of drug in the colon because it is secreted by the intestines and biliary tract into the colon. Combination therapy may ensure that antibiotic delivery to the colon is optimized.

Unfortunately, recurrent *C. difficile* disease occurs in about one-quarter of the patients treated. The options to treat recurrent disease are similar to the options for the first episode. In addition, rifaximin and fidaxomicin are two new options that may prove to be more useful for the treatment of recurrent infections.

Infectious Diarrhea

Infectious diarrhea generally is associated with either the consumption of contaminated food, exposure to pets, or travel. When you book your dream cruise trip on that luxurious ocean liner, the last thing you want to think about is your risk of acquiring infectious diarrhea. Now that we have you thinking of your dream cruise vacation, we do not want to spoil your thoughts just yet so we will discuss food-borne infectious diarrhea first.

infectious diarrhea: infection of the gastrointestinal tract that involves the stomach and small intestine

It has been estimated that there are approximately 200,000 cases of food-borne illness each year resulting in 1.8 million hospitalizations, 3,100 deaths, and $6.5 billion in excess medical costs. These illnesses primarily affect individuals who are very young or old, pregnant, or immunocompromised. These diseases continue to cause problems in the United States because of changing demographics, the way food is produced and distributed, lack of public health resources, and microorganism adaptation. Consumption of certain foods places an individual at higher risk of acquiring disease (Table 8-9).

TABLE 8-9 Foods Associated with Illness

Fresh produce	Raw/unpasteurized milk
Runny eggs	Unpasteurized apple juice/cider
Ready-to-eat meats	Pink chicken*
Raw shellfish	Pink turkey*
Raw fresh fish	Pink hamburgers*
Alfalfa sprouts	Pink ground pork*

*Undercooked

Several different types of bacteria, parasites, and viruses may cause infectious diarrhea. Table 8-10 provides a summary of the various causative microorganisms. In general, patients with infectious diarrhea will complain of stomach cramps, diarrhea, and watery or bloody stools. Fever may be present in some cases but not all. The good news is that most of these cases are self-limiting and require treatment with only fluids to prevent dehydration. Antibiotics are generally not indicated and may even make the disease worse in some cases. The increasing prevalence of antibiotic resistance is another reason for rationing antibiotic use in patients with infectious diarrhea.

The pathogens discussed in Table 8-10 are the same ones implicated as the cause of travelers' diarrhea. High-risk parts of the world for acquiring travelers' diarrhea include Central America, South America, Africa, the Middle East, and South Asia. Cruise ship travel is another way of becoming ill with infectious diarrhea. Food is more often the source than water. Because antibiotics are rarely indicated and symptomatic treatment with antipyretics and antidiarrheals have limited effectiveness, prevention is key. Hand washing and cautious food and beverage consumption are key prevention measures.

TABLE 8-10 Microorganisms Causing Infectious Diarrhea

Pathogen	Source	Symptoms
Campylobacter (C. jejuni, C. coli)	Raw poultry, unpasteurized milk, meat	Bloody diarrhea, abdominal cramps, fever, vomiting
Salmonella (S. typhi)	Poultry, reptiles, livestock, pets, raw eggs	Fever, nausea, vomiting, diarrhea
Shigella	Milk, dairy products, food/water contaminated with fecal matter	Abdominal cramps, fever, bloody/mucus diarrhea
Escherichia coli	Undercooked hamburger, fresh/prepackaged produce	Watery or bloody diarrhea, fever
Giardia	Contaminated water	Sudden onset of explosive watery stools, abdominal cramps, nausea, bloating, flatulence
Cryptosporidiosis/Cyclosporiasis	Contaminated water, produce	Abdominal pain, watery diarrhea
Norovirus	Fecal-oral contaminants	Diarrhea
Rotavirus	Fecal-oral contaminants	Diarrhea

Food for Thought
"Boil It, Peel It, Cook It, or Forget It"

Because the vast majority of diarrheal illness comes from food, here are some tips on how to eat safely while traveling:

Safe: steaming-hot foods, dry bread, peeled fruits, foods with high sugar content, citrus juices, and carbonated drinks

Unsafe: room-temperature food, buffet items, hamburgers that are not steaming hot, and fruits, vegetables, and berries with intact skin

8-4
Stop and Review

1. _____ and _____ are types of skin infections that rarely produce cultures with organisms.

2. If a patient develops severe diarrhea after a course of antibiotic treatment, you might suspect _____ as the possible infectious organism.

3. _____ is an anaerobic organism that can cause serious skin infections in patients who have had surgery or trauma.

Genitourinary Tract Infections

We deviate a bit from our format for discussing infectious diseases in this section on **genitourinary tract infections**. The first few diseases are transmitted by sexual contact and may initially involve just the sex organs but left untreated may expand to other areas of the body. That is why we discuss sexually transmitted diseases from a bug rather than organ system perspective. However, we get back on track discussing infections occurring in the bladder and kidney.

genitourinary tract infection: group of infections of the male and female genitalia and infections of the urinary tract

Sexually Transmitted Diseases

Sexually transmitted diseases (STDs), also known as sexually transmitted infections (STIs) account for a large number of cases worldwide. In most cases they can be preventable with safe sex practices.

sexually transmitted diseases (STDs): group of diseases transmitted through sexual contact that can be caused by bacteria, viruses, protozoans, fungi, and parasites

Chlamydia

Chlamydia [klah MID ee ah]: bacterial disease that causes genital infections in men and woman

There are an estimated 3 million new **Chlamydia** infections each year in the United States. Infection is transmitted by either the genital or anal route after exposure to an infected partner. The incubation period prior to becoming symptomatic is 7–21 days. Because many infected individuals are asymptomatic, a large reservoir of individuals without symptoms exists in the population, which is largely responsible for the high reinfection rate. In males, the most common site of infection is the urethra, causing painful urination and a mucoid discharge from the penis. The majority of infections in males are asymptomatic. Infections in women can result in cervicitis, urethritis, salpingitis, endometritis, or pelvic inflammatory disease (PID). Symptoms in women may include a mucopurulent cervical/vaginal discharge (cervicitis), painful urination (urethritis), and frequent urge to urinate (urethritis). Because PID may be caused by other organisms in addition to Chlamydia, it will be discussed later.

It is not possible to reliably diagnose Chlamydia infections based on history and physical examination alone. Nucleic acid amplification tests (NAATs) have largely replaced other tests to diagnose Chlamydial infections. Urine in men and women, urethral swabs in men, and endocervical swabs in women are recommended for testing using this technology.

Treatment of uncomplicated Chlamydial infections with either azithromycin or doxycycline usually results in a cure. To date there has been no clinically important drug resistance among *C. trachomatis* strains. Patients and their sex partners should be instructed to abstain from sexual intercourse for at least 7 days after a single dose of azithromycin or until completion of a 7-day regimen of doxycycline.

Gonorrhea

gonorrhea: a sexually transmitted disease caused by a gram-negative diplococcus, *Neisseria gonorrhoeae*

Gonorrhea is second only to Chlamydia in the number of cases reported to public health authorities. Unlike Chlamydia, antibacterial resistance is increasing, making treatment decisions more difficult. Gonorrhea can be transmitted by sexual contact through either vaginal, anal, or oral routes. *Neisseria gonorrhoeae* can cause urogenital, pharyngeal, and rectal infections in males and females and conjunctivitis in very young children and adults. Depending on the site of infection, symptoms may include painful urination, purulent urethral discharge, testicular pain and swelling, lower abdominal pain, sore throat, and anal irritation and pruritus. Asymptomatic infection is common in both men and women, and these individuals serve as disease reservoirs in the community.

The laboratory diagnosis of gonorrhea may include culture or non-culture methods or both. The non-culture methods rely on bacterial DNA detection and consist of both amplified and non-amplified options. The test used may depend on local laboratory availability and the specimen to be tested because not all tests are FDA approved to test every clinical specimen.

Antimicrobial resistance is an increasing problem and complicates treatment decisions. The CDC recommends ceftriaxone intramuscularly or cefixime orally for uncomplicated gonococcal infections of the cervix, urethra, and rectum in adults. For patients allergic to penicillin, azithromycin is a useful option. It is important to instruct patients and partners that they should refrain from having sexual intercourse until treatment is completed and symptoms have resolved. All patients diagnosed with gonorrhea should be screened for Chlamydia infection because coinfection is common.

Herpes Simplex Virus (HSV)

There are two types of **herpes simplex viruses**: type 1 (HSV-1) and type 2 (HSV-2). Most genital herpes infections are caused by the type 2 virus. It is estimated that about 16.2% of the U.S. population between the ages of 14 and 49 years is infected with HSV-2. Because most infected individuals have minimal or no symptoms of infection, reservoirs in the community exist that can easily spread the virus from person to person during sexual contact. When the virus does cause symptoms, it generally produces blisters around the rectum or genitals. These blisters rupture, causing sores that take 2 to 4 weeks to heal. Because the herpes virus cannot be eliminated from the body, recurrent outbreaks of blisters occur with decreasing frequency and duration over time. Herpes infections can cause serious illness in patients with weakened immune systems, and if transmitted to a baby during birth, death of the infant.

Because other diseases such as syphilis can cause genital ulcers, it is important to confirm the clinical diagnosis of herpes. This can be done by culturing fluid from the lesion, testing the fluid for viral DNA using polymerase chain reaction (PCR), testing the specimen for virus using a direct fluorescent antibody (DFA) test, or obtaining a blood sample and testing it for viral antibodies specific for the herpes virus.

There are several antiviral agents available to help decrease the duration, number, and severity of genital herpes virus ulcers. Patients presenting with a primary infection are usually offered treatment because the first outbreak is usually the most severe, and antiviral therapy started within 3 days of a primary infection may decrease the duration and severity of illness. Acyclovir, famciclovir, and valacyclovir all have similar effectiveness in treating primary and recurrent infections. Patients may choose to take one of the three medications on a daily basis, or they may choose to initiate treatment at the time of a symptomatic recurrence of infection. No drug treatment is an option for some patients who have infrequent mild recurrences.

herpes simplex virus: human DNA virus that causes repeated painful vesicular eruptions on the genitals and other surfaces on the skin

Human Immunodeficiency Virus (HIV)

Untreated, HIV infection progresses to the acquired immunodeficiency syndrome (AIDS), which is a progressively fatal disease caused by the retrovirus human immunodeficiency virus (HIV). We are discussing this viral infection under the category of sexually transmitted diseases, but this virus can also be found in injection drug users, recipients of blood products, and health care workers via needlestick or other sharps-related injuries. Once the virus enters the body, it sets up residence in the host's immune system.

Once a person is infected with HIV, the initial symptoms are very similar to a common viral syndrome consisting of fever, swollen lymph nodes, and sore throat. If left untreated, HIV infection continues to weaken the host's immune system leaving the individual susceptible to a host of infections from opportunistic pathogens that otherwise would cause no harm.

HIV infection is usually diagnosed by using serological tests that detect antibodies in the serum. Because it takes 3 to 6 weeks for these antibodies to appear after infection, a diagnosis of HIV infection could be missed in this time window. New tests that combine antibody and antigen detection are useful to diagnose infection during the window period when antibody testing only may miss the diagnosis.

Treatment of HIV comprises several different drugs to suppress the virus. These drugs are termed *antiretrovirals*. Pharmacological classes include nucleoside reverse transcriptase inhibitors, non-nucleoside reverse transcriptase inhibitors, protease inhibitors, integrase strand transfer inhibitors, fusion inhibitors, and CCR5 antagonists (Table 8-11). In addition, several HIV vaccines are undergoing clinical testing.

TABLE 8-11 Common Antiretrovirals*

	Generic Name	**Brand Name**
Nucleoside reverse transcriptase inhibitors (NRTIs)	abacavir	Ziagen
	didanosine (ddl)	Videx
	lamivudine (3TC)	Epivir
	zidovudine (AZT)	Retrovir
Non-nucleoside reverse transcriptase inhibitors (NNRTIs)	efavirenz	Sustiva
	nevirapine	Viramune
Protease inhibitors	indinavir	Crixivan
	ritonavir	Norvir
	atazanavir	Reyataz

*For a more complete listing, visit www.aidsinfo.gov.

Urinary Tract Infections

Infections of the urinary tract can be broken down into lower and upper tract infections. **Cystitis** (inflammation of the bladder) is the medical term for a lower tract infection and **pyelonephritis** (inflammation of the kidney) is the medical term used for an upper tract infection. These infections are most common in sexually active young women. These infections occur much more often in women than men because of the ability of the fecal flora to gain access to the urethra due to the close proximity of the anus to the vagina and urethra. The bacteria then migrate to the bladder and possibly to the kidney causing an infection. In men, these infections are much less common due to the longer urethral length making it more difficult for bacteria to migrate north against the flow of urine and antibacterial substances found in prostatic fluid.

When bladder infections occur in men or women, complaints of dysuria, frequency, urgency, and possibly even bloody urine are common. If the infection involves the kidney then fever, chills, flank pain that may radiate to the back, nausea and vomiting, and low blood pressure may also be found. Laboratory studies may be done to confirm the diagnosis and guide treatment. A urinalysis to detect pyuria (white blood cells in the urine) and nitrite (common uropathogens can convert nitrate to nitrite) may be done to confirm the diagnosis. Urine cultures may not be necessary in young women with simple bladder infections since the organisms and their responsiveness to commonly used antibiotics may be predictable. However, reasons to obtain a culture prior to starting empiric antibiotics include a suspected kidney infection (blood cultures may also be obtained if the patient is admitted to a hospital), a recurrence of symptoms within 3 months of treatment or if a complicated infection is suspected. Urine cultures are recommended for all males to confirm the diagnosis of urinary tract infection in men. Common uropathogens in men and women include *Eschericia coli*, *Proteus mirabilis*, and *Klebsiella pneumoniae*.

For cystitis, oral treatment with trimethoprim-sulfamethoxasole or a fluoroquinolone (ciprofloxacin or levofloxacin) is usually effective. Antimicrobials for 3 days in women and 7 days in men usually result in a good clinical response. Kidney infections are usually treated with intravenous antibiotics in a hospital first, followed by oral therapy, depending on patient response. For mild to moderate kidney infections, ceftriaxone, cefepime, ciprofloxacin, or levofloxacin are good empiric choices, while piperacillin-tazobactam or meropenem should be used for severe infections, especially in immunocompromised patients who have abnormalities of their urinary tract. A duration of 5 to 14 days is usually sufficient, and once the organism and susceptibilities are known, oral therapy may be used to complete the treatment course.

cystitis: bladder inflammation usually occurring as a result of an urinary tract infection

pyelonephritis [PYE eh loh neh FRY tis]: inflammation of kidney and upper urinary tract

Bone and Joint Infections

Infections of the bone, called osteomyelitis, and joint, called septic arthritis will be discussed in this section.

Osteomyelitis

osteomyelitis [OSS tee oh MY eh LYE tis]: a bone infection, almost always caused by bacteria; over time, the result can be destruction of the bone itself

Infections located in one or more bones of the body are called **osteomyelitis**. These infections are treated in a similar fashion as our previous discussion about intra-abdominal infections. This means they are usually treated with a combination of both antibiotics and surgical debridement of dead bone. Bone infections can arise from bacteria in the bloodstream that take up residence in bone, usually because of an abnormality in the bone. Alternatively, a patient may develop this infection from adjacent skin soft tissue infections that spread to the bone, or they may occur because of trauma or direct inoculation from an injury to the bone (e.g., bone exposed to the environment as a result of an automobile accident that becomes contaminated with bacteria). Patients with these infections usually complain of pain at the site of infection. They may also have redness, warmth, fever, swelling, and chills.

The diagnosis is usually made by combining radiographic studies and laboratory data and obtaining cultures of the blood and bone to identify the organism(s) responsible for the infection. Staphylococci, gram-negative rods, enterococci, streptococci, mycobacteria, and anaerobes may be found depending on how the infection developed.

In addition to possible surgery to remove dead bone, antibiotics are selected depending on the organism(s) identified from a bone culture. Infections caused by *Staphylococcus aureus* are treated with nafcillin or cefazolin if methicillin-susceptible or vancomycin if methicillin-resistant. Fluoroquinolones such as ciprofloxacin or levofloxacin are preferred for gram-negative organisms if they are susceptible because of excellent penetration into the bone. The treatment duration is usually for at least 6 weeks.

Septic Arthritis

septic arthritis: a form of joint inflammation caused by infection

Septic arthritis is an infection occurring in one or more joints of the body. These infections usually occur in patients who have one or more risk factors such as diabetes, steroid use, recent surgery or trauma to the joint, rheumatoid arthritis, intravenous drug use, or being elderly. Patients will typically complain of a painful swollen joint. Swelling, warmth, pain on movement of the joint, and fever with chills may also be present (Figure 8-8).

The diagnosis of this infectious disease is made by aspirating the joint fluid and sending it for Gram stain, white blood cell count, and culture and susceptibility. *Staphylococcus aureus* (both MSSA and MRSA) are the most common organisms followed closely by streptococci.

Once the joint (synovial) fluid has been aspirated and Gram stained, antibiotic therapy can be started based on the Gram stain while awaiting final culture and susceptibility results. If the Gram stain results shows gram-positive cocci suggestive of staphylococcus, vancomycin should be started. If gram-negative bacilli are recovered on Gram stain, a third-generation cephalosporin such as ceftazidime would be appropriate empiric therapy. Antibiotic therapy is then adjusted once the organism is definitively identified and the susceptibility is known.

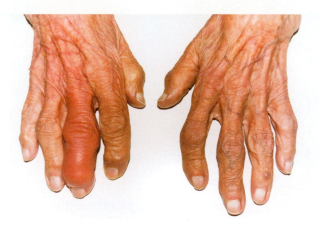

FIGURE 8-8 Septic arthritis of the fingers. ©iStock.com/iMay.

Chapter Summary

- This chapter discussed the clinical presentation, diagnosis, and treatment of common nonrespiratory infections using a body systems approach.

- We emphasized infections that health care professionals are likely to encounter frequently.

- Some of these infections are so serious that treatment may begin before the actual identification of the microorganism. As we learned in Chapter 2, this is called empiric therapy.

- Once the organism is known along with its susceptibility, then therapy may be directed or targeted to the microbe using an appropriate anti-infective.

- We continue along our infectious diseases journey in the next chapter, which focuses on the respiratory system.

Case Study

Mr. Jones is a 69-year-old man who was admitted to the hospital 10 days earlier with a diagnosis of acute diverticulitis. He was given intravenous fluids and empiric antibiotic coverage with ceftriaxone and metronidazole. His antibiotics were stopped after 7 days, and he continued to do well until today when he developed abdominal pain, fever, and diarrhea. A diagnosis of *Clostridium difficile* colitis was made, and antibiotic treatment was initiated. What diagnostic test would confirm the diagnosis? What risk factors did Mr. Jones have to acquire a *Clostridium difficile* infection? Why is oral but not intravenous vancomycin a potential treatment option for this infection?

Chapter Review

Match the term with its description.

1. _____ conjunctivitis

2. _____ otitis media

3. _____ endocarditis

4. _____ meningitis

5. _____ catheter-related bloodstream infection

6. _____ keratitis

7. _____ cellulitis

8. _____ parotitis

9. _____ cholecystitis

10. _____ chlamydia

11. _____ septic arthritis

12. _____ osteomyelitis

a. inflammation of the covering of the brain

b. also known as *pink eye*

c. infection of the middle ear

d. swollen and red facial features

e. inflammation of the cornea

f. inflammation of the heart valves

g. a hospital acquired infection caused by invasive therapy

h. infection of the skin

i. inflammation of the gallbladder

j. sexually transmitted disease

k. infection of the bone

l. infection of the joint

Discuss the answers to the following questions with your instructor.

13. What viral form of encephalitis is fatal if not treated?

14. List several risk factors for otitis media.

15. List the three most common pathogens in acute otitis media.

16. What is the initial antibiotic treatment for parotitis?

17. What are the microbial causes of keratitis?

18. What is the treatment for bacterial conjunctivitis?

19. Contrast erysipelas and cellulitis in terms of diagnosis and treatment.

20. Describe several precautions one could take to prevent getting infectious diarrhea.

21. Contrast the diagnosis and treatment of the sexually transmitted diseases discussed in this chapter.

Fill in the blanks.

22. The treatment for many intra-abdominal infections requires _____ in addition to surgery.

23. The most common organism for septic arthritis is _____.

Additional Activities

1. Research the various common diseases in this chapter and see how much you can add to your classroom's body of knowledge.

2. Research other infectious diseases of each of the systems discussed in this chapter. List and describe the diseases you found along with causative agents and possible treatments.

3. Invite an infectious disease specialist to come to your class for further discussion.

4. Investigate the CDC website to describe frequency of occurrence of some diseases discussed in this chapter.

Media Connection

Go to the accompanying online resources and have fun learning as you play games, view animations and videos, and take practice tests to help reinforce key concepts you learned in this chapter.

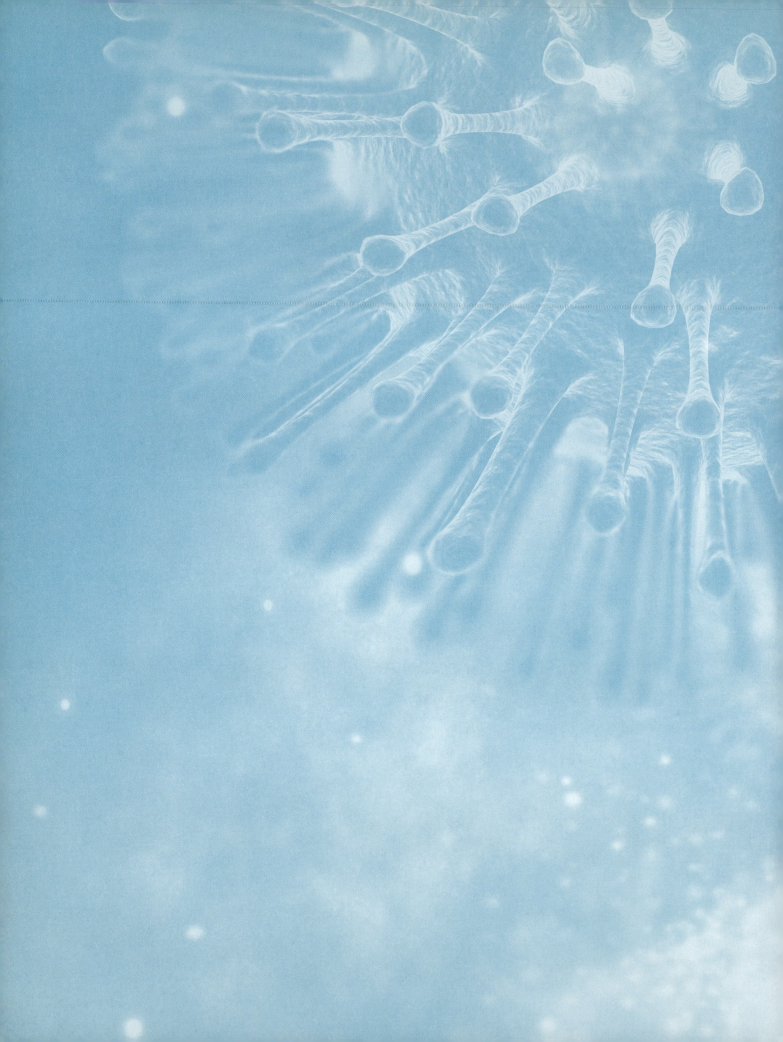

CHAPTER 9

Respiratory-Related Microbiological Diseases

OBJECTIVES

After studying this chapter, the learner will be able to:

- Explain why the respiratory system is prone to a host of infectious diseases.

- Discuss the types of organisms causing infection, clinical presentation, and possible antimicrobial treatments of upper respiratory infections to include sinusitis, pharyngitis, epiglottitis, and croup.

- Discuss why a throat culture should be obtained in a patient with a sore throat and a negative rapid antigen detection test.

- List the four "Ds" of epiglottitis.

- Discuss the types of organisms causing infection, clinical presentation, and possible antimicrobial treatments of lower respiratory infections to include acute bronchitis, bronchiolitis, pneumonia, tuberculosis, and avian influenza.

- Discuss acute bronchitis and why antibiotics are not indicated in its treatment.

- Compare and contrast the various types of pneumonias with respect to the common causative bacteria and the empiric antibiotics for each type.

- List general categories of risk factors that predispose patients to health care–associated pneumonias.

- Discuss why directly observed therapy (DOT) for the treatment of tuberculosis may be important to limit the development of antibiotic resistance.

- Discuss bioterrorism and its relationship to antimicrobial therapy.

KEY TERMS

acute bronchitis

aspiration pneumonia

atypical pneumonia

avian flu

bioterrorism

bronchiolitis
[BRONG kee oh LIGHT is]

(Continues)

KEY TERMS (Continued)

community–acquired
  pneumonia (CAP)

croup

epiglottitis [EP ih glot EYE tis]

health care-associated
  pneumonia (HCAP)

pharyngitis [FAR in JIGH tis]

pneumonia

sinusitis [SIGH nuh SIGH tis]

tracheobronchitis
  [TRAY kee oh brong KYE tis]

tuberculosis

ventilator-associated
  pneumonia (VAP)

Introduction

Because of the nature of the respiratory system, it can serve as host to a large number of infectious diseases. Not only is it a warm, moist environment that facilitates microbiological growth, it is constantly sampling via inhalation whatever is in the outside environment. While it has many layers of defense, it has several locations where microbiological infections can inhabit, thrive, and spread if not properly treated. Figure 9-1 shows the upper airway infections discussed in this chapter and where respiratory-related diseases can originate and spread.

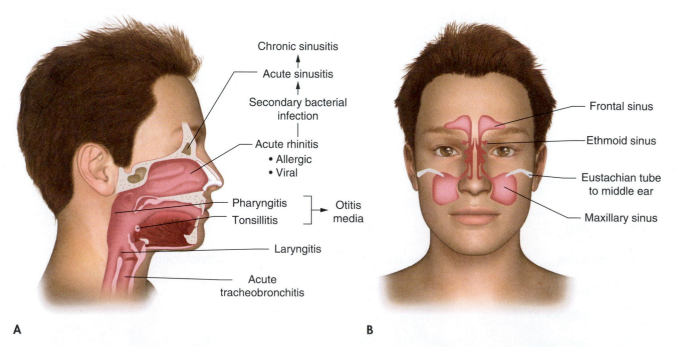

A

B

FIGURE 9-1 A. The upper airway and related diseases. **B.** Note the contiguous nature of the sinuses, structures of the ear, and the respiratory system making the spread of infection relatively easy. © 2016 Cengage Learning®.

Upper Respiratory Airway Infections

The upper respiratory system is composed of the nose, mouth, and larynx. Its primary function is to heat and humidify inspired gases to body temperature and 100% humidity. It also serves to assist in the sense of smell and taste and conducts the inspired gas to the lower respiratory system where gas exchange will take place.

Sinusitis

One of the first places disease can occur is in the hollow sinuses located in the nasal cavity. Most patients with **sinusitis** complain of nasal stuffiness, nasal discharge, and pain or pressure in the face that worsens when bending forward. Severe sinus infections can cause high fever and facial pain with swelling and redness. It is often difficult to tell whether the cause is viral or bacterial, but symptoms suggestive of a bacterial cause include facial or tooth pain, nasal discharge that is yellow or green in color, or symptoms that continue to get worse without treatment.

> **sinusitis [SIGH nuh SIGH tis]:** inflammation of a sinus caused by various agents, including viruses, bacteria, or allergy

Cultures are usually not helpful, and most patients should be observed for at least 10 days before considering antibiotic therapy. This is because most viral and even bacterial sinus infections resolve within 10 days even without antibiotics.

Treatment usually consists of oral or topical decongestants, nasal steroids, and analgesics. When antibiotic therapy is necessary, it is directed at the most common causes such as *Streptococcus pneumoniae, Haemophilus influenzae,* and *Moraxella catarrhalis.* Amoxicillin, trimethoprim-sulfamethoxazole, and azithromycin are good first choices for patients requiring antibiotic treatment.

Pharyngitis

Pharyngitis, or in lay terminology a sore throat, is a relatively common occurrence. This makes sense because the oral cavity represents the large opening of the respiratory system to inhaled or ingested microbes. Pharyngitis is medically described as an inflammation of the pharynx and surrounding lymphoid tissue that may be caused by bacteria or viruses (Figure 9-2). The evaluation, diagnosis, and treatment of patients with pharyngitis is a common problem in primary care. The occurrence of a sore throat is associated with more than 10% of physician office visits, while less than 20% of those patients who experience a sore throat actually seek care.

> **pharyngitis [FAR in JIGH tis]:** inflammation or infection of the pharynx, usually causing a sore throat

Pathogens that cause pharyngitis can be both viral and bacterial; however, viruses cause most of the pharyngitis cases. These viruses are generally

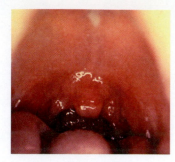

FIGURE 9-2 Pharyngitis. The cause of the sore throat cannot be determined by visual inspection. Courtesy of the CDC.

the same ones that cause the common cold and consist of the rhinovirus, coronavirus, adenovirus, and parainfluenza virus. Other viral causes include herpes simplex virus, influenza virus, coxsackie virus, Epstein-Barr virus, and cytomegalovirus (CMV).

Some pharyngitis (10% to 30%) is the result of bacterial infection, most commonly with group A β-hemolytic streptococci such as *Streptococcus pyogenes*. Acute bacterial pharyngitis can also be caused by groups C and G streptococci, *Arcanobacterium hemolyticum*, and possibly *Mycoplasma pneumoniae* or *Chlamydophila pneumoniae*.

Most often, pharyngitis is self-limiting, lasting from 2 to 7 days. The diagnosis is relatively straightforward. The major symptom is sore throat, with or without associated dysphagia (difficulty swallowing). Fever is typically present. Examination usually reveals erythema and possible exudate appearing as white patches, and mucosal congestion is present. The presence of an exudate with fever usually suggests a bacterial infection, but a culture or rapid antigen detection test ("quick strep test") should be obtained to confirm the causative organism. The rapid antigen detection test allows the diagnosis of group A β-hemolytic streptococcus (GAS) infection within 5 minutes. This test is very specific for group A β-hemolytic streptococcus, and patients with a positive test can be treated immediately without waiting for culture results. Unfortunately, a negative test does not exclude the possibility of a GAS infection, and a throat culture may be necessary. Bacterial eradication occurs within 24 to 72 hours of treatment, which is important in decreasing transmission.

Complications of untreated pharyngitis include spread of the infection to the tonsils, retropharyngeal abscess, otitis media, sinusitis, and mastoiditis. Another complication from group A β-hemolytic streptococcus pharyngitis is acute rheumatic fever (common before the second half of the twentieth century and the advent of antibiotics). The most serious outcome of acute rheumatic fever is heart valve damage. Penicillin has long been the antibiotic of choice for pharyngitis. Even with the development of antimicrobial resistance, group A streptococcus remains susceptible to penicillin, and penicillin remains the drug of choice for this infection. Children younger than 12 years of age should receive 50 mg/kg/day, divided into three doses, of penicillin V for 10 days, or an injection of benzathine penicillin, 50,000 units/kg IM, as a single dose. For adolescents and adults, penicillin V, 500 mg twice daily for 10 days, should be given. In the penicillin-allergic patient, azithromycin 500 mg orally on day 1, followed by 250 mg daily on days 2 through 5 (12 mg/kg/day in children under 27 kg) or clindamycin are acceptable alternatives.

Epiglottitis

The epiglottis, sitting above the trachea, serves as the gatekeeper for the respiratory and gastrointestinal systems. It functions to close over the opening to the trachea (glottis) when swallowing to prevent food from entering the lungs (aspiration). Because of its location, swelling and inflammation of the epiglottis, or **epiglottitis**, is an airway emergency that can cause acute airway obstruction. *Haemophilus influenzae* type B is the major causative microbe involved.

Airway maintenance (keeping the airway open) is the critical initial treatment, with antibiotic therapy empirically selected against *H. influenzae* type B, although other pathogens can still cause the disease such as penicillin-resistant *pneumococcus,* β-hemolytic *Streptococci,* and *Staphylococcus aureus* (including MRSA).

Onset is fast, and fever and sore throat are usually the first symptoms. Epiglottitis is nonseasonal, and recurrence is rare. Respiratory distress, drooling, dysphagia (difficulty swallowing), and dysphonia (difficulty speaking) are the four Ds of this dangerous disease.

It is most prevalent in children ages 2 to 6 and requires rapid recognition and treatment. Since the introduction of the universal *Haemophilus influenza* type B (Hib) vaccine, the incidence is decreasing. The preferred antibiotic treatments are cefotaxime or ceftriaxone $\pm$ clindamycin or vancomycin (added in severely ill patients for staphylococcal coverage).

epiglottitis [EP ih glot EYE tis]: an infection of the epiglottis, which can lead to severe airway obstruction

Croup

Croup is different from epiglottitis but also results from infections of the laryngeal area. It too can cause airway obstruction and is characterized by noisy breathing, especially on inspiration. Clinical presentation of croup is that of a barking cough and inspiratory stridor (harsh high-pitched sound heard on inspiration).

Croup is usually caused by viruses such as parainfluenza virus types 1 and 2, influenza types A and B, adenovirus, and respiratory syncytial virus. Bacterial infection may occur after a previous viral infection. Bacterial causes include *Staphylococcus aureus*, group A β-hemolytic streptococci, and pneumococci while milder cases may be caused by Mycoplasma.

Croup progresses slowly, usually at night. Fever is uncommon. It is most common in late spring and late fall. Children younger than 3 years old most commonly get croup. It is characterized by stridor and no drooling. Treatment consists of air humidification and oxygen.

croup: viral infection of the larynx (voice box); associated with mild upper respiratory symptoms such as a runny nose and cough (usually in children)

Pharmacological therapy starts with nebulized epinephrine and corticosteroids to decrease swelling and inflammation regardless of the microbial cause. If a laryngotracheitis develops, empiric antibiotic treatment for the bacteria may be necessary after appropriate cultures are obtained with a regimen that would be similar to the one recommended for epiglottitis.

Now that we have discussed upper respiratory tract infections, we move down to lower respiratory tract infections, including bronchitis, bronchiolitis, pneumonia, and tuberculosis.

Clinical Application
Whooping Cough

Bordetella pertussis, or whooping cough, is a highly contagious infection that is often not considered as a cause of upper respiratory tract infections. It should be considered as a potential cause of a prolonged upper respiratory infection and cough that fails to resolve after 2 weeks. This is true even if the childhood whooping cough vaccination was given. Azithromycin for 5 days or clarithromycin for 7 days have replaced erythromycin as the drugs of choice for treatment because of better tolerability and shorter treatment courses.

9-1
Stop and Review

Match the disease with a common causative organism:

1. sinusitis   a. *Haemophilus influenzae*
2. pharyngitis   b. adenovirus
3. epiglottitis   c. *Streptococcus pyogenes*
4. croup   d. *Streptococcus pneumoniae*

Infectious Diseases of the Lower Respiratory System

The lower respiratory system begins at the vocal cords and ends at the blind alveolar sacs where gas exchange takes place. The main function of the lower respiratory system is conduction of inhaled atmospheric gas to the peripheral respiratory regions for gas exchange to facilitate oxygen entering the capillaries and carbon dioxide being exhaled with the breath.

Acute Bronchitis and Bronchiolitis

Acute bronchitis and **bronchiolitis** are inflammatory conditions of the large and small airways of the tracheobronchial tree and do not extend downward to the peripheral alveoli. They are usually associated with a respiratory infection. Acute bronchitis occurs in all ages and is seen most commonly in the winter months, following a pattern very similar to that of other acute respiratory tract infections. Damp, cold climates, the presence of respiratory pollutants in the air, or cigarette smoke can precipitate acute attacks. Bronchiolitis is the term for this disease in infants.

Acute bronchitis is usually a self-limiting illness and rarely leads to further complications. Acute bronchitis generally begins in the upper airways, and patients present with nonspecific complaints including headache, malaise, and sore throat. In general, infection in the trachea and bronchi leads to increased bronchial secretions along with thick secretions that impair the ability to clear these tenacious secretions from the lung. Cough is the hallmark symptom that distinguishes bronchitis from other upper airway infections such as pharyngitis. The cough may develop slowly or rapidly and usually progresses, becoming productive with mucopurulent sputum. Fever is not usually present. Breath sounds reveal rhonchi and coarse crackles bilaterally, and the chest x-ray is usually normal. This respiratory condition is almost always caused by a virus, so cultures are not useful. Most infants have symptoms suggestive of an upper respiratory tract infection for 2 to 7 days before the onset of bronchiolitis. These infants are usually irritable and restless, with a mild fever. Again, the most common clinical sign is cough. As the infection progresses, the infant may experience vomiting, diarrhea, noisy upper airway breathing, and an increased respiratory rate. Infants who require hospitalization have noisy, labored breathing with tachypnea and tachycardia. Many of these infants have a mild conjunctivitis,

acute bronchitis: a short, severe attack of bronchitis, with fever and a productive cough

bronchiolitis [BRONG kee oh LIGHT is]: inflammation of the membranes lining the bronchioles

Learning Hint

What Is in a Term?

The ending *-iole* means small or little. For example, the bronchi are the larger airways while the bronchioles are the smaller airways (1 mm in diameter or less). The same can be said for an artery versus an arteriole.

and 5% to 10% may also have otitis media. Because of their increased work of breathing and coughing, combined with fever, the infants are frequently dehydrated.

In the adult, acute bronchitis is almost always self-limiting, and the goals of therapy should be to provide comfort to the patient. Guidelines from the Centers for Disease Control and Prevention state that the only indication for antibiotics is acute bronchitis as a result of pertussis. Unfortunately, antibiotic prescriptions for this condition are common. In the well infant, bronchiolitis is also usually a self-limiting disease, and all that is necessary is to wait for the underlying viral infection to resolve. Hospitalization is necessary for a child suffering from respiratory failure or dehydration.

Viruses are the most common infectious agents that cause bronchitis. The common cold viruses (coronavirus and rhinovirus), influenza virus, adenovirus, and respiratory syncytial virus (RSV) are most often involved. In infants and children, the same pathogens are usually involved. Even though it has been suggested that the same bacterial pathogens that cause pneumonia such as *Streptococcus pneumoniae, Moraxella catarrhalis, Haemophilus influenzae,* and *Staphylococcus aureus* can cause bronchitis, there is no convincing evidence that this is the case.

Bronchiolitis is an acute viral infection of the lower respiratory tract of infants. The peak attack age for children is between 10 months and 2 years of age. Incidence spikes in the winter months and persists through the spring. Bronchiolitis is one of the major reasons that infants under the age of 6 months require hospitalization. RSV is the most common cause of bronchiolitis, accounting for over 50% of cases. Certain times of the year can bring almost epidemic incidence of RSV, with over 80% of bronchiolitis cases during those times caused by the virus. Parainfluenza virus types 1, 2, and 3 cause most of the rest of the cases of bronchiolitis. Bacteria only rarely cause this disease.

Patients with acute bronchitis frequently self-medicate with over-the-counter cough and cold remedies. The most common medications used are for symptomatic therapy. Analgesics, antipyretics, or acetaminophen are helpful in reducing the malaise, lethargy, and fever in adults. Persistent cough may require nighttime suppression with cough-suppressing mixtures. Please note that one should avoid suppressing a productive cough except when it is persistent enough to disrupt sleep.

Because bacteria rarely cause bronchiolitis, antibiotics should not be used routinely. The aerosolization and inhalation of the antiviral agent ribavirin may offer benefit to a small number of bronchiolitis cases. This agent is effective against a variety of RNA and DNA viruses, including influenza, parainfluenza, and respiratory syncytial virus (RSV). Use of the aerosolized drug requires special nebulizer equipment (small-particle aerosol generator) and specifically trained personnel for administration via an oxygen hood or mist tent. Special care must be taken to avoid drug particle deposition and clogging of respiratory tubing and valves in mechanical ventilators.

Most experts recommend reserving ribavirin for severely ill patients, especially those with serious underlying disorders such as bronchopulmonary dysplasia, congenital heart disease, prematurity, or immunodeficiency disorders.

pneumonia: an acute or chronic disease marked by inflammation of the lungs and caused by viruses, bacteria, or other microorganisms and sometimes by physical and chemical irritants

Pneumonia

Pneumonia is the ninth leading cause of death in the United States and one of the most common causes of hospitalization. It is defined as an inflammation of the lung tissue and may be caused by bacteria, viruses, fungi, or even noninfectious agents such as drugs or chemicals. The principal site of infection is in the alveoli and surrounding interstitial tissue.

Individuals with pneumonia classically present with high white blood cell counts, high fevers, crackles, rhonchi, bronchial breath sounds, and dullness to percussion over the involved areas of the lung. Patients with pneumonia may have pleural effusions, and their chest x-rays usually reveal infiltrates or signs of consolidation (Figure 9-3). Patients with pneumonia are far more likely to experience complications such as hypoxia (lack of oxygen to tissues), cardiopulmonary failure, and possible spread of infection to other organs by way of the bloodstream. There are several well-defined categories of pneumonia that help to define appropriate therapy, and we will review this disease according to these subclassifications.

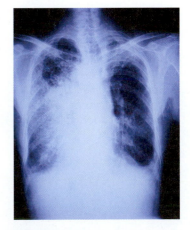

FIGURE 9-3 Chest x-ray of pneumonia. © joloei/Shutterstock.com.

Community-Acquired Pneumonia (CAP)

Community-acquired pneumonia (CAP) is an infection of the lung tissue that, in its purest definition, is contracted outside the institutional setting (institutional meaning nursing homes, hospitals, or any other place that might encourage the transmission of bacteria between compromised

community-acquired pneumonia (CAP): most common type of pneumonia that occurs outside hospitals or other health care facilities

individuals). This definition by setting has evolved to be more a description of the likely pathogens than a delineation of where the disease was contracted. *Streptococcus pneumoniae, Haemophilus influenzae, Mycoplasma pneumoniae, Chlamydophila pneumoniae,* and *Legionella* spp. account for the majority of cases of bacterial CAP, with *S. pneumoniae* responsible for a majority of the cases of acute CAP. Gram-negative bacteria and *Staphylococcus aureus* are uncommon causes of CAP but are more likely in patients who have taken antibiotics or have underlying respiratory diseases.

The most significant problem in the treatment of CAP is the growing resistance of *Streptococcus pneumoniae* to antimicrobials. This increasing resistance, combined with the much wider variety of organisms causing the disease, has made diagnosis and treatment a much greater therapeutic challenge.

Atypical Pneumonia

The term *atypical* was used to describe organisms that were not detectable on Gram stain and were not able to be grown on standard culture media but were causes of pneumonia. Over the years, organisms such as *Chlamydophila pneumoniae, Mycoplasma pneumoniae,* and *Legionella pneumophila* have been found to cause pneumonia yet could not be cultured using standard media. Viral causes of pneumonia are also included in this group. Except for *Legionella,* these organisms are common causes of pneumonia, especially in outpatients. All of these causes were lumped into the classification of **atypical pneumonia**. One of the most recent bacterial additions to this class was the outbreak and identification of a new organism, *Legionella pneumophila,* at the 1976 Philadelphia convention of the American Legion.

The term *atypical pneumonia* has been in use in the medical literature for over a century to refer to a subset of CAP organisms (e.g., *Legionella* spp., *Chlamydophila pneumoniae,* and *Mycoplasma pneumoniae*). However, some suggest we should no longer use this term because there is no way to distinguish typical versus atypical CAP pathogens clinically. However, for the purpose of this book, we will still use this term for contrasting purposes.

Current recommendations from the Infectious Diseases Society of America and the American Thoracic Society for the treatment of CAP recommend that empiric therapy should cover both the typical and atypical causative organisms.

Mycoplasma pneumoniae infections tend to follow epidemic patterns, with outbreaks every 4 to 8 years, making it hard to define its true incidence. *Legionella* tends to infect older and more immunocompromised patients. It also has a more seasonal occurrence, tending to break out in the spring, when air conditioning is started. *Chlamydophila* tends to infect young people such as college students and military recruits.

atypical pneumonia: organisms that cannot be cultured with standard microbiological media or techniques, and do not respond to treatment with penicillins or other antibiotics classically used for typical pneumonia

When you analyze the signs, symptoms, and chest x-rays of patients infected with these three atypical pathogens, very little difference can be seen between atypical and typical pneumonia. *Mycoplasma* may be more slow and insidious and *Legionella* more rapidly progressive, but that is not standard for all. Keep in mind as stated before, the only real difference between the atypical organisms—*Chlamydophila, Legionella,* and *Mycoplasma*—and the typical pneumonia organisms—*S. pneumoniae, M. catarrhalis,* and *H. influenzae*—is that the atypical organisms cannot be cultured with standard microbiological media or techniques, and they do not respond to treatment with penicillins or other antibiotics classically used for typical pneumonia.

In the past, antibiotic therapy for CAP was fairly simple. It was quite likely that *S. pneumoniae* was the causative organism, and the pneumococcus responded very well to treatment with penicillin. However, as early as 1967, resistant pneumococcus began to show up. We are now faced with 20% to 40% of *S. pneumoniae* strains showing resistance to penicillin. *S. pneumoniae* still accounts for the majority of CAP cases, but other organisms are creeping up in incidence. Because eradication of the offending organism is one of our major treatment goals in pneumonia, appropriate empiric antibiotic therapy is a major challenge.

The first priority in the treatment of pneumonia is to evaluate the patient's respiratory function and to determine if the patient requires hospitalization or can be treated as an outpatient. Patients may require intravenous fluids, oxygen, bronchodilators, chest physiotherapy with postural drainage, or even temporarily a breathing machine (mechanical ventilator). The second priority in hospitalized patients is to obtain cultures of the sputum and blood and to use other diagnostic procedures to determine the microbiological cause of the acute disease. Assessing the patient's clinical setting can help the choice of empiric therapy once you understand what pathogens are likely in specific patient populations. Table 9-1 can help you consider these circumstances.

Empiric therapy is guided by local resistance patterns in addition to considering the patient's clinical setting, prior exposure to antibiotics, clinical condition, chest x-ray, and underlying state of health.

Guidelines for the treatment of CAP continue to be revised, and the clinician must be careful to review current literature for the most up-to-date recommendations. The American Thoracic Society and the Infectious Diseases Society of America published a joint guideline in 2007 that continues to be periodically updated. They recommend macrolides (erythromycin, clarithromycin, or azithromycin) or doxycycline (or tetracycline) for children aged 8 years or older or an oral beta-lactam with good antipneumococcal activity (cefuroxime axetil, amoxicillin, or amoxicillin clavulanate) as the first-line therapies for CAP. An oral fluoroquinolone with improved activity against *S. pneumoniae* (levofloxacin, moxifloxacin, or gatifloxacin) may be used for the treatment of adults for whom one of these regimens has already failed, who are allergic to the alternative agents, or who have a documented infection with a highly drug-resistant pneumococcus. The fluoroquinolones should not be used in children because of serious potential side effects. For children younger than 5 years in whom atypical pathogens are uncommon and for whom doxycycline and fluoroquinolone should be avoided, beta-lactams are the best choice.

TABLE 9-1 Empiric Antibiotic Choices for Adult Pneumonias

Clinical Setting	Likely Pathogen	Therapy
Elderly patient, from nursing home or other care facility (health care–associated pneumonia)	*Streptococcus pneumoniae* *Moraxella catarrhalis* *Haemophilus influenzae* *Klebsiella pneumoniae* *Staphylococcus aureus* Gram-negative bacilli	Piperacillin tazobactam, third- or fourth-generation cephalosporin, imipenem–cilastatin, or meropenem
History of chronic bronchitis	*Streptococcus pneumoniae*	Amoxicillin, doxycycline, cefprozil, amoxicillin/clavulanate, clarithromycin, azithromycin, fluoroquinolone
Alcoholic	*Streptococcus pneumoniae* *Klebsiella pneumoniae* *Staphylococcus aureus* *Haemophilus influenzae* Possibly anaerobes from the oral cavity	ampicillin–sulbactam, piperacillin–tazobactam, plus aminoglycoside; imipenem–cilastatin or meropenem, fluoroquinolone, vancomycin (if MRSA suspected)
Previously healthy, ambulatory patient (CAP)	*Streptococcus pneumoniae*, *Mycoplasma pneumoniae*	Clarithromycin, azithromycin, or doxycycline
Aspiration pneumonia	Anaerobes from the oral cavity *Staphylococcus aureus*, gram-negative enteric organisms	Penicillin, clindamycin, ampicillin–sulbactam
Ventilator–associated (VAP) or health care–associated (HCAP) pneumonia	Gram-negative bacilli such as *Klebsiella pneumoniae*, *Enterobacter* sp., *Pseudomonas aeruginosa*, *Staphylococcus aureus*	Piperacillin–tazobactam, imipenem-cilastatin, meropenem, expanded-spectrum cephalosporins such as ceftazidime or cefepime plus an aminoglycoside, fluoroquinolone

✋ **9-2**
Stop and Review

1. _____ was a microorganism discovered after a number of people attending a convention in Philadelphia developed pneumonia.

2. _____ is the most common cause of community-acquired pneumonia.

3. *Legionella pneumophila, Mycoplasma pneumoniae,* and *Chlamydophila pneumoniae* are commonly called _____.

4. _____ is the ninth leading cause of death in the United States.

5. Increasing antibiotic resistance to the pathogen _____ is a big problem because it is a common cause of CAP.

Viral Pneumonias

In some studies looking at patients with community-acquired pneumonia, viruses were a cause in up to one-third of the cases. Viruses are difficult to culture and therefore are infrequently reported as causes in most clinical settings. Some hospitals are beginning to use molecular diagnostic methods such as polymerase chain reaction (PCR) tests for viral diagnosis.

The difficulty for the clinician is distinguishing between viral colonization and infection. Because viruses may be present in our upper airways without causing disease, a bacterial cause must be ruled out before deciding to withhold antibiotics in a patient with pneumonia. At times, both bacteria and a virus may coinfect a patient with pneumonia, and this usually results in a more severe disease.

Table 9-2 lists viruses commonly implicated as a cause of pneumonia and risk factors contributing to infection.

Tracheobronchitis

Tracheobronchitis is a pneumonia-like infection associated with patients who require breathing machines (mechanical ventilators). The breathing tube inserted into the trachea bypasses the normal defenses of the upper airway and lungs and makes the patient more prone to infection (Figure 9-4). Patients with this infection have a fever, new or increased sputum production, but no evidence of pneumonia on a chest x-ray.

tracheobronchitis [TRAY kee oh brong KYE tis]: inflammation of the mucous membrane of the trachea and bronchi

TABLE 9-2 Viral Causes of Pneumonia

Virus	At-Risk Populations
Influenza virus	Elderly, patients with chronic diseases especially lung disease, children younger than 2 years
Avian influenza (H5N1) (bird flu)	Populations living in close quarters with poultry
Parainfluenza	Immunocompromised adults
Respiratory syncytial virus	All ages
Adenovirus	Military recruits
Human metapneumovirus	Young children and older adults
Severe acute respiratory syndrome (SARS)*	All ages
Coronaviruses	All ages
Hantavirus	Spread to humans from infected mice
Varicella zoster virus	Adults
Middle East respiratory syndrome virus (MERS-CoV)*	People living in the Arabian peninsula

*SARS and MERS-CoV are of the coronavirus family

© 2016 Cengage Learning®.

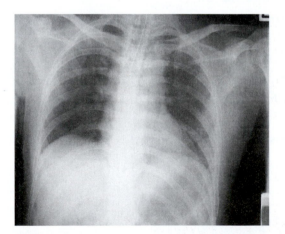

FIGURE 9-4 A chest film showing endotracheal tube placement above the bifurcation of the right and left lung.
© Santibhavank P/Shutterstock.com.

health care–associated pneumonia (HCAP): pneumonia acquired as a result of exposure in a health care setting

A sputum sample is obtained from the breathing tube (endotracheal tube) and sent to the microbiology laboratory for Gram staining and culture. The bacteria that are usually found as causes of this infection include *Staphylococcus aureus*, *Enterobacteriaceae*, and *Pseudomonas aeruginosa*.

Once the causative agent is identified by the microbiology laboratory, therapy can be directed at the pathogen found. Local antibiotic susceptibility patterns are important in determining therapy because differences in antibiotic resistance patterns can be found both regionally and nationally.

Health Care–Associated (HCAP), Ventilator-Associated (VAP), or Hospital-Acquired (HAP) Pneumonia

The common thread for **health care–associated pneumonia (HCAP)** is exposure to or frequent contact with various health care settings. Pneumonia is the second most common hospital-acquired infection in the United States and is associated with substantial morbidity and mortality.

Learning Hint

Immune Defense Bypass

Because intubation and mechanical ventilation bypass and therefore alter first-line patient respiratory defenses of the upper airway, they greatly increase the risk for health care–associated bacterial pneumonia.

Clinical Application

Precautions to Prevent Pneumonias

Pneumonias caused by *Legionella* sp., *Aspergillus* sp., and influenza virus are often caused by inhalation of contaminated aerosols. RSV infection usually occurs after viral inoculation of the conjunctivae or nasal mucosa by contaminated hands, again stressing the need for proper hand hygiene. Traditional preventive measures for VAP, HCAP, and HAP include taking precautions to decrease aspiration by the patient, preventing cross-contamination or colonization via hands of personnel, appropriate disinfection or sterilization of respiratory therapy devices, use of available vaccines to protect against particular infections, and education of hospital staff and patients. Figure 9-5 describes the pathogenesis of pneumonia acquired from health care settings.

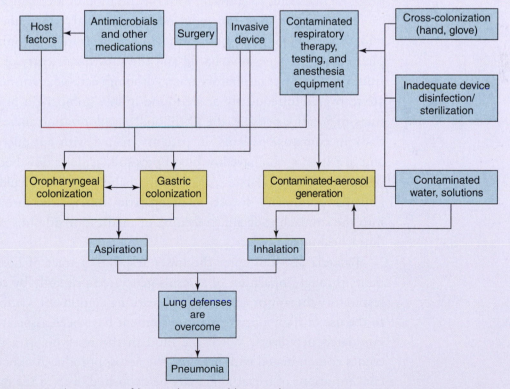

FIGURE 9-5 Pathogenesis of hospital-acquired bacterial pneumonia. © 2016 Cengage Learning®.

ventilator-associated pneumonia (VAP): pneumonia acquired as a result of being intubated and placed on a mechanical ventilator

Most patients who have so-called **ventilator-associated pneumonia (VAP)**, hospital-acquired pneumonia (HAP), or HCAP are persons who have severe underlying disease, are immunosuppressed, are comatose, or are otherwise incapacitated and who have cardiopulmonary disease. In addition, some health care–associated pneumonia patients are persons who have had thoracic or abdominal surgery. Although patients receiving mechanical ventilation do not represent a major proportion of patients who have pneumonia, they are at highest risk for acquiring a VAP.

Recent epidemiological studies have identified other subsets of patients who are at high risk for acquiring health care–associated bacterial pneumonia. Such patients include persons older than 70 years; persons who have endotracheal intubation and/or mechanically assisted ventilation, a depressed level of consciousness (particularly those with closed-head injury), or underlying chronic lung disease; and persons who have previously had an episode of a large-volume aspiration. Other risk factors include presence of a nasogastric tube, severe trauma, and recent bronchoscopy.

HCAP, HAP, and VAP have been associated with mortality rates of 20% to 50%. Patients receiving mechanically assisted ventilation have higher mortality rates than patients not receiving ventilation support; however, other factors (e.g., the patient's underlying disease and organ failure) are stronger predictors of death in patients who have pneumonia. VAP is difficult to diagnose but seems to correlate with the duration of mechanical ventilation.

The high incidence of gram-negative bacillary pneumonia in hospitalized patients might result from factors that promote colonization of the pharynx by gram-negative bacilli and the subsequent entry of these organisms into the lower respiratory tract. Although aerobic gram-negative bacilli are recovered infrequently or are found in low numbers in pharyngeal cultures of healthy persons, the likelihood of colonization increases substantially in comatose patients, in patients treated with antimicrobial agents, and in patients who have low blood pressure, acidosis (low body pH), high blood urea nitrogen lab test, alcoholism, diabetes mellitus, leukocytosis, leukopenia, pulmonary disease, or nasogastric (tube placed through the nose into the stomach to facilitate feeding or medication administration) or endotracheal tubes in place.

Bacteria also can enter the lower respiratory tract of hospitalized patients through inhalation of aerosols generated primarily by contaminated respiratory therapy or anesthesia or breathing equipment. Outbreaks related to the use of respiratory therapy equipment have been associated with contaminated nebulizers. When the fluid in the reservoir of a nebulizer becomes contaminated with bacteria, the aerosol produced may contain high concentrations of bacteria that can be deposited deep in the patient's lower respiratory tract. Contaminated aerosol inhalation is particularly hazardous for intubated patients because endotracheal and tracheal tubes provide direct access to the lower respiratory tract.

Several large studies have examined the potential risk factors for bacterial pneumonias acquired in a health care setting. Although specific risk factors have differed among study populations, they can be grouped into the following general categories:

1. Host factors (e.g., extremes of age and severe underlying conditions, including immunosuppression)

2. Factors that enhance colonization of the oropharynx and/or stomach by microorganisms (e.g., administration of antimicrobials, admission to an ICU, drugs that suppress stomach acid secretion or production, underlying chronic lung disease, or coma)

3. Conditions that favor aspiration or reflux (e.g., endotracheal intubation, insertion of a nasogastric tube, or supine position)

4. Conditions that require prolonged use of mechanical ventilation support with potential exposure to contaminated respiratory equipment and/or contact with contaminated or colonized hands of health care workers (HCWs)

5. Factors that impede adequate pulmonary toilet (cleaning) (e.g., undergoing surgical procedures that involve the head, neck, thorax, or upper abdomen, or being immobilized as a result of trauma or illness)

By sorting out these risk categories, the clinician can better define the likely pathogens and then choose the most appropriate empiric antibiotic therapy. Each patient is different, and individual analyses must be made. In general, selection of antibiotics for a patient with HCAP, VAP, or HAP requires an antibiotic to cover gram-negative pathogens, methicillin-resistant *Staphylococcus aureus* (MRSA), as well as the more common pneumonia pathogens. Most patients require more than one antibiotic to cover the entire spectrum of likely organisms. If a culture is obtained and the pathogenic organisms are isolated, the antibiotic regimen may be simplified or narrowed to specifically cover the isolated organisms.

Antibiotic Therapy Recommendations for the Treatment of Pneumonia Acquired in a Health Care Setting (HCAP, VAP, HAP)

Patients with pneumonia acquired in a health care setting require many supportive and symptomatic therapies. They may be mechanically ventilated, they may be in an ICU, and they may be very sick. It is not possible to go over all of their potential therapies in detail; you will need to use your clinical knowledge of respiratory illness to help the prescriber know what symptomatic therapies will be needed. We will focus on the antibiotic therapies at this point.

Antibiotic resistance in hospitals is variable, and specific institutions have their own guidelines. The newer antibiotics for resistant cases tend to be expensive and restricted in use. The 2007 joint American Thoracic Society/Infectious Diseases Society of America guideline recommends that empiric therapy should cover MRSA, *Pseudomonas aeruginosa,* gram-negative bacilli, and *Legionella.* Empiric therapy decisions can be modified based on local data indicating the most frequent bacterial pathogens isolated and their respective susceptibility patterns. Moderately ill patients with pneumonia may receive intravenous ceftriaxone, levofloxacin, or ertapenem. Alternatively, in patients who have been hospitalized for more than five days and have been receiving antibiotics previously, intravenous cefepime or ceftazidime, meropenem or doripenem, or piperacillin-tazobactam plus either gentamicin or tobramycin should be considered along with a drug that has activity against MRSA such as vancomycin or linezolid.

Aspiration Pneumonia

aspiration pneumonia: bronchopneumonia that develops due to entrance of foreign materials into the tracheobronchial tree; usually consists of oral or regurgitated gastric contents

Aspiration pneumonia can be either chemical (exposure to stomach acid) or bacterial. Bacteria can invade the lower respiratory tract by aspiration of oropharyngeal organisms or inhalation of aerosols containing bacteria. In addition, bacterial translocation from the gastrointestinal tract has been hypothesized recently as a mechanism for infection.

Aspiration pneumonia brings a different set of possible pathogens. If the pneumonia is because of the acid exposure, antibiotics won't help. Only symptomatic therapy can be used as the lungs heal. Empiric antibiotic therapy generally consists of agents with anaerobic and gram-negative coverage in their spectrums of activity.

Patients who develop aspiration pneumonia in the community setting should be treated with an antibiotic that is effective against gram-positive anaerobes. Such antibiotics include clindamycin or penicillins. If the patient

Clinical Application
Causes of Aspiration

In radioisotope tracer studies, 45% of healthy adults were found to aspirate during sleep. Persons who swallow abnormally (e.g., those who have depressed consciousness, neuromuscular disease, respiratory tract instrumentation and/or mechanically assisted ventilation, or GI tract instrumentation or diseases) or who have just undergone surgery are particularly likely to aspirate.

aspirated while hospitalized or is significantly debilitated by coexisting disease, broader-spectrum therapy should be used to expand the coverage to gram-negative pathogens. Generally, clindamycin or a penicillin combined with a beta-lactamase inhibitor (such as piperacillin-tazobactam) plus an aminoglycoside (tobramycin, gentamicin, or amikacin) should be considered.

Pneumocystis jiroveci Pneumonia

Pneumocystis jiroveci pneumonia (PJP), formerly known as *Pneumocystis carinii*, is a complication of HIV infection. In the past, this organism was classified as a protozoan, but recent genetic studies have now classified it as a fungus. It should be noted that it can also occur in non–HIV-infected patients. Patients with organ or bone marrow transplants and patients taking certain medications that suppress immunity such as glucocorticoids (often called *steroids*, e.g., medicines like prednisone) are also at risk of developing pneumonia from this organism. The common thread between these diseases and medications is they cause defects in cell-mediated immunity. Like tuberculosis, *Pneumocystis* can be asymptomatic and latent and live in our bodies without causing disease until we develop a problem with our cell-mediated immune defense.

Symptoms, when present, may include fever, cough, tachypnea, and dyspnea. Arterial blood gases are one of the key factors in therapy decisions. The disease can be classified as mild, moderate, or severe on the basis of arterial oxygenation.

Factors to consider when starting drug therapy for PJP are whether it is a first episode, arterial blood gases, history of drug reaction, and route of therapy. Drugs used for treatment are IV trimethoprim–sulfamethoxazole (TMP–SMX), dapsone, IV clindamycin, primaquine, atovaquone, or IV pentamidine. These drugs are toxic. For example, more than 50% of patients who receive trimethoprim-sulfamethoxazole may develop rash, fever, leukopenia, hepatitis, or thrombocytopenia. Pentamidine can cause azotemia, pancreatitis, hypocalcemia, or leukopenia, to name a few complications.

Learning Hint

Learn How to Keep Up to Date

Because care of patients with pneumonia is quite common, therapeutic guidelines for the care of pneumonia patients are published and updated frequently. Individual institutions may have guidelines as well. It is important to stay updated with the current recommendations. The American Thoracic Society, the British Thoracic Society, the Canadian Infectious Diseases Society, and the Infectious Diseases Society of America all publish sets of guidelines (some jointly), and each of these societies updates them regularly.

Tuberculosis

Even though we discussed antitubercular drugs in the previous chapter, no respiratory infectious disease chapter would be complete without a short discussion of **tuberculosis**. Tuberculosis (TB) is a chronic disease caused by *Mycobacterium tuberculosis*. Although it can affect any part of the body, it most commonly affects the lungs. While there has been a gradual decline in the number of active cases over the years, there are still millions of people with TB infection that have not progressed to active TB. TB is spread by microscopic droplets and is an airborne disease. It can be spread when an infected person coughs or sneezes. Once the droplet is inhaled, it becomes encapsulated, and the infection is latent.

When the infection droplets called bacilli escape, the disease becomes active. Symptoms of active TB can range from none to weight loss, fever, night sweats, or bloody sputum. Diagnosis is made with a skin test (Mantoux) or purified protein derivative (PPD) test (Figure 9-6), sputum sample, and chest x-ray. Drug therapy of TB is aimed at preventive therapy for latent infection or treatment of active TB disease.

Preventive therapy is usually with isoniazid for 6–12 months, which will decrease the risk that the infection will progress to disease. Research is always in progress to determine the easiest yet most effective method of prophylaxis. Certain

tuberculosis: an infectious airborne disease caused by tubercle bacteria that most commonly affects the respiratory system but other parts of the body can also be affected

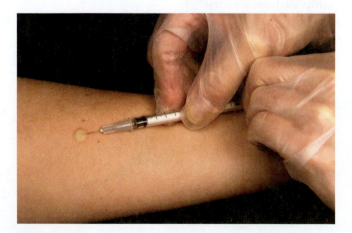

FIGURE 9-6 Mantoux tuberculin skin test being used to evaluate the patient for TB infection. Source: CDC/ Gabrielle Benenson. Photo credit: Greg Knobloch.

people are at a higher risk for developing TB; this group includes people who are in close contact with others with TB, people with a chest x-ray suggesting previous TB that has not been treated, persons with HIV, and people who are substance (drug) abusers. Patients on corticosteroids also may be at increased risk of disease progression.

Treatment of active TB takes 6 to 24 months. Drug treatment must be in combination because resistance is a problem. Drugs used are isoniazid, rifampin, pyrazinamide, ethambutol, and streptomycin. Because of resistance, adherence to the drug regimen is the key point for TB. One way to try to reduce tuberculosis treatment failures is to use directly observed treatment (DOT) to make sure a patient is medication compliant.

Bioterrorism

Pulmonary irritants such as chlorine and phosgene have been used since World War I. Through biochemical reactions, these irritants can cause laryngospasm and pulmonary edema. Anthrax acts as a biological weapon through skin contact or inhalational exposure and has been used for **bioterrorism**. Spore inhalation is transported to the lymphatic system where spores germinate and toxins are produced (Figure 9-7). Anthrax is best treated prophylactically with antibiotics such as ciprofloxacin.

Plague is a potential bioweapon because it is contagious with close contact and aerosol transmission is possible. Systemic illness warrants parenteral antibiotic therapy with agents such as streptomycin or gentamicin. Postexposure prophylaxis is usually oral treatment with doxycycline and ciprofloxacin. Vaccination was discontinued in 1999.

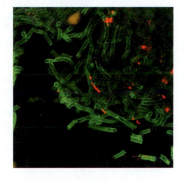

FIGURE 9-7 *Bacillus anthracis*; notice the cell walls are green and the spores are red. Source: CDC/ Dr. Sherif Zaki; Dr. Kathi Tatti; Elizabeth White.

bioterrorism: the use of biological warfare agents against civilian populations

Avian Influenza

Avian flu, also known as bird flu is a type of influenza virus carried in the intestines of wild birds. The first avian influenza virus to infect humans occurred in Hong Kong in 1997. The epidemic was linked to chickens and classified as avian influenza A (H5N1). Figure 9-8 shows the genetic evolution of another strain called the H7N9 strain. Notice how the multiple reassortment of genes can lead to a new emerging virus.

Though the wild birds themselves may not get sick, they transmit the virus to domestic birds. Poultry industry conditions make it possible for humans to be exposed and a humanized mutated strain to evolve. The avian flu virus (H5N1) has been shown to survive in the environment for long

avian flu: highly contagious viral disease caused by influenza A virus subtypes H5 and H7; also known as bird flu

Genetic Evolution of H7N9 Virus in China, 2013

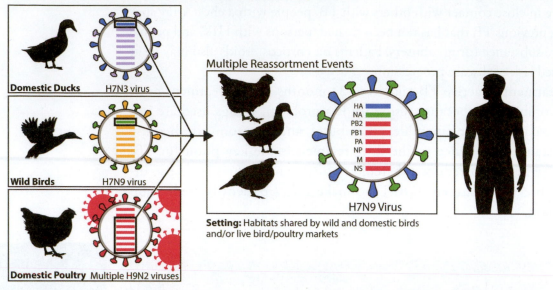

The eight genes of the H7N9 virus are closely related to avian influenza viruses found in domestic ducks, wild birds and domestic poultry in Asia. The virus likely emerged from "reassortment," a process in which two or more influenza viruses co-infect a single host and exchange genes. This can result in the creation of a new influenza virus. Experts think multiple reassortment events led to the creation of the H7N9 virus. These events may have occurred in habitats shared by wild and domestic birds and/or in live bird/poultry markets, where different species of birds are bought and sold for food. As the above diagram shows, the H7N9 virus likely obtained its HA (hemagglutinin) gene from domestic ducks, its NA (neuraminidase) gene from wild birds, and its six remaining genes from multiple related H9N2 influenza viruses in domestic poultry.

FIGURE 9-8 The genetic evolution of the H7N9 virus in China in 2013. Source: CDC/Douglas E. Jordan. Illustrator: Dan Higgins.

periods of time. Infection may be spread simply by touching contaminated surfaces. Birds who were infected with this flu can continue to release the virus in their feces and saliva for as long as 10 days.

Because the immune system of humans has not been exposed, it does not have any antibodies, allowing a potentially devastating outbreak. Some of the clinical features that may present after an incubation period of 2 to 5 days are high fever, cough, rhinorrhea, diarrhea, vomiting, abdominal pain, shortness of breath, myalgia, and headache. Some patients may have lymphopenia, thrombocytopenia, or pulmonary infiltrates. Symptoms appear like a viral pneumonia, with progression to acute respiratory distress syndrome a possibility. Treating avian influenza is difficult, making prophylaxis and supportive treatment imperative.

In general, treatment with the antiviral medication oseltamivir (Tamiflu) or zanamivir (Relenza) may make the disease less severe if the patient starts taking the medicine within 48 hours after symptoms start. Oseltamivir may also be prescribed for persons who live in the same house as those diagnosed with avian flu.

Chapter Summary

- This chapter discussed the clinical presentation, diagnosis, and treatment of common infections affecting the respiratory tract.

- Health care professionals frequently encounter patients with respiratory tract infections so this chapter should provide a good foundation for understanding these diseases.

- We started with a discussion of upper respiratory tract infections and then worked our way down to discuss pneumonia, tuberculosis,

- agents of bioterrorism, and finally avian influenza.

- It is important to remember that many upper respiratory tract infections are caused by viruses, and with the exception of influenza, are not treatable with antimicrobials.

- Knowing when antimicrobials are useful is vitally important because treating viral infections with antibiotics promotes the development of resistance in bacteria.

Case Study

Mrs. Ida May, a 75-year-old woman, activated 911 because of difficulty breathing, shaking chills, and cough productive of a thick green sputum. She has been in the hospital twice in the last 2 months. The first time was for a total right hip replacement, and the second time was for a blood clot in her right femoral vein. Upon arrival the paramedics noted Mrs. May was unable to speak in full sentences, and her pulse oximetry reading was 80% (measures the saturation of hemoglobin with oxygen, normal values are >92%). She is immediately placed on oxygen delivered via a face mask and transported to the local emergency department. A chest radiograph revealed diffuse lung infiltrates consistent with bilateral pneumonia. What type of pneumonia does Mrs. May have? What are her risk factors for developing this particular type of pneumonia? What empiric antibiotic treatment would you recommend?

Chapter Review

Match the term with its distinguishing feature or definition.

1. _____ community-acquired pneumonia
2. _____ bronchiolitis
3. _____ aspiration pneumonia
4. _____ sinusitis
5. _____ pharyngitis
6. _____ health care–associated pneumonia
7. _____ tracheobronchitis
8. _____ tuberculosis
9. _____ acute bronchitis
10. _____ epiglottitis

a. nasal stuffiness, nasal discharge, and pain or pressure in the face

b. caused by group A streptococcus or virus

c. lung infection acquired outside the hospital

d. pneumonia acquired by patients who are hospitalized

e. infection occurring in patients with breathing tubes

f. treatment started with four drugs

g. pneumonia that may occur after vomiting

h. airway emergency

i. antibiotics are not useful

j. infection with RSV in infants

Fill in the blanks.

11. _____ is a rare but serious complication from group A *Streptococcal* pharyngitis.

12. Influenza may be treated with an oral neuraminidase inhibitor called _____.

13. PCR testing may identify _____ as a cause of pneumonia because the organisms are difficult to culture.

14. _____ is a lung infection that may occur in patients infected with HIV.

15. _____ is a way of making sure patients who have tuberculosis take their medications.

16. _____ is the second most common health care–associated infection.

17. The most common bacterial cause of community-acquired pneumonia is _____.

18. Acute bronchitis could be treated with antimicrobials if caused by _____, which is only responsible for 1% of U.S. cases.

Additional Activities

1. Visit the Hospital Compare Web site, which is the official website maintained by the Department of Health and Human Services, to view the infection rates of hospitals in your area. How are the hospitals in your area performing compared with the national benchmarks and each other?

2. Speak with local health care providers concerning their use of antimicrobials for infections that are commonly caused by viruses. How well are physicians doing in your community to prevent antimicrobial resistance?

3. Divide your class into at least two groups. Make up note cards with each respiratory tract infection on one side and the potential etiological agents and treatment on the other. Choose a game show host and have this individual ask questions concerning these infections of each team using the information found on the note cards. The team earns a point for each correct answer.

4. Find images of x-ray and CT pictures of lungs with different types of pneumonias on the Internet.

Media Connection

Go to the accompanying online resources and have fun learning as you play games, view animations and videos, and take practice tests to help reinforce key concepts you learned in this chapter.

APPENDIX A

Answers to Chapter Stop and Review Questions

Chapter 1

Stop and Review 1-1

1. Flora
2. Virulence
3. Mitochondria
4. Nucleus

Stop and Review 1-2

1. None, these body fluids should never contain microorganisms
2. Normal flora, pathogens
3. *Clostridium difficile, Salmonella typhi,* or *Giardia lamblia*

Stop and Review 1-3

1. Innate
2. Cellular, antibody
3. Present
4. Humoral or antibody
5. Cell-mediated

Chapter 2

Stop and Review 2-1

1. Binary fission
2. Immunology
3. Nosocomial

Stop and Review 2-2

1. Bacteriology—studies bacteria

   Virology—studies viruses

   Mycology—studies yeasts and molds

   Parasitology—studies parasites

2. Hand washing

3. Bacteria have two names. The first name is the genus (similar to your last name), and the second name is the species (similar to your first name).

4. The morphology, or shape, of bacteria consists of three basic shapes: cocci—round, bacilli—rod-shaped, and spirilla—spiral shaped.

Stop and Review 2-3

1. Bacteria that retain a purple color after the decolorizing rinse is applied are termed gram-positive. The organisms that turn red or pink after the red dye is applied are termed gram-negative.

2. Culture, Susceptibility

3. Bacteriostatic refers to an agent that inhibits the replication of microorganisms. Bactericidal refers to an agent that actively kills bacteria.

4. Antibiotics are not effective against viral infections, the patient may develop adverse effects, and it promotes the development of resistant bacteria.

Chapter 3

Stop and Review 3-1

1. The HIV virus must be treated with at least three medicines at once to slow the development of resistance.

2. If you could identify a virus as the cause of an illness, then you could avoid the unnecessary prescription of antibiotics because they don't work against viruses.

3. Liver cirrhosis or cancer

4. Viruses

Stop and Review 3-2

1. Protozoa

2. Hookworm

3. Bed bugs

Stop and Review 3-3

1. *Candida*

2. Onychomycosis

3. *Aspergillus* may cause allergic reactions or a lung infection that spreads throughout the body. Patients who are immunocompromised (e.g., low white blood cell counts and organ or bone marrow transplant patients) are the most susceptible to serious, life-threatening infections.

Chapter 4

Stop and Review 4-1

1. Cleaning—the physical removal of foreign matter; sanitization—a process that reduces the total bacterial load to a safe level; disinfection—a process that eliminates vegetative, pathogenic microorganisms from an inanimate object; sterilization—the complete destruction or inactivation of all forms of microorganisms.

2. Health care–associated infections

3. Chain, infection

Stop and Review 4-2

1. 10

2. Pasteurization

3. Isopropyl, ethyl

Stop and Review 4-3

1. The combination of steam (water) and pressure is an effective way to sterilize items. Boiling water alone cannot sterilize an item.

2. Gas concentration, temperature, humidity, and time

3. Alcohol—denatures proteins and disrupts plasma membrane; quaternary ammonium—disrupts membranes; glutaraldehydes—inactivates enzymes by alkylation; phenols—denature proteins and disrupt the plasma membrane

Chapter 5

Stop and Review 5-1

1. Portals of entry

2. Direct contact

3. Vectors

Stop and Review 5-2

1. Properly washing your hands is the best way to prevent the spread of infection.
2. Gowns are worn to protect your skin and clothing during any activity that may generate splashes or spray of blood, body fluids, secretions, or excretions.
3. Soap and water should be used when caring for patients with diarrhea.

Stop and Review 5-3

1. Influenza
2. Sharps container
3. Droplet precautions

Chapter 6

Stop and Review 6-1

1. Infectious waste
2. Sharps
3. Gloves

Stop and Review 6-2

1. Medical, surgical
2. Three
3. One inch

Stop and Review 6-3

1. Swab
2. Povidone-iodine (Betadine)
3. Nasal or nasopharyngeal

Chapter 7

Stop and Review 7-1

1. Mortality
2. Morbidity
3. Epidemiology

4. Antibiotics

5. Broad spectrum

Stop and Review 7-2

1. Antibiotics may be classified as bacteriostatic vs. bactericidal, broad- vs. narrow-spectrum, or based on mechanism of action.

2. Broad-spectrum means the antibiotic would be effective against a wide range of bacteria. Broad-spectrum antibiotics are extremely useful for empiric (initial) therapy of very ill or immunocompromised patients because the specific pathogen or pathogens causing the infection may not be known to the treating clinician.

3. As you move from first to later generations of cephalosporins, gram-positive activity is generally better than gram-negative activity with earlier generations. Gram-negative activity is enhanced with later generations.

4. Carbapenems, doripenem

5. Monobactams, aztreonam

6. Cephalosporin, ceftazidime

7. Penicillin, ampicillin

Stop and Review 7-3

1. Bactericidal because the organisms would be killed instead of inhibited as with a bacteriostatic antibiotic.

2. Beta-lactams inhibit cell wall synthesis. Fluoroquinolones block two enzymes responsible for DNA synthesis.

3. Tetracyclines, minocycline

4. Macrolides, clarithromycin

5. Glycopeptides, vancomycin

6. Aminoglycosides, tobramycin

Stop and Review 7-4

1. Viruses replicate in a living host cell. This makes it difficult to kill the virus without harming the host cell.

2. Viruses are classified by whether they contain DNA or RNA.

Match the following drug and disease:

3. Herpes simplex, acyclovir

4. Tuberculosis, rifampin

5. Influenza, oseltamivir

6. *Clostridium difficle*, metronidazole

Chapter 8

Stop and Review 8-1

1. Meningitis is an infection of the meninges causing inflammation. Encephalitis is an inflammation of the brain tissue. With meningitis the patient may feel tired and have a headache. Patients with encephalitis, on the other hand, have those symptoms and abnormal brain function such as memory deficits, seizures, paralysis, and abnormal movements.

2. Herpes

3. *Neisseria meningitidis*

4. West Nile

Stop and Review 8-2

1. Symptomatic treatment should be tried before prescribing antibiotics.

2. Initial therapy should cover *Staphylococcus aureus* and anaerobes. If it develops in the hospital, coverage should also include gram-negative organisms.

Stop and Review 8-3

1. Conjunctivitis

2. Catheter-related bloodstream infection

3. Endocarditis

Stop and Review 8-4

1. Cellulitis, erysipelas

2. *Clostridium difficile*

3. *Clostridium perfringens*

Chapter 9

Stop and Review 9-1

1. d

2. c

3. a

4. b

Stop and Review 9-2

1. *Legionella pneumophila*
2. *Streptococcus pneumoniae*
3. Atypical organisms
4. Pneumonia
5. *Streptococcus pneumoniae*

Stop and Review 9-3

1. Viruses
2. Tracheobronchitis
3. Heath care–associated pneumonia
4. Aspiration pneumonia

APPENDIX B

Clinical Laboratory–Related Abbreviations and Acronyms

μg, mcg	Microgram
μL, μl	Microliter
μmol	Micromole
A	Absorbance
Ab	Antibody
ABGs	Arterial blood gases
ac	Before meals
ACT	Activated clotting time
AFB	Acid-fast bacillus
Ag	Antigen
AHG	Anti-human globulin
AIDS	Acquired immunodeficiency syndrome
ALL	Acute lymphocytic leukemia
ALP, AP	Alkaline phosphatase
ALT	Alanine aminotransferase (formerly SGPT)
am, AM	Morning
AML	Acute myelogenous leukemia
amt	Amount
ANA	Antinuclear antibody
AP	Anteroposterior
aPTT	Activated partial thromboplastin time
ARDS	Acute respiratory distress syndrome
AST	Aspartate aminotransferase (formerly SGOT)
BA	Blood agar
bacti	Bacteriology

BBP	Bloodborne pathogen
bid	Twice a day
BM	Bowel movement
BP	Blood pressure
BS	Bowel sounds
BSI	Body substance isolation
BSN	Bachelor of science in nursing
BT	Bleeding time
BUN	Blood urea nitrogen
$\overline{c}$	With
C	Centigrade, Celsius
C&S	Culture and sensitivity
CBC	Complete blood count
cc, ccm	Cubic centimeter
CC	Critical care
CCU	Coronary care unit
CD4	Protein on helper T-cell lymphocyte
CDC	Centers for Disease Control and Prevention
CFU	Colony-forming unit
CGL	Chronic granulocytic leukemia
chol	Cholesterol
CK	Creatine kinase
Cl	Chloride
CLL	Chronic lymphocytic leukemia
CLS	Clinical laboratory scientist
CLT	Clinical laboratory technician
cm	Centimeter
CMA	Certified medical assistant
CNA	Certified nurse aide
CNS	Central nervous system
CO	Carbon monoxide
CO$_2$	Carbon dioxide
COPD	Chronic obstructive pulmonary disease
COTA	Certified occupational therapy assistant

CPK	Creatine phosphokinase
crit	Hematocrit
CRNP	Certified registered nurse practitioner
CRP	C-reactive protein
CRT	Certified respiratory therapist
CSF	Cerebrospinal fluid
cu mm	Cubic millimeter, mm^3
CXR	Chest X-ray
DAT	Direct antiglobulin test
DDM	Doctor of dental medicine
DIC	Disseminated intravascular coagulation
diff	White blood cell differential count
dL	Deciliter
DO	Doctor of osteopathy
DOB	Date of birth
EBV	Epstein-Barr virus
E. coli	*Escherichia coli*
EDTA	Ethylenediaminetetraacetic acid
EHR	Electronic health records
EIA	Enzyme immunoassay
ELISA	Enzyme-linked immunosorbent assay
EMB	Eosin-methylene blue
EMT-B	Emergency medical technician–basic
EMT-I	Emergency medical technician–intermediate
EMT-P	Emergency medical technician–paramedic
ESR	Erythrocyte sedimentation rate
ET	Endotracheal
E.U.	Ehrlich units
F	Fahrenheit
FBS	Fasting blood sugar
FDA	Food and Drug Administration
FDP	Fibrinogen degradation products
fL	Femtoliter
FUO	Fever of unknown origin

g	Gram
GC	Gonococcus, gonorrhea
GFR	Glomerular filtration rate
GGT	Gamma-glutamyltransferase
GI	Gastrointestinal
gt	Drop
gtt	Drops
GTT	Glucose tolerance test
GU	Genitourinary
H&H	Hemoglobin and hematocrit
HAV	Hepatitis A virus
Hb, HgB	Hemoglobin
HbA1c	Hemoglobin A1c
HBV	Hepatitis B virus
hCG	Human chorionic gonadotropin
HCL	Hydrochloric acid
HCO$_3^-$	Bicarbonate
Hct	Hematocrit
HCV	Hepatitis C virus
HDL chol	High-density lipoprotein cholesterol
HIV	Human immunodeficiency virus
HLA	Human leukocyte antigen
H$_2$O	Water
HPF	High-power field
HPV	Human papillomavirus
hs-CRP	High-sensitivity C-reactive protein
HSV	Herpes simplex virus
ICU	Intensive care unit
Ig	Immunoglobulin
IgA	Immunoglobulin A
IgE	Immunoglobulin E
IgG	Immunoglobulin G
IgM	Immunoglobulin M
IM	Infectious mononucleosis

IM, i.m.	Intramuscular
inj	Injection
I&O	Intake and output
ITP	Immune thrombocytopenic purpura
IU	International unit
IV, i.v.	Intravenous
K	Potassium
kg	Kilogram
L	Liter
LDL chol	Low-density lipoprotein cholesterol
LP	Lumbar puncture
LPF	Low-power field
LVN	Licensed vocational nurse
m	Meter
M	Molar
MAR	Medication administration record
MCH	Mean cell hemoglobin
MCHC	Mean cell hemoglobin concentration
MCV	Mean cell volume
MD	Doctor of medicine, muscular dystrophy
mEq	Milliequivalent
mg	Milligram
MI	Myocardial infarction
MIC	Minimum inhibitory concentration
mIU	Milli-international unit
mL	Milliliter
MLS	Medical laboratory scientist
MLT	Medical laboratory technician
mm	Millimeter
mmol	Millimole
mol	Mole
MPV	Mean platelet volume
MRI	Magnetic resonance imaging
MRSA	Methicillin-resistant *Staphylococcus aureus*

MSDS	Material safety data sheet
MSN	Master of science in nursing
MT	Medical technologist
N	Normal, normality
Na	Sodium
NaCl	Sodium chloride
NG	Nasogastric (tube)
nm	Nanometer
npo	Nothing by mouth
O&P	Ova and parasites
O.D.	Optical density
OGTT	Oral glucose tolerance test
oint.	Ointment
OPIM	Other potentially infectious material
OT	Occupational therapy
OTR	Occupational therapist
PCV	Packed cell volume
PDR	*Physician's Desk Reference*
pg	Picogram
pH	Hydrogen ion concentrate
PharmD	Doctor of pharmacy
PLT	Platelet
PMN	Polymorphonuclear neutrophil
po	By mouth
POC	Point of care
POCT	Point of care test(ing)
POL	Physician office laboratory
pp	Postprandial (after meals)
PPD	Purified protein derivative (tuberculin test)
PPE	Personal protective equipment
PPM	Parts per million
Preop, pre-op	Preoperative
prot	Protocol
PSA	Prostate specific antigen

PT	Prothrombin time, protime
PTA	Physical therapy assistant
q	Every
QA	Quality assessment
QC	Quality control
qh	Every hour
qhs	Every night
qns	Quantity not sufficient
qs	Quantity sufficient
RA	Rheumatoid arthritis
RBC	Red blood cell
RD	Respiratory disease, registered dietitian
RDH	Registered dental hygienist
REEGT	Registered electroencephalography technologist
RF	Rheumatoid factors
RHIA	Registered health information administrator
RhIG	$Rh_o(D)$ immune globulin
RHIT	Registered health information technician
RIA	Radioimmunoassay
RN	Registered nurse
RNA	Ribonucleic acid
RPh	Registered pharmacist
rpm	Revolutions per minute
RPR	Rapid plasma reagin
RRT	Registered radiologic technologist, registered respiratory therapist
sed rate	Erythrocyte sedimentation rate
SEM	Scanning electron microscope
SGOT	Serum glutamic oxaloacetic transaminase
SGPT	Serum glutamic-pyruvic transaminase
SI	International unites (Le Systeme International d'Unites)
SICU	Surgical intensive care unit
sl	Sublingual (under the tongue)
SP	Standard Precautions

sp. gr.	Specific gravity
staph	*Staphylococcus*
stat	Immediately
STD	Sexually transmitted disease
STI	Sexually transmitted infection
strep	*Streptococcus*
STS	Serological tests for syphilis
TB	Tuberculosis
TEM	Transmission electron microscope
TIA	Transient ischemic attack
tid	Three times a day
TSH	Thyroid-stimulating hormone
UA	Urinalysis
UP	Universal precautions
URI	Upper respiratory infection
UTI	Urinary tract infection
UV	Ultraviolet
VD	Venereal disease
VDRL	Venereal disease research laboratory
VRE	Vancomycin-resistant *Enterococcus*
WBC	White blood cell

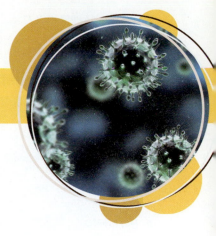

APPENDIX C

Select Viral, Bacterial, Fungal, and Protozoa Conditions and Their Causative Agents

Viral Conditions

Disease	Representative Virus
Acquired immunodeficiency syndrome (AIDS)	Human immunodeficiency virus (HIV)
Chickenpox (varicella) and shingles (herpes zoster)	Varicella zoster virus (VZV)
Common cold and upper respiratory infections (URIs)	Rhinoviruses
Fever blisters and herpes	Herpes simplex 1 and 2
Hantavirus pulmonary syndrome	Hantavirus
Hepatitis	Hepatitis A virus, Hepatitis B virus, Hepatitis C virus
Infectious mononucleosis	Epstein-Barr virus (EBV)
Influenza	Influenza A, B, C, etc.
Measles	Rubeola virus
Mumps	Paramyxovirus
Poliomyelitis	Poliovirus 1, 2, and 3
Rabies	Rabies virus
Rubella (German measles)	Rubella virus
Viral encephalitis	Herpes, Herpes simplex, West Nile virus
Warts, genital warts, and cervical cancer	Human papillomaviruses (HPV)

Bacterial Conditions

Disease	Causative Organism
Acute conjunctivitis	*Staphylococcus, Haemophilus,* and other organisms
Anthrax	*Bacillus anthracis*
Botulism	*Clostridium botulinum* (bacillus)
Brucellosis	*Brucella* species (bacilli)
Cholera	*Vibrio cholerae* (curved)
Dental caries	*Streptococcus mutans* (coccus) and other organisms
Diarrhea	*Campylobacter jejuni* and many others
Diphtheria	*Corynebacterium diphtheria* (bacillus)
Epiglottitis	*Haemophilus influenza*
External otitis (swimmer's ear)	*Pseudomonas aeruginosa, Staphylococcus aureus, Streptococcus pyogenes,* etc.
Gonorrhea	*Neisseria gonorrhoeae* (coccus)
Legionnaries' disease	*Legionella pneumophila* (bacillus)
Lyme disease	*Borrelia burgdorferi* (spirochete)
Meningitis	*Streptococcus pneumoniae, Neisseria meningitides, Haemophilus influenzae,* and other organisms
Parrot fever (psittacosis)	*Chlamydia psittaci*
Pelvic inflammatory disease (PID)	*Neisseria gonorrhoeae* (coccus), *Chlamydia trachomatis,* and other organisms
Peptic ulcer	*Helicobacter pylori*
Pertussis (whooping cough)	*Bordetella pertussis* (bacillus)
Pharyngitis (strep throat)	*Streptococcus pyogenes*
Pneumonia	*Streptococcus pneumoniae, Pseudomonas aeruginosa,* and other organisms
Rheumatic fever	Group A beta-hemolytic streptococci (cocci)
Rocky Mountain spotted fever (RMSF)	*Rickettsia rickettsii*
Salmonellosis	*Salmonella* species (bacilli)
Shigellosis or bacillary dysentery	*Shigella* species (bacilli)
Skin infections	*Staphylococcus* species (cocci)
Syphilis	*Treponema pallidum* (spirochete)
Tetanus	*Clostridium tetani* (bacillus)
Toxic shock syndrome (TSS)	*Staphylococcus aureus* (cocci)
Trachoma (chlamydial conjunctivitis)	*Chlamydia trachomatis*
Tuberculosis	*Mycobacterium tuberculosis*
Typhoid fever	*Salmonella typhi* (bacillus)
Urinary tract infections	*E. coli, Proteus* sp., enterococcus

Mycotic (Fungal) and Protozoa Conditions

Disease	Causative Organism
Amebiasis and amebic dysentery	*Entamoeba histolytica*, *Entamoeba polecki*, and other organisms (ameba)
Aspergillosis	*Aspergillus* species
Blastomycosis	*Blastomyces dermatitidis*
Candidiasis (thrush)	*Candida albicans* and other species
Coccidioidomycosis (San Joaquin fever)	*Coccidioides immitis*
Histoplasmosis	*Histoplasma capsulatum*
Giardiasis (travelers' diarrhea)	*Giardia lamblia* (flagellate)
Isosporiasis	*Isospora belli* (sporozoan)
Malaria	*Plasmodium* species (sporozoan)
Tinea (includes athlete's foot and jock itch)	*Epidermophyton*, *Microsporum*, and *Trichophyton* species
Toxoplasmosis	*Toxoplasma gondii* (sporozoan)
Trichomoniasis	*Trichomonas vaginalis* (flagellate)

APPENDIX D

Patient Education on Preventing Health Care–Associated Infections (HAIs)

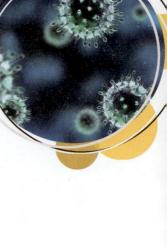

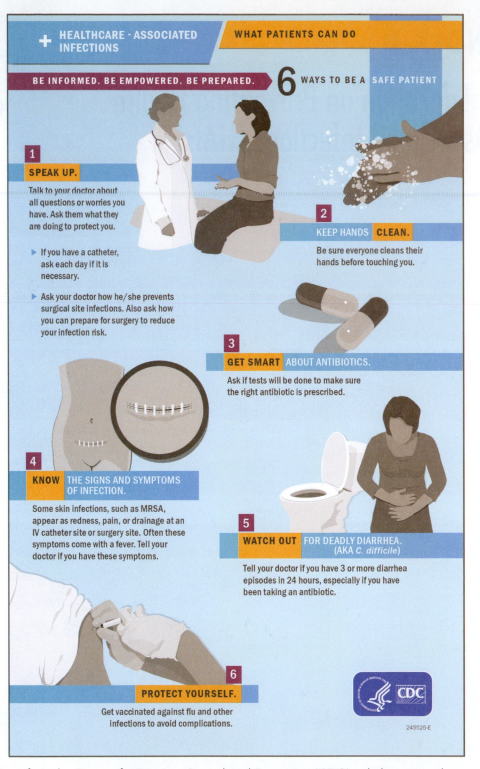

Informational poster from the Centers for Disease Control and Prevention (CDC) to help patients become more informed about their medical condition. According to the CDC, approximately 1 in 25 U.S. patients has at least one infection contracted during the course of hospital care, adding up to about 722,000 infections in 2011.

Courtesy of the Centers for Disease Control and Prevention.

GLOSSARY

A

acetic acid [uh SEE tic]—a clear, colorless organic acid, CH_3COOH, with a distinctive pungent odor, used as a solvent and in the manufacture of rubber, plastics, acetate fibers, pharmaceuticals, and photographic chemicals. Also known as vinegar.

acid-fast (Ziehl-Neelsen) stain—a bacterial staining procedure in which application of acid-alcohol does not cause decolorization, maintaining a dark stain.

acquired immunodeficiency syndrome (AIDS)—a late-stage infection with the human immunodeficiency virus (HIV).

active immunity—a type of immunity that can be produced artificially by vaccination or naturally by a person becoming ill with a particular disease.

acute bronchitis—a short, severe attack of bronchitis, with fever and a productive cough.

acute cholecystitis [KOH luh sis TYE tis]—inflammation of the gallbladder.

adaptive immune response—immune mechanisms that "learn" to deal with specific invaders.

aerobic [air ROW bick]—in the presence of oxygen.

airborne precautions—set of precautions to prevent transmission of infectious agents that remain infectious over long distances when suspended in the air.

airborne transmission—a transmission mechanism in which the infectious agent is spread as an aerosol and usually enters a person through the respiratory tract.

amebiasis [ah me BUY uh sis]—an infection of the intestines caused by the parasite *Entamoeba histolytica* invading the colon causing colitis, acute dysentery, or long-term (chronic) diarrhea; may also spread to other areas of the body.

aminoglycosides [a ME noh GLY koh sides]—a group of antibiotics used to treat certain bacterial infections; primarily aerobic, gram-negative bacteria.

anaerobic [an uh ROW bick]—in the absence of oxygen.

antibiotic—a natural or synthetic substance that destroys microorganisms or inhibits their growth to prevent or treat infection in plants, animals, and humans.

antibody—a substance produced by a B lymphocyte in response to a unique antigen, which it can then combine with to destroy or control it.

antifungal drugs—destructive to fungi, or suppressing their reproduction or growth; effective against fungal infections.

antigen-presenting cells (APCs)—a group of immunocompetent cells that mediate cellular immune response by engulfing, processing, and presenting antigens to the T-cell receptor. Traditional antigen-presenting cells include macrophages, dendritic cells, Langerhans cells, and B lymphocytes.

antitubercular drugs [AN tee too BER kyu ler]—any agent or group of drugs used to treat tuberculosis; at least two drugs, and usually three, are required in various combinations in pulmonary tuberculosis therapy.

antiviral drug—a drug that can destroy viruses and help treat illnesses caused by them.

appendicitis—inflammation and infection of the appendix.

artificial immunity—deliberate exposure of antigen to develop immunity such as in immunizations.

asepsis—a condition free from germs, infection, and any form of life.

asexual reproduction—without sex; a mode of reproduction in which offspring arise from a single parent and inherit the genes of that parent only, making the offspring a genetic copy.

Aspergillus—a genus of fungi comprising more than 600 species of molds, some of which can cause human disease.

aspiration pneumonia—bronchopneumonia that develops due to entrance of foreign materials into the tracheobronchial tree; usually consists of oral or regurgitated gastric contents.

atypical pneumonia—organisms that cannot be cultured with standard microbiological media or techniques, and do not respond to treatment with penicillins or other antibiotics classically used for typical pneumonia.

autoclave—a strong, pressurized, steam-heated vessel, as for laboratory experiments, sterilization, or cooking.

automated—to install automatic procedures.

avian flu—highly contagious viral disease caused by influenza A virus subtypes H5 and H7; also known as bird flu.

B

bacilli [bah SILL eye]—a genus of gram-positive, spore-forming, often aerobic, rod-shaped bacteria in the family *Bacillaceae* that exist singly or in chains and mostly inhabit soil or water.

bactericidal [back TEER ih SIGH dul]—capable of killing bacteria.

bacteriology—scientific study of bacteria.

bacteriostatic [BACK teer ee oh STAT ik]—inhibiting the growth of bacteria.

B cell—a type of lymphocyte, developed in bone marrow, that circulates in the blood and lymph and, upon encountering a particular foreign antigen, differentiates into a clone of plasma cells that secrete a specific antibody and a clone of memory cells that make the antibody on subsequent encounters.

beta-lactams—any of a class of antibiotics that is structurally and pharmacologically related to the penicillins and cephalosporins.

binary fission [BI nuh ree FISH un]—method of asexual reproduction in which DNA is replicated and the cell splits into two genetically identical daughter cells.

biological liquid waste—a liquid that contains or has been contaminated by a biohazardous agent.

biological vector—a vector that is essential in the life cycle of a pathogenic organism.

bioterrorism—the use of biological warfare agents against civilian populations.

blastomycosis [blas toe my KOH sis]—a rare infection caused by inhalation of the fungus *Blastomyces dermatitidis* which may produce inflammatory lesions of the skin or lungs or a generalized invasion of the skin, lungs, bones, central nervous system, kidneys, liver, and spleen.

Bloodborne Pathogen Standard—extensive, detailed regulations to be practiced by employers and employees to prevent occupational exposure to harmful pathogens.

blood cultures—a microbiological culture of blood employed to detect infections that are spreading through the bloodstream.

broad-spectrum drug—drug that acts on a wide range of disease-causing bacteria.

bronchiolitis [BRONG kee oh LIGHT is]—inflammation of the membranes lining the bronchioles.

broth dilution—process of taking a known concentration and doing several serial dilutions to determine the lowest concentration needed to inhibit or kill bacteria.

C

capsid—the protein covering around the central core of a virus that protects the nucleic acids in the core and promotes attachment of the virus to susceptible cells.

capsule or slime layer—a sheath or continuous enclosure around an organ or structure.

carbapenem [kahr buh PEN um]—a subtype of beta-lactam antibiotics, including imipenem and meropenem, which are effective against a wide range of bacteria.

catheter-related bloodstream infections (CRBSIs)—bloodstream infections related to the invasive introduction of a peripheral or central catheter.

cell membrane—a semipermeable phospholipid bilayer that separates the interior of cells from the outside environment and controls movement into and out of the cell.

cellulitis—inflammation of skin and subcutaneous tissues.

Centers for Disease Control and Prevention (CDC)—federal agency under the Department of Health and Human Services that serves to protect public health through the control and prevention of disease.

cephalosporin [SEF uh loh SPORE in]—a subtype of beta-lactam antibiotic that kills bacteria or prevents its growth; used to treat infections in different parts of the body, such as the ears, nose, throat, lungs, sinuses, and skin.

cerebral spinal fluid (CSF)—the fluid surrounding the brain and spinal cord; a lumbar puncture or spinal tap can be performed to sample CSF fluid to test for the presence of microorganisms.

cerebrospinal fluid (CSF) cultures—a laboratory test (by spinal tap) to look for bacteria, fungi, and viruses in the normally sterile fluid that moves in the space surrounding the spinal cord.

chain of infection—process by which an agent leaves its reservoir or host through a portal of exit, and is conveyed by some mode of transmission, then enters through an appropriate portal of entry to infect a susceptible host.

chief complaint or concern (CC)—the main sign or symptom that caused an individual to seek health care.

Chlamydia [klah MID ee ah]—bacterial disease that causes genital infections in men and woman.

chlorine—a chemical element with the atomic number 17; a disinfectant, decolorant, and irritant poison used for disinfecting, fumigating, and bleaching.

chromosome—a linear strand made of DNA that carries genetic information (genes).

cilia [SILL ee ah]—threadlike projections from the free surface of certain epithelial cells used to propel or sweep materials across a surface.

cleaning—the process of physically removing all foreign material from an object.

clindamycin [KLIN duh MY sin]—a semisynthetic derivative of lincomycin used systemically, topically, and vaginally as an antibacterial, primarily against gram-positive bacteria.

Clostridium difficile [klos TRID ee um dif us SEEL]—gram-positive anaerobe bacteria that causes watery diarreha, fever, appetite loss, and abdominal pain; sometimes accompanied by pseudomembraneous colitis.

cocci [KOK sigh]—a bacterial type that is spherical or ovoid.

coccidioidomycosis [KOK sid ee oy dough my KOH sis]—infection with the pathogenic fungus, *Coccidioides immitis,* whose spores, when inhaled, may cause the development of active or subclinical infection.

common vehicle transmission—the mode of transmission of infectious pathogens from a source that is common to all the cases of a specific disease, by means of a vehicle such as water, food, air, or the blood supply.

community-acquired pneumonia (CAP)—most common type of pneumonia that occurs outside hospitals or other health care facilities.

comparative research—a research methodology in the social sciences that aims to make comparisons across different countries or cultures.

conjunctivitis—an inflammation or redness of the lining of the white part of the eye and the underside of the eyelid (conjunctiva) that can be caused by infection, allergic reaction, or physical agents such as infrared or ultraviolet light.

contact precaution—a type of isolation used when a patient is infected with or carrying an epidemiologically important organism that can be spread by body-to-body contact.

contact transmission—occurs when microorganisms are transferred from one infected person to another.

contamination—the presence of extraneous, especially infectious, material that renders a substance or preparation impure or harmful.

croup—viral infection of the larynx (voice box); associated with mild upper respiratory symptoms such as a runny nose and cough (usually in children).

culture and sensitivity [C&S] test—a diagnostic lab procedure used to identify the type of bacteria or fungi and to determine which antimicrobials can successfully fight an infection by collecting urine, blood, or other body fluid to culture in a medium and analyze for antimicrobial susceptibility.

cystitis—bladder inflammation usually occurring as a result of a urinary tract infection.

cytoplasm [SIGH toh plazm]—a gel-like matrix contained within the cell membrane that holds all of the cell's internal substructures.

D

daptomycin [DAP toe MY sin]—a miscellaneous anti-infective used to treat complicated skin and skin structure infections caused by *Staphylococcus aureus, S. agalactiae, S. dysgalactiae,* and *Enterococcus faecalis.*

decontamination—the process of making a person, object, or environment free of microorganisms, radioactivity, or other contaminants.

denatured—to deprive a substance of its natural qualities.

dependent variable—a variable (often denoted by y) whose value depends on that of another; what is being observed in an experiment.

dermatophytes [der MAT uh fites]—fungal parasites that grow in or on the skin.

descriptive research—used to describe characteristics of a population or phenomenon being studied. It does not answer questions about how/when/why the characteristics occurred.

diagnose—determine the cause of the patient's symptoms and signs.

dimorphic [di MORE fic]—occurring in two distinct forms.

direct contact—mutual touching of two individuals or organisms; many communicable diseases may be spread by direct contact between an infected and a healthy person.

disinfection—using specialized cleansing techniques that destroy or prevent growth of organisms capable of infection.

disk diffusion—test that uses antibiotic-impregnated wafers to test whether particular bacteria are susceptible to specific antibiotics.

diverticulitis [DYE ver tick you LYE tis]—inflammation of the diverticulum in the intestinal tract causing possible pain, anorexia, and fever.

droplet precautions—measures to reduce the risk of droplet transmission of infectious agents.

E

Ebola virus—causative microorganism of Ebola hemorrhagic fever (EHF), a disease with a high mortality rate.

echinocandins [ee KYE noh KAN dins]—antifungal drugs that inhibit the synthesis of glucan in the cell wall.

ectoparasite [eck toe PAIR uh site]—any parasite that thrives on the skin, such as fleas, lice, maggots, mites, or ticks.

empiric therapy—use of antimicrobials to treat an infection before the specific causative organism has been identified with laboratory tests.

encephalitis [EN sef ah LYE tis]—an inflammation of the brain, usually caused by a direct viral infection or a hypersensitivity reaction to a virus or foreign substance.

endemic—a condition or disease related to a specific population or region of the world.

endocarditis [EN doh kar DYE tis]—inflammation of the endocardium, when microorganisms from the bloodstream can become lodged on the heart valves or heart lining.

endoplasmic reticulum (ER)—organelle that consists of a network of channels that transport materials within the cell.

endotoxin—a lipopolysaccharide that is part of the cell wall of gram-negative bacteria released after the cell's death.

epidemic—an outbreak of a disease that suddenly affects a large group of people in a geographical region or a defined population group.

epidemiology—the study of the origin, distribution, and determinants of diseases.

epiglottitis [EP ih glot EYE tis]—an infection of the epiglottis, which can lead to severe airway obstruction.

ergosterol—the primary sterol found in the cell membrane of some fungi; it stabilizes the membrane, as does cholesterol in human cells.

erysipelas [ER i SIP eh les]—an infection of the skin that is marked by a bright red, swollen, sharply defined rash on the face, scalp, arms, legs, or trunk.

ethanol (ethyl alcohol)—a primary alcohol formed by microbial fermentation of carbohydrates or by synthesis from ethylene; excessive ingestion results in acute intoxication, and ingestion during pregnancy can harm the fetus; also known as alcohol.

ethylene oxide (ETO)—a colorless flammable gas with a slightly sweet odor and taste that is used to sterilize objects.

etiology—the specific cause of the disease.

eukaryote [you CARE ee oat]—organism in which the cell nucleus is surrounded by a membrane.

exacerbation—a worsening or flare-up of a disease process.

exotoxin—a poisonous substance produced by certain bacteria.

experimental research—experiment where the researcher manipulates one variable, and controls/randomizes the rest of the variables.

eye protection—recommended safety glasses, chemical splash goggles, or face shields to be used when handling a hazardous material.

F

face masks— a personal protective device (PPE) to shield the facial area from contamination.

flagella [fla JEL ah]—threadlike structures that provide motility for certain bacteria, protozoa, and spermatozoa.

folate inhibitor—agent that inhibits folic acid synthesis.

fomite [FO might]—object that may harbor microorganisms and is capable of transmitting them.

G

gamma irradiation—a type of radiation therapy that uses short wavelengths of light that ionize water molecules for sterilization.

genitourinary tract infections—groups of infections of the male and female genitalia and infections of the urinary tract.

genus [JEE nus]—in taxonomy, the classification between the family and the species.

germicidal [JUR muh side ul]—preventing infection by inhibiting the growth or action of microorganisms.

Giardia [jee ARE dee uh]—a genus of protozoa that is pear shaped, has two nuclei and four pairs of flagella, and inhabits the small intestine of humans and other animals to which it attaches and absorbs nourishment.

gloves—sterile or clean fitted coverings for the hands, usually with a separate sheath for each finger and thumb.

glutaraldehyde [glue tuh RAL duh hide]—a disinfectant used in aqueous solution for sterilization of non–heat-resistant equipment; also used as a tissue fixative for light and electron microscopy.

glycocalyx—a thin layer of glycoprotein and oligosaccharides on the outer surface of cell membranes that contributes to cell adhesion and forms antigens involved in the recognition of "self."

glycopeptide [GLY koh PEP tide]—any of a class of peptides that contain carbohydrates, including those that contain amino sugars.

Golgi apparatus [GOAL jee app ah RA tuss]—stacks of membrane-bound structures that package proteins inside the cell before they are sent to their destination; important in the processing of proteins for secretion.

gonorrhea—a sexually transmitted disease caused by a gram-negative diplococcus, *Neisseria gonorrhoeae*.

gown—a robe or smock worn in operating rooms and other parts of hospitals as a guard against contamination.

Gram stain—a method of differentiating bacterial species into two large groups (gram-positive and gram-negative) based on chemical and physical properties of the cell wall.

H

hand hygiene—the removal of visible soil and the removal or killing of transient microorganisms from the hands accomplished by using soap and running water or an alcohol-based hand rub.

health care–associated infections (HAIs)—infections patients get while receiving medical treatment.

health care–associated pneumonia (HCAP)—pneumonia acquired as a result of exposure in a health care setting.

helminth [HELL minth]—a wormlike animal; any animal, either free-living or parasitic, belonging to the phyla *Platyhelminthes, Acanthocephala, Nemathelminthes,* or *Annelida.*

hepatitis C virus (HCV)—a small, enveloped, positive-sense single-stranded RNA virus of the family *Flaviviridae* responsible for hepatitis C disease in humans.

herpes simplex virus—human DNA virus that causes repeated painful vesicular eruptions on the genitals and other surfaces on the skin.

histoplasmosis [his toe plaz MO sis]—a systemic fungal respiratory disease caused by *Histoplasma capsulatum.*

hookworm—a parasitic nematode belonging to the family *Strongyloidea* that can cause hookworm disease.

human immunodeficiency virus (HIV)—a retrovirus of the subfamily *Lentivirus* that causes acquired immunodeficiency syndrome (AIDS).

humoral immune response [hu MORE al]—immunity associated with circulating antibodies.

hydrogen peroxide—a colorless, heavy, strongly oxidizing liquid capable of reacting explosively with combustibles and used principally in aqueous solution as a mild antiseptic, a bleaching agent, an oxidizing agent, and a laboratory reagent.

I

immunity—the protection against infectious disease conferred either by the immune response generated by immunization or previous infection or by other nonimmunological factors.

immunization—the protection of individuals or groups from specific diseases by vaccination or the injection of immunoglobulins.

immunoglobulins [IM you noh GLOB you lins]—protein of animal origin with known antibody activity, synthesized by lymphocytes and plasma cells and found in serum and in other body fluids and tissues; abbreviated Ig; there are five distinct classes based on structural and antigenic properties—IgA, IgD, IgE, IgG, and IgM.

incubation—the interval between exposure to infection and the appearance of the first symptom.

independent variable—a variable (often denoted by *x*) whose variation does not depend on that of another; what is being tested or changed in an experiment.

indirect contact—achieved through some intervening medium, such as prolongation of a communicable disease through the air or by means of fomites.

infection—a disease caused by microorganisms, especially those that release toxins or invade body tissues.

infection control and prevention—policies and procedures used to minimize the risk of spreading infections, especially in hospitals and human or animal health care facilities.

infectious diarrhea—infection of the gastrointestinal tract that involves the stomach and small intestine.

infectious waste—hazardous waste with infectious characteristics, including contaminated animal waste and human blood and blood products.

inflammation—a localized reaction that produces redness, warmth, swelling, and pain as a result of infection, irritation, or injury.

influenza—an acute contagious respiratory infection marked by fever, chills, muscle aches, headache, prostration, runny nose, watering eyes, cough, and sore throat.

innate immune response—the ability to protect oneself from pathogens; the immunity you have when you are born.

inoculum—a substance or microorganism introduced by inoculation.

isopropyl [eye sah PRO pil]—a colorless, flammable, water-soluble liquid; used chiefly in the manufacture of antifreeze and rubbing alcohol and as a solvent.

K

keratitis [KER ah TYE tis]—an inflammation of the cornea, the transparent membrane that covers the iris (colored part) and pupil of the eye.

L

latency—state of being concealed, delayed, dormant, or inactive.

lysosome [LIE soh soam]—cell organelle containing hydrolytic enzyme capsules used to break down proteins and carbohydrates to aid in intracellular digestion.

M

macrolides—a class of antibiotics discovered in *Streptomyces,* characterized by molecules made up of large-ring lactones.

macrophage [MACK roh fayj]—a monocyte that has left the circulation and settled and matured in a tissue such as the spleen, lymph nodes, alveoli, and tonsils.

malaria—a febrile hemolytic disease caused by infection with protozoa of the genus *Plasmodium.*

mechanical vector—a vector that simply conveys pathogens to a susceptible individual and is not essential to the development of the organism.

medical asepsis—procedures used to reduce the number of microorganisms and prevent their spread such as hand "no touch" dressing technique.

medical microbiology—a branch of medicine and microbiology that deals with the study of microorganisms including bacteria, viruses, fungi, and parasites that are of medical importance and are capable of causing infectious diseases in human beings.

meningitis [MEN in JIGH tis]—a serious inflammation of the meninges, the thin, membranous covering of the brain and the spinal cord, most commonly caused by infection (by bacteria, viruses, or fungi), although it can also be caused by bleeding into the meninges, cancer, diseases of the immune system, and an inflammatory response to certain types of chemotherapy or other chemical agents.

metronidazole [MET roh NYE duh zole]—an antiprotozoal and antibacterial effective against obligate anaerobes; used as the base or the hydrochloride salt and also used as a topical treatment for rosacea.

microbiology—the scientific study of microorganisms, that is, of bacteria, fungi, intracellular parasites, protozoans, viruses, and some worms.

mitochondria [MITE oh KAHN dree ah]—cell organelles of rod or oval shape that contain the enzymes for the aerobic stages of cell respiration and are the site of most ATP synthesis.

mitosis—type of cell division of somatic cells in which each daughter cell contains the same number of chromosomes as the parent cell.

mold—one of the parasitic or saprophytic fungi that grow in a mycelium pattern; a fuzzy coating due to growth of a fungus on the surface of decaying vegetable matter or on an inorganic object.

monobactam [MAHN oh back tam]—a class of synthetic antibiotics with a cyclic beta-lactam nucleus; may be useful in patients with severe beta-lactam allergies.

monocyte—a mononuclear phagocytic white blood cell derived from myeloid stem cells that circulate in the bloodstream and act as the first line of defense in the inflammatory process.

mononuclear phagocyte system (MPS)—the system of fixed macrophages and circulating monocytes that serves as phagocytes, engulfing foreign substances in a wide variety of immune responses.

morbidity—state of being diseased.

morphology [more FALL oh gee]—the science of structure and form of organisms without regard to function.

mortality—condition of being dead or the number of deaths in a given population.

mucormycosis [mu core my KOH sis]—an invasive and frequently fatal infection with fungi of the family *Mucoraceae* and the class *Zygomycetes*.

mucous membranes—linings of mostly *endodermal* origin, covered in *epithelium,* which are involved in *absorption* and *secretion*.

multidrug-resistant (MDR) TB—a lack of expected therapeutic response in tuberculosis patients to several disease-specific pharmaceutical agents, especially antibiotics.

mycology [my CALL uh jee]—the science and study of fungi.

N

narrow-spectrum drug—drug that is effective against specific families of bacteria.

nasal specimens—a specimen obtained using a cotton swab on a stick, passed up the nostril to obtain a sample of exudate and epithelial debris for microbiological or cellular examination; not recommended unless testing for viruses.

natural active immunity—an active immunity acquired by experiencing and having recovered from a disease.

necrotizing fasciitis [NECK roh TIZE ing FAS ee EYE tis]—bacterial infection that can destroy the deep layers of skin; also known as flesh eating disease.

necrotizing skin and soft tissue infections—usually rare but very severe type of bacterial infection that can destroy the muscles, skin, and underlying tissue.

neutrophils [NEW troh fills]—granular white blood cells responsible for much of the body's protection against infection; they play a primary role in inflammation and are readily attracted to foreign antigens, destroying them by phagocytosis.

nonsharp—does not contain pointed edges that can easily penetrate other objects.

nonsterile gloves—gloves not put through the process of sterilization.

normal flora—mixture of bacteria normally found at specific body sites.

nosocomial infection [nos uh KOH mee al]—infection resulting from treatment in a hospital or a health care service unit; older term that is replaced with health care–associated infections (HAIs) by the Centers for Disease Control and Prevention (CDC).

nucleolus [new clee OL us]—a spherical structure in the nucleus of a cell made of DNA, RNA, and protein; the site of synthesis of rRNA.

nucleus [NEW clee us]—the structure within a cell that contains the chromosomes and is responsible for the cell's metabolism, growth, and reproduction.

O

Occupational Safety and Health Administration (OSHA)—a government agency in the Department of Labor that strives to maintain a safe and healthy work environment.

opportunistic infection—any infection that results from a defective immune system that cannot defend against pathogens normally found in the environment.

osteomyelitis [OSS tee oh MY eh LYE tis]—a bone infection, almost always caused by bacteria; over time, the result can be destruction of the bone itself.

otitis media—an infection of the middle ear space, behind the eardrum (tympanic membrane) characterized by pain, dizziness, and partial loss of hearing.

oxazolidinones [ock SAY zoh LYE di nohns]—heterocyclic organic compounds containing both nitrogen and oxygen in a 5-membered ring; antibiotic used against gram-positive pathogens.

P

pandemic—disease or condition that affects many people worldwide.

parasitology [pair uh sigh TALL uh jee]—the study of parasites and parasitism.

parotitis [PAH roh TYE tis]—inflammation or infection of one or both parotid salivary glands.

passive immunity—immunity acquired by the introduction of preformed antibodies into an unprotected individual.

pasteurization [PASS tuh rise aye shun]—partial sterilization of foods at a temperature that destroys harmful microorganisms without major changes in the chemistry of the food.

pathogen [PATH oh jen]—a microorganism capable of producing a disease.

pathogenic [PATH oh JEN ick]—productive of disease.

pathological waste—waste material consisting of only human or animal remains, anatomical parts, and/or tissue, the bags/containers used to collect and transport the waste material, and animal bedding.

penicillins—any group of antibiotics biosynthesized by several species of molds.

personal protective equipment (PPE)—specialized clothing or equipment worn by employees for protection against health and safety hazards; designed to protect many parts of the body, for example, eyes, head, face, hands, feet, and ears.

phagocyte [FAG oh sight]—white blood cell that can ingest and destroy microorganisms, cell debris, and other particles in the blood or tissues.

pharyngitis [FAR in JIGH tis]—inflammation or infection of the pharynx, usually causing a sore throat.

phenol [FEE nowl]—extremely poisonous compound that is caustic and disinfectant; used as a pharmaceutical preservative and in dilution as an antimicrobial and topical anesthetic and antipruritic.

pinocytic vesicle [PIN o sit ik VES ih kul]—compartment made when cells ingest extracellular material and its contents by invaginating the cell membrane and pinching off.

pinworm—any of numerous long, slender nematode worms that parasitize humans.

pneumonia—an acute or chronic disease marked by inflammation of the lungs and caused by viruses, bacteria, or other microorganisms and sometimes by physical and chemical irritants.

portal of entry—the area in which a microorganism enters the body such as cuts, lesions, injection sites, or natural body orifices.

prion [PRI on]—a small proteinaceous infectious particle that is believed to be responsible for central nervous system diseases in humans and other mammals.

prognosis—the predicted outcome of a disease.

prokaryotes [pro CARE ee oats]—in taxonomy, the kingdom of organisms with prokaryotic cell structure; that is, they lack membrane-bound cell organelles and a nuclear membrane around the chromosome.

protists [PRO tists]—any member of the kingdom *Protista*; organisms that include the protozoa, unicellular and multicellular algae, and the slime molds.

protozoa [pro tah ZOE uh]—unicellular protists with animal-like behavior.

pyelonephritis [PYE eh loh neh FRY tis]—inflammation of kidney and upper urinary tract.

Q

quaternary ammonium compounds [KWOT er ner ee uh MOH nee uhm]—a group of compounds used as disinfectants that are bactericidal to many organisms.

quinolones [KWIN oh lohns]—a class of broad-spectrum antibacterial drugs.

quinupristin-dalfopristin [kwin YOU pris tin dal FOE pris tin]—a combination of two antibiotics used to treat infections by staphylococci and by vancomycin-resistant *Enterococcus faecium*.

R

relapse—a reoccurrence of a disease or symptoms after an apparent recovery.

remission—a lessening of severity or disappearance of symptoms.

reservoir of infection—a continuous source of infectious disease; people, animals, and plants may be reservoirs of infection.

resident flora—species of microorganisms that are always present on or in the body and are not easily removed by mechanical friction.

resistance—a lack of response of a pathogen to treatment such as antibiotic therapy.

respiratory syncytial virus (RSV) [sin SISH ul]—virus that causes infection of the lungs and breathing passages.

route of transmission—the passing of a communicable disease from an infected host individual or group to a nonspecific individual or group, regardless of whether the other individual was previously infected.

S

sanitization—the process whereby pathogenic organisms are reduced to safe levels on inanimate objects, thereby reducing the likelihood of cross-infection.

science—knowledge about or study of the natural world based on facts learned through experiments and observation.

scientific hypothesis—the initial building block in the scientific method; many describe it as an "educated guess," based on prior knowledge and observation, as to the cause of a particular phenomenon.

scientific inquiry—the activities through which individuals develop knowledge and understanding of scientific ideas, as well as an understanding of how scientists study the natural world.

scientific theory—a well-substantiated explanation of some aspect of the natural world that is acquired through the scientific method and repeatedly tested and confirmed through observation and experimentation.

septic arthritis—a form of joint inflammation caused by infection.

serology—the scientific study of fluid components of the blood, especially antigens and antibodies.

severe acute respiratory syndrome (SARS)—a highly contagious, potentially lethal viral respiratory illness characterized by a fever, cough, difficulty breathing, or hypoxia.

sexually transmitted diseases (STDs)—group of diseases transmitted through sexual contact that can be caused by bacteria, viruses, protozoan, fungi, and parasites.

sharps—any needles, scalpels, or other articles that could cause wounds or punctures to personnel handling them.

sharps container—container in every clinic that is designed for the disposal of sharps; required and regulated by the Occupational Safety and Health Administration (OSHA).

sign—any objective evidence or manifestation of an illness or disordered function of the body.

sinusitis [SIGH nuh SIGH tis]—inflammation of a sinus caused by various agents, including viruses, bacteria, or allergy.

social ethics—the philosophical or moral principles that, in one way or another, represent the collective experience of people and cultures.

species [SPEE seas]—a category of classification for living organisms; group is just below the genus.

spirilla [spih RILL uh]—flagellated aerobic bacteria with an elongated spiral shape, of the genus *Spirillum*.

spore—cell produced by fungi for reproduction; a resistant cell produced by bacteria to withstand extreme heat or cold or dehydration.

sputum culture—a test to find and identify the microorganism causing an infection of the lower respiratory tract by obtaining a sample of sputum (mucus coughed up from the lungs) from the mouth.

standard precautions—guidelines recommended by the Centers for Disease Control and Prevention for reducing the risk of transmission of bloodborne and other pathogens in hospitals; the standard precautions synthesize the major features of universal precautions (designed to reduce the risk of transmission of bloodborne pathogens) and body substance isolation (designed to reduce the risk of pathogens from moist body substances) and apply them to all patients receiving care in hospitals regardless of their diagnosis or presumed infection status.

sterile field—a specified surgical area that is free of microorganisms.

sterile gloves—clean, germ-free gloves.

sterile principles—a set of guidelines designed to determine the areas and items that are considered sterile and what actions might cause contamination especially in surgical procedures.

sterilization—a technique for destroying microorganisms on inanimate objects using heat, water, chemicals, or gases.

stool specimens—a test to identify bacteria in patients with a suspected infection of the digestive tract by taking a sample of the patient's feces and placing it in a special medium where the bacteria is then grown.

superinfection—infection occurring after or on top of an earlier infection, especially following treatment with broad-spectrum antibiotics.

surgical asepsis—the exclusion of all microorganisms before they can enter an open surgical wound or contaminate a sterile field during surgery; measures taken include sterilization of all instruments, drapes, and all other inanimate objects that may come in contact with the surgical wound; all personnel coming in contact with the sterile field perform a surgical hand scrub with an antimicrobial agent and put on a surgical gown and gloves.

symptom—any change in the body or its functions as perceived by the patient.

syndrome—a set of symptoms and signs associated with, and characteristic of, one particular disease.

T

tapeworm—species of worms of the class Cestoda, which are intestinal parasites of humans and animals.

T cell—a type of white blood cell that matures in the thymus, contains a T-cell receptor, and plays a central role in cell-mediated immunity.

tetracyclines [TET ruh SIGH kleens]—a class of broad-spectrum bacteriostatic antibiotics.

throat culture—a technique for identifying disease bacteria in material taken from the throat; most throat cultures are done to rule out infections caused by beta-hemolytic streptococci, which cause strep throat.

tracheobronchitis [TRAY kee oh brong KYE tis]—inflammation of the mucous membrane of the trachea and bronchi.

transient flora—microorganisms that may be present in or on the body under certain conditions and for certain lengths of time; they are easier to remove by mechanical friction than resident flora.

transmission-based precautions—safeguards designed for patients documented or suspected to be infected with highly transmissible or epidemiologically important pathogens for which additional precautions beyond standard precautions are needed to interrupt transmission in hospitals.

tuberculosis—an infectious airborne disease caused by tubercle bacteria that most commonly affects the respiratory system but other parts of the body can also be affected.

U

urinary tract infection (UTI)—infection of the kidneys, ureters, or bladder by microorganisms that either ascend from the urethra or that spread to the kidney from the bloodstream.

urine specimens—clean-catch, midstream urine specimen for routine urinalysis and culture.

V

vaccines—any suspension containing antigenic molecules derived from a microorganism, given to stimulate an immune response to an infectious disease.

vector—carrier of disease.

vector borne—transmitting a pathogenic microorganism from an infected individual to another individual by an arthropod or other agent, sometimes with other animals serving as intermediary hosts.

vegetative organisms—microorganisms that can grow and reproduce in rich, moist soil where many nutrients are available.

ventilator-associated pneumonia (VAP)—pneumonia acquired as a result of being intubated and placed on a mechanical ventilator.

viral load—a measure of the total body burden of viral particles present in human blood; the greater the number, usually, the sicker the patient.

virology [vear RALL oh jee]—the study of viruses and viral diseases.

virulence [VEAR you lence]—the relative power and degree of pathogenicity possessed by organisms.

virus—a pathogen composed of nucleic acid within a protein shell that can grow and reproduce only after infecting a host cell.

vital signs—medical assessment during a physical examination in which the temperature, pulse, and respirations (TPR), as well as the blood pressure, are measured.

W

wound culture—a laboratory test in which micro-organisms from a wound are grown in a special growth medium to find and identify the microorganism causing an infection in a wound or an abscess.

Y

yeasts—any of several unicellular fungi, for example, *Candida,* that reproduce by budding.

INDEX

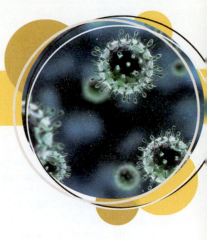

Note: Photos/figures are noted with *f*; tables are noted with *t*.

A

Abacavir, 195*t*, 226*t*
Acalculous cholecystitis, 217
Acetaminophen, otitis media and, 207
Acetic acid
    defined, 100
    infection prevention/control and,
        100–101
Acid-fast (Ziehl-Neelsen) stain, 49
ACIP. *See* Advisory Committee on
        Immunization Practices
Acne, 183
Acquired immunodeficiency syndrome
        (AIDS), 64, 65, 70–71. *See also*
        Human immunodeficiency virus
        (HIV), 193, 226
Active immunity, 66, 169
Acute bronchitis, 239–241
    defined, 239
    treatment for, 240
Acute cholecystitis, 217
Acute conditions, 168
Acyclovir, 70, 190, 193*t*, 204, 225
Adaptive immune response, 20
Adenosine triphosphate, 13
Adenovirus, 236
    bronchitis and, 240
    conjunctivitis and, 209
    croup and, 237
    pneumonia and, 246*t*
Adenovirus respiratory disease, DNA
        viruses and, 189
Adult parasites, 73
Adverse reactions, true allergies *versus,* 188
Advisory Committee on Immunization
        Practices, 170
Aerobic bacteria, 57
Aerosol inhalation, contaminated, hospital-
        acquired pneumonia and, 248–249

Agar culture, 51, 51*f*
AIDS. *See* Acquired immunodeficiency
        syndrome (AIDS)
Airborne precautions, 130–131
    chart, 130*f*
    defined, 122
    for herpes zoster, 131
    patient candidates for, 130–131
Airborne route of transmission, 26, 116, 116*f*
Albendazole, 76
Alcohol
    effect, mode of action, and uses for, 105*t*
    infection prevention and control
        and, 100
Alcohol-based hand rubs, when to use,
        122–123
Algae, defined, 9*t*
Alkylating agents, effect, mode of action,
        and uses for, 105*t*
Allergies, medication-related, 188
Altitude, pressure and, 99
Amantadine, 70, 191, 193*t*
Ambisome, 197*t*
Amebiasis, 74
American Academy of Family
        Physicians, 207
American Academy of Pediatrics, 207
American Thoracic Society, 251
    CAP treatment recommendations of,
        242, 243
    empiric therapy guidelines of, 250
Amikacin, 181, 251
Amikin, 181
Aminoglycosides, 171, 181
Aminopenicillins, 176, 177*t*
Amoeba, 118*f*
Amoxicillin, 177, 177*t*, 214*t*, 215
    community-acquired pneumonia treated
        with, 243

    otitis media treated with, 208
    sinusitis treated with, 235
Amoxicillin-clavulanate, 177*t*, 208,
        214*t*, 243
Amoxil, 177*t*
Amphotericin B, 83, 85, 197*t*
Amphotericin B deoxycholate, 196
Ampicillin, 177*t*, 213*t*
Ampicillin-sulbactam, 177*t*, 212*t*
Anaerobes, 18
Anaerobic bacteria, 57
Ancef, 178*t*
Anidulafungin, 196, 197*t*
Anthrax, 253
Antibacterial agents, 43, 176–186
    aminoglycosides, 181
    beta-lactams, 176
    carbapenems, 179
    cephalosporins, 177–178, 178*t*
    clindamycin, 186
    daptomycin, 185
    folate inhibitors, 184
    glycopeptides, 182
    macrolides, 182–183
    metronidazole, 186
    monobactams, 179
    oxazolidinones, 184–185
    penicillins, 176, 177*t*
    quinolones, 180–181
    quinupristin-dalfopristin, 185
    resistance to, 11
    tetracyclines, 183
Antibacterial drug classification, 174–176
    bacteriostatic *versus* bactericidal,
        174, 175*t*
    mechanism of action and, 175–176
    spectrum of activity: broad *versus*
        narrow, 175, 175*t*
Antibiotic era, beginning of, 56

Antibiotic resistance, 57
  description of, 172
  in hospitals, variance in, 250
  otitis media and, 207
  simplified model of, 173*f*
Antibiotics, 171
  bactericidal *versus* bacteriostatic, 175*t*
  broad-spectrum *versus* narrow-spectrum,
    57, 175
  classification of, 56–57
  defined, 56
  development of, history behind, 33*t*–35*t*
  empiric therapy and, 54
  fungal infections and, 79
  otitis media and, 207
  prudent use of, 241
  testing susceptibility to, 52–55
Antibiotic therapy, general principles of,
    56–57
Antibodies, 21, 22, 23*f*, 27, 169
Antifungal agents, 194–197, 197*t*
Antifungal creams, 195
Antifungal drugs, 79
  classes of, 196
  defined, 166
Antigen-presenting cells, 20, 21*f*
Antigens, 20, 23*f*
Antimicrobials
  classifying, 176
  patient and family education about, 172
  wise use of, 166
Antimicrobial soap and water, when to
    use, 122
Antimicrobial therapy, monitoring, 170–171
Antiretrovirals, 71, 71*t*, 193
  common, 195*t*, 226*t*
  HIV treatment with, 226
Antiseptic hand sanitizers, 112*f*, 120
Antiseptic surgery, 38
Antithymocyte globulin, 169*t*
Antitubercular drugs, 186, 252
Antituberculosis agents, 186–188
Antiviral agents, 69–72
Antiviral drugs, 67, 188–195
  common, 193*t*
  defined, 166
  hepatitis C virus treated with, 192–193
  herpes virus infections treated with, 190
  HIV infection treated with, 194
  influenza virus treated with, 190–192
  initial infection with HIV and, 190
  respiratory syncytial virus treated
    with, 192
APCs. *See* Antigen-presenting cells
Appendectomy, 217
Appendicitis, 216–217
Appendix, 216

Armpit, yeast infection of, 81*f*
Arthropods, 118*f*
Arthropod vectors, 116, 116*f*
Artificial active immunity, 66
Artificial immunity, 66
Artificial passive immunity, 67
Asepsis, 147–148
Asexual reproduction, 41
Aspergillus, 85*f*
  defined, 84
  treatment for infections caused by, 85
Aspiration, causes of, 250
Aspiration pneumonia
  defined, 250
  empiric antibiotic choices for, 244*t*
  treatment for, 250–251
Aspirin, Reye syndrome in children and, 207
Atazanavir, 195*t*, 226*t*
Atgam, 169*t*
Athlete's foot (tinea pedis), 80, 83*t*, 195,
    196*f*, 214
Atovaquone, 251
Atovaquone-proguanil, 74
ATP. *See* Adenosine triphosphate
Atypical pneumonia
  defined, 242
  treatment of, 243–244
Augmentin, 177*t*, 208
Autoclave, 141
  defined, 99
  steam and heat used for sterilizing in,
    99–100, 100*f*
Automated methods, 54
Avelox, 181
Avian influenza (H5N1, bird flu),
    253–255
  defined, 253
  pneumonia and, 246*t*
Avian influenza H7N9 virus strain, 253
  genetic evolution of, in China (2013),
    253, 254*f*
Azactam, 176, 179
Azithromycin, 183
  chlamydia treated with, 224
  gonorrhea treated with, 225
  pharyngitis treated with, 236
  pneumonia treated with, 243
  sinusitis treated with, 235
Azoles, 196
AZT, 195*t*, 226*t*
Aztreonam, 179

B

BabyBIG, 169*t*
Bacilli, structure and morphology of, 44, 45
Bacillus anthracis bacteria, 253*f*

  spores from Sterne strain of, 44*f*
  three-dimensional image of, 8*f*
Bacteremia, 45
Bacteria, 11, 25, 39
  aerobic and anareobic, 57
  beneficial, 43
  coryneform, 119
  defined, 9*t*
  friendly, 17
  growing and testing, 50–55
  naming, 43
  structure and morphology of, 43–46
Bacterial cell, structures of, 42*f*
Bacterial disease, 55–56
Bacterial infection, signs and symptoms
    of, 56
Bacterial meningitis
  community-acquired, common causes
    of, 203*t*
  symptoms of, 203
Bacterial pneumonia, 65
Bacterial pumps, 172
Bacterial staining, 47
  differential stains, 49
  simple stains, 47
Bactericidal, defined, 174
Bactericidal drugs, 56
Bacteriology, 39, 41–56
  bacterial disease, 55–56
  bacterial structure and morphology,
    43–46
  growing and testing bacteria, 50–55
  naming bacteria, 43
  specimen collection, 46–49
Bacteriostatic, defined, 100, 174
Bacteriostatic agents, 56
Bacteroides fragilis, diverticulitis and, 219
Bactrim, 184
Basophils, 19
B cells, 21, 22, 22*t*
"Beaver fever," 73
Bedaquiline, 188
Bed bugs, 78, 79*f*
Beef or pork tapeworm, 75, 75*t*
Beta-lactamase inhibitor + aminoglycoside,
    aspiration pneumonia treated
    with, 251
Beta-lactamase inhibitors, penicillins
    combined with, 176, 177*t*
Beta-lactams, 175*t*
  defined, 176
  pneumonia in children and treatment
    with, 244
B-hemolytic *Streptococci,* epiglottitis and, 237
B-lactamase, 57, 172
Biaxin, 183
Binary fission, 41

Biohazard bags/containers, 134, 134*f*, 140–141, 155*f*
Biological liquid waste, 141*t*
Biological vector, 25–26, 116
Bioprosthetic valves, heart, 210
Bioterrorism, defined, 253
Blastomyces dermatidis, 83
Blastomycosis, 83, 83*t*
Blood, 16
Blood agar, streaking and inoculating patterns on, 51, 51*f*
Blood and body substances, cleaning, 128
Bloodborne Pathogen Standard, 132–134
Blood culture
  defined, 152
  obtaining, technique for, 152
Blood draws, safe injection practices for, 127
Blood specimen containers, 46*f*
Bloodstream response, immune system and, 17, 19
B lymphocytes, 23*f*
Boceprevir, 71, 192, 193*t*
Boiling water, disinfecting and sterilizing with, 99
Bone and joint infections, 228–229
  osteomyelitis, 228
  septic arthritis, 228–229
Bordetella pertussis, 12*f*
  acute bronchitis and, 241
  droplet precautions and, 131
Botulism, 45
Botulism immune globulin, 169*t*
Bowel infections, stool specimens and, 155–157
Brain infection, symptoms of, 82
Bread, mold on, 80*f*
British Thoracic Society, 251
Broad-spectrum antibiotics, 175, 175*t*
Broad-spectrum drugs, 57, 172
Bronchiolitis, 239–241
  defined, 239
  treatment for, 240–241
Bronchitis. *See* Acute bronchitis; Tracheobronchitis
Broth dilution, 53
Bugs, 118*f*

C

Campylobacter, infectious diarrhea and, 222*t*
Canadian Infectious Diseases Society, 251
Cancer cell, cytotoxic T-cell activation and actions on, 21, 22*f*
Cancidas, 196, 197*t*
Candida albicans, 195, 196*f*
Candida infections, invasive, 82*t*
Candida species, 81, 82*t*

CAP. *See* Community-acquired pneumonia
Capsid, 65
Capsule (or slime layer), 11, 43
Carbacephems, 176
Carbapenem, 176, 179
  acute cholecystitis and, 217
  spectrum of activity for, 175*t*
Cardiovascular infections, 210–213
  catheter-related bloodstream infections, 211–212
  endocarditis, 210–211
Carriers of disease, 113
Caspofungin, 196, 197*t*, 213*t*
Catheter-related bloodstream infections, 211–212
  defined, 212
  organisms related to and antimicrobial treatment of, 213*t*
CC. *See* Chief complaint or concern
CCR5 antagonists, 194, 226
CDC. *See* Centers for Disease Control and Prevention
CD4 T cells, 70
Ceclor, 178*t*
Cefaclor, 178*t*
Cefazolin, 178*t*, 214*t*, 215, 228
Cefdinir, 208
Cefepime, 178*t*, 213*t*
  kidney infections treated with, 227
  pneumonia treated with, 250
Cefixime, 178*t*
Cefotetan, 178*t*
Cefoxitin, 178*t*
Cefpodoxime proxetil, 208
Ceftaroline, 178, 178*t*
  spectrum of activity for, 175*t*
Ceftazidime, 178*t*
  pneumonia treated with, 250
  septic arthritis treated with, 229
Ceftin, 178*t*, 208
Ceftriaxone, 178*t*, 212*t*, 214*t*, 215
  gonorrhea treated with, 225
  kidney infections treated with, 227
  pneumonia treated with, 250
Ceftriaxone +/- gentmicin, 212*t*
Ceftriaxone + metronidazole
  acute cholecystitis and, 217
  appendicitis and, 217
  diverticulitis and, 219
Cefuroxime, 178*t*
Cefuroxime axetil, 208, 243
Cell culture, 67
Cell lysis, 65
Cell-mediated immune response, 20, 23*f*
Cell-mediated immunity, 22*t*
Cell membrane, 13
Cellular anatomy and physiology, 9–14

  eukaryotes, 9, 13–14
  prokaryotes, 9, 11–12
Cellular function and structure, 15*t*
Cellulitis
  causative microbes and treatment for, 214*f*
  defined, 213
  diagnosis of, 214
  of leg, 214*f*
  treatment of, 214–215
Centers for Disease Control and Prevention, 67, 95, 96, 168, 194
  acute bronchitis guidelines of, 240
  in Atlanta, Georgia, 40*f*
  FluView, 38, 38*f*
  Get Smart campaign, 172
  on health care-associated infections, 39
  National Healthcare Safety Network and, 96
  standards precautions recommended by, 96, 121
  vaccine and immunization recommendations by, 170
Centers for Medicare and Medicaid Services, 96
Central catheters, 212
Centrosomes, function of, 15*t*
Cephalexin, 178*t*, 214*t*, 215
Cephalosporins, 176
  commonly used, 178*t*
  defined, 177
  generations of, 178
  inactivation of, 172
Cerebrospinal fluid, 16, 47, 203, 204
  cultures, 153
  defined, 151
Cervicitis, chlamydia and, 224
Chain of infection, 91, 112
  components of, and ways it can be broken, 95*f*
  defined, 94
Chickenpox, 64, 190
Chief complaint or concern, defined, 168
Childbed fever, 37
Chlamydia, 224
  gonorrhea coinfection with, 225
  tetracyclines and, 183
Chlamydophila, 183
Chlamydophila pneumoniae
  atypical pneumonia and, 242, 243
  community-acquired pneumonia and, 242
Chlorine, infection prevention/control and, 101
Chloroquine, 74
Chromatin, function of, 15*t*
Chromosomes, 10, 10*f*, 13
Chronic conditions, 168

Cilia, 11
Ciliate, 118*f*
Cipro, 181
Ciprofloxacin, 181, 204
  anthrax exposure treated with, 253
  kidney infections treated with, 227
  osteomyelitis treated with, 228
  plague treated with, 253
Circulatory response, immune system and, 17, 19
CJD. *See* Creutzfeldt-Jakob disease
Clarithromycin, 183, 243
Clean-catch midstream collection technique, 156*t*
Cleaning, 94, 96. *See also* Infection prevention and control
Clindamycin, 74, 175*t*, 186, 214*t*, 215, 216
  aspiration pneumonia treated with, 250, 251
  diverticulitis and, 219
  IV, *Pneumocystis jiroveci* pneumonia treated with, 251
  pharyngitis treated with, 236
Closed method, applying and removing sterile gloves with, 142, 146*f*–147*f*, 146*t*
Clostridium difficile, 129, 155, 186
Clostridium difficile colitis, 219–221
  defined, 220
  diagnosis of, 220
  medical history and, 219
  micrograph of bacterial cells, 220*f*
  recurrence of, 221
  treatment of, 220–221
Clostridium perfringens, necrotizing skin infections and, 216
CMS. *See* Centers for Medicare and Medicaid Services
CMV. *See* Cytomegalovirus
Coagulase-negative staphylococci, 118
Cocci, structure and morphology of, 44–45
Coccidioides antigen, positive skin test for, 84*f*
Coccidioidomycosis, 83
Coccidionides immitis, 83
Cold sores, 65, 190
Colon
  with diverticula in lining of, 218*t*
  healthy, endoscopic view of, 218*t*
Common cold, 65, 67, 190, 236
Common vehicle transmission, 26
Communicable diseases, controlling transmission of, 94
Community-acquired pneumonia, 185, 241–242

Comparative research, 36, 37
Compound microscope, 7*f*
Confocal laser microscope, 8*f*
Conjunctivitis (pink eye), 209, 209*f*
Contact precautions
  chart, 129*f*
  Clostridium difficile colitis and, 220
  defined, 122
  hand hygiene, 129
  for herpes zoster, 131
  personal protective equipment, 128–129
Contact transmission, 25
Contamination, defined, 95
Coronavirus, 236
  bronchitis and, 240
  pneumonia and, 246*t*
Corticosteroids, croup treated with, 238
Coryneform bacteria, 119
Cough
  acute bronchitis and, 239, 241
  etiquette and respiratory hygiene, 124
  suppressants, 240
Cowpox, 36
Coxsackie virus, 236
Crackles
  acute bronchitis and, 239
  pneumonia and, 241
Cradle cap, 83*t*
CRBSIs. *See* Catheter-related bloodstream infections
Creutzfeldt-Jakob disease, signs and symptoms of, 86–87
Crixivan, 195*t*, 226*t*
Croup
  defined, 237
  treatment of, 238
Cruise ship travel, infectious diarrhea and, 221, 222
Cryptococcus neoformans, 82
Cryptosporidiosis, infectious diarrhea and, 222*t*
CSF. *See* Cerebrospinal fluid
Cubicin, 185
Culture and sensitivity (C&S) test, 51
Culturing, 51–52
Cyclosporiasis, infectious diarrhea and, 222*t*
Cyst, of parasites, 73
Cystitis, treatment of, 227
CytoGam, 169*t*
Cytomegalovirus, 194, 236
Cytomegalovirus immune globulin, 169*t*
Cytoplasm, 13
Cytotoxic T-cell activation, against cancer cell, 21, 22*f*

D

Dapsone, 251
Daptomycin, 175*t*, 185, 212*t*, 213*t*
Debridement, of dead bone, 228
Decongestants, 235
Decontamination, defined, 96
Deer flies, as vectors of disease, 116*f*
Denatured, defined, 95
Dendritic cells, 21
Deoxyribonucleic acid. *See* DNA
Dependent variables, 38
Dermatophyte infections, common, 83*t*
Dermatophytes, 82
Descriptive research, defined, 35
Diagnosis, defined, 167
Diagnostic procedure, 167–168
Dialysis, 211
Diarrhea
  infectious, 221–222
  travelers', 222
Dicloxacillin, 177*t*, 215
Didanosine (ddl), 195*t*, 226*t*
Differential stains, 49
Diflucan, 196, 197*t*
Digestive system, protective barriers in, 18
Dimorphic, defined, 83
Diphtheria, 45
Direct contact
  defined, 115
  disease transmission and, 25
Direct fluorescent antibody (DFA) test, 225
Directly observed treatment, tuberculosis patients and, 253
Disease outbreaks, modeling, 38
Disease(s)
  bacillus-type, 45
  bacterial, 55–56
  defined, 167
  direct and indirect transmission of, 25–26
  prion-related, 86
  protozoans and, 74*t*
  signs and symptoms of, 167–168
  viruses and causes of, 65
Disinfection
  defined, 96
  of patient care rooms, 128
Disinfection of medical equipment and facilities, 98–104, 104*t*–105*t*
  boiling water and, 98, 99
  gas sterilization and, 98, 103
  heat and, 98–99
  pasteurization and, 98, 99
  radiation and, 98, 104
  steam and pressure and, 98, 99–100
  various liquids and compounds and, 98, 100–102

Disk diffusion (Bauer-Kirby test), 52, 53*f*
Diskhaler, 191
Disseminated herpes zoster, 131
Diverticulitis, 218–219
    defined, 218
    endoscope view of colon with
        diverticula, 218*t*
DNA, 11, 13, 52
DNA viruses, 65, 189
Doribax, 179
Doripenem, 179, 250
DOT. *See* Directly observed treatment
Doxycycline, 74, 183, 214*t*, 215
    chlamydia treated with, 224
    plague treated with, 253
    pneumonia treated with, 243
Dracunculiasis, 77*f*
Dracunculus medinensis, life cycle of, 77*f*
Drooling, epiglottitis and, 237
Droplet precautions, 122, 126, 126*f*, 131
Drug names, learning, 84
Dry heat
    for disinfecting and sterilizing, 98, 99
    effect, mode of action, and uses for, 104*t*
Dynapen, 177*t*
Dysphagia, epiglottitis and, 237
Dysphonia, epiglottitis and, 237
Dysuria, 227

E

Ears, tympanostomy tubes in, 207
Ebola hemorrhagic fever, 72
Ebola virus, 67
Echinocandins, 196
Echocardiogram, 211
Ectoparasites, 78
    defined, 78
    examples of, 79*f*
Efavirenz, 195*t*, 226*t*
Effusions, 207
EHF. *See* Ebola hemorrhagic fever
EIA. *See* Enzyme immunoassay
ELISA. *See* Enzyme-linked
        immunosorbent assay
Empiric therapy, 54
    for adult pneumonias, 243, 244*t*
Employers, Bloodborne Pathogen Standard
        and, 132–134
E-Mycin, 183
Encephalitis, 65
    defined, 204
    RNA viruses and, 189
    viral causes of, 204*t*
Endemic, defined, 168
Endocarditis
    defined, 210

microbial causes and treatment of, 212*t*
    petechiae on fingernail of patient
        with, 211*f*
    symptoms of, 210–211
    vegetative growth in, 211*f*
Endometritis, chlamydia and, 224
Endoplasmic reticulum, 14, 15*t*
Endotoxins, 24, 56
Endotracheal intubation, health
        care-associated pneumonia
        and, 248, 249
Endotracheal tube placement, above
        bifurcation of right and left
        lung, 246*f*
Engineering controls, Bloodborne
        Pathogen Standard and, 133
Entamoeba histolytica, 73, 73*f*, 74
    route of transmission, and disease
        condition related to, 74*t*, 117*t*
Enterobacter, acute cholecystitis and, 217
Enterobacteriaceae, tracheobronchitis
        and, 246
Enterococcus, acute cholecystitis and, 217
Enteroviruses, detecting, 157
Entry inhibitors, 71*t*
Enzyme immunoassay, 68, 69, 220
Enzyme-linked immunosorbent assay, 69
Eosinophils, 19
Epidemic, defined, 168
Epidemiology, defined, 168
Epiglottitis, defined and treatment for, 237
Epinephrine, nebulized, croup treated
        with, 238
Epivir, 195*t*, 226*t*
Epstein-Barr mononucleosis, DNA viruses
        and, 189
Epstein-Barr virus, 236
ER. *See* Endoplasmic reticulum
Eraxis, 196, 197*t*
Ergosterol, in fungi, 79, 195
Ertapenem, 179
    acute cholecystitis and, 217
    pneumonia treated with, 250
Erysipelas
    causative microbes and treatment
        for, 214*f*
    defined, 213
    treatment for children, 215
Erythromycin, 183, 215
    eye ointment, 210
    pneumonia treated with, 243
Escherichia coli (E. coli), 12*f*, 18, 45, 115
    acute cholecystitis and, 217
    diverticulitis and, 219
    effectiveness of germicides on, 102*f*
    gram negative, 50*f*
    infectious diarrhea and, 222*t*

parotitis and, 208
    urinary tract infections and, 227
Esophagitis, 82*t*
Ethambutol, 187–188, 253
Ethanol, defined, 100
Ethionamide, 187
Ethylene oxide
    effect, mode of action, and uses for, 105*t*
    in gas sterilization, cautionary note
        on, 103
Etiology, defined, 168
ETO. *See* Ethylene oxide
Etravirine, 195*t*
Eukaryotes, 8, 9, 13–14
Eukaryotic human cell, with organelles, 10*f*
Eustachian tube, otitis media and, 206
Exacerbation, defined, 168
Exotoxins, 24, 55–56
Experimental research, 38
Exposure control plan, Bloodborne
        Pathogen Standard and, 132
Extended-spectrum penicillins, 176, 177*t*
Eye infections, 209–210
    conjunctivitis, 209–210, 209*f*
    keratitis, 210
Eye protection
    Bloodborne Pathogen Standard and, 133
    defined, 123

F

Face masks, 123, 124*f*
Face shields, 123, 124*f*, 131
Famciclovir, 70, 190, 193*t*, 225
Famvir, 70, 190, 193*t*
Fatal familial insomnia, 86
FDA. *See* Food and Drug Administration
Fecal-oral route of transmission,
        Clostridium difficile colitis and, 220
Fever, inflammatory response and, 27
Fidaxomicin, 221
Fifth-generation cephalosporins, 178
First-generation cephalosporins, 178
First-generation protease inhibitors, 193
Flagella, 12, 43, 44*f*
Flagellate, 118*f*
Flagyl, 186
Flare up, 168
Fleas, 78, 79*f*, 116*f*
Flies, 118*f*
Flora
    on hands, types of, 118–119
    meaning of, 6
    resident, 118, 119, 152
    transient, 119, 148
Flu. *See* Influenza
Fluconazole, 83, 196, 197*t*, 213*t*
Flucytosine, 83

Flucytosine + liposomal amphotericin, 212t
Flukes, 118f
Flumadine, 70, 191, 193t
Fluoroquinolones, 175t, 180, 181
    oral, pneumonia treated with, 243–244
    osteomyelitis treated with, 228
Flu syndrome, 167
FluView (CDC), 38, 38f
Folate inhibitors, 184
Fomites
    defined, 114
    disease transmission and, 25
Food and Drug Administration, 55, 68
    Nonprescription Drugs Advisory
        Committee, 43
Food-borne illness, infectious diarrhea
    and, 221
Food safety, travel and, 223
Formaldehyde, effect, mode of action, and
    uses for, 105t
Fortaz, 178t
Fournier, Jean-Alfred, 215
Fournier's gangrene, 215
Fourth-generation cephalosporins, 178
Fungal diseases, types of, 196f
Fungal infections
    from annoying to life threatening, 194
    examples of, 81f
    identifying, 79–80
    impaired immune function and, 195
    opportunistic, 79
Fungal spores, 80
Fungi, 25, 39, 79, 195
    defined, 9t
    dimorphic, 83
    molds, 79, 84–85
    mushrooms, 79, 80f
    yeasts, 79, 81–83
Fungizone, 196, 197t
Fusion inhibitor, 71t, 194, 226

G

Gallbladder infections, 217
Gammagard, 169t
Gamma irradiation, sterilization with, 104
Gamma rays, effect, mode of action, and
    uses for, 105t
Garamycin, 181
GAS infection. See Group A β-hemolytic
    streptococcus infection
Gas sterilization, disinfecting and
    sterilizing with, 103
Gastrointestinal (GI) tract, parasites in, 74
Gatifloxacin, 181, 244
Genital herpes, 70, 190
Genital herpes virus ulcers, antiviral agents
    for, 225

Genitourinary tract, protective barriers in,
    18–19
Genitourinary tract infections, 223–226
Genotypes, hepatitis C and, 71
Gentamicin, 181
    aspiration pneumonia treated with, 251
    pneumonia treated with, 250
Genus, 43
Germicidal, defined, 96
Germicidal susceptibility, of various
    microorganisms, 97t
Germicides, effectiveness of, for various
    pathogens, 102f
Gerstmann-Straussler-Scheinker
    syndrome, 86
Giardia lamblia, 73, 74t
    route of transmission, and disease
        condition related to, 117t
    stool specimens evaluated for, 155
Gloves, 123, 124f, 128
    airborne precautions and, 131
    Bloodborne Pathogen Standard and, 133
    droplet precautions and, 131
    hand hygiene performed after removal
        of, 129
    nonsterile, 140, 141–142
    sterile, 140
Glutaraldehyde
    effect, mode of action, and uses for, 105t
    infection prevention and control
        and, 102
Glycocalyx, 43
Glycopeptides, 182
Gnosis, meaning of, 168
Goggles, 124f, 131
Golgi, Camillo, 14
Golgi apparatus (or Golgi bodies), 10f,
    14, 15t
Gonorrhea
    antimicrobial resistance and treatment
        of, 224, 225
    chlamydia coinfection with, 225
    defined, 224
    diagnosis of, 224–225
Gowns, 123, 124f, 129
    Bloodborne Pathogen Standard and, 133
    droplet precautions and, 131
Gram-negative bacillary pneumonia, in
    hospitalized patients, 248
Gram-negative bacilli, 119
Gram-negative infections, treating, 57
Gram-positive infections, treating, 57
Gram's iodine, 49
Gram stain, 49
Gram stain procedure, steps in, 49f
Gram stain reaction, of medically related
    bacteria, 55t

Grass mold, 80f
Group A β-hemolytic streptococci
    croup and, 237
    pharyngitis and, 236
Group A streptococcus
    necrotizing fasciitis and, 216
    necrotizing skin infections and, 216
Guinea worm disease, 77, 78f

H

Haemophilus influenzae
    bronchitis and, 240
    community-acquired pneumonia
        and, 242
    conjunctivitis and, 209
    otitis media and, 207
    sinusitis and, 235
Haemophilus influenzae type B, epiglottitis
    and, 237
Haemophilus influenzae type B (Hib)
    vaccine, 205, 237
HAIs. See Health care-associated infections
Hand hygiene/hand washing, 91, 94, 112,
    118–121, 147, 222
    Clostridium difficile colitis and, 220
    compliance issues with, 120
    contact precautions and, 128, 129
    defined, 118, 148
    description of, 39
    droplet precautions and, 126, 131
    gloving and, 141, 142
    history behind, 37
    proper technique for, 119–120f
    as standard precaution, 122–123
    for surgical asepsis, 148
Hantavirus, pneumonia and, 246t
HAP. See Hospital-acquired pneumonia
Hazards, labels and signs for, 134
HCAP. See Health care-associated
        pneumonia
HCV. See Hepatitis C virus
Head and neck, infectious diseases of,
        202–208
Health care-associated infections, 39, 40,
        95–96
    Clostridium difficile colitis, 219
    data on, 96
    hand hygiene and reduction in, 119
Health care-associated pneumonia, 185, 246
    antibiotics for, 249–250
    empiric antibiotic choices for, 244t
    morbidity and mortality attached to,
        246, 248
Heart, infections of, 210–212
Heat, disinfecting and sterilizing with, 98
Helicobacter pylori, 183, 186

Helminths, 72, 75–76, 75*t*, 118*f*
  examples of, 76*f*
  main groups of, 75, 75*t*
Helper T cells, 20
Hemodialysis, 211
HepaBam B, 169*t*
HEPA-filtered masks, 131, 131*f*
Hepatitis B immune globulin, 169*t*
Hepatitis B vaccinations, Bloodborne
      Pathogen Standard and, 133
Hepatitis B virus, 69
Hepatitis C virus, 67, 69, 71, 189*f*
  antivirals in treatment of, 192–193, 193*t*
Heredity, 13
Herpes infection, example of, 190*f*
Herpes simplex virus-1, 70
Herpes simplex virus(es), 67, 189*f*, 236
  antivirals in treatment of infections, 70,
      190, 193*t*
  defined and treatment for, 225
  DNA viruses and, 189
  encephalitis and, 204, 204*t*
Herpes simplex virus type 1, 190, 225
Herpes simplex virus type 2, 190, 225
Herpes zoster virus
  airborne and contact precautions for, 131
  chickenpox, shingles, and, 190
Hexachlorophene, 101, 102*f*
H5N1. *See* Avian influenza A (H5N1)
      strain
High-level disinfectants, 97
Histoplasma capsulatum, 83
Histoplasmosis, 83
HIV. *See* Human immunodeficiency
      virus (HIV)
HIV medications, classifying, 176
HIV vaccines, 71, 226
Hooke, Robert, 36
Hookworms, 75*t*, 76*f*
  route of transmission, and disease
      related to, 75*t*, 117*t*
  treatment for, 76
Hospital-acquired pneumonia, 248
  antibiotics for, 249–250
  pathogenesis of, 247*f*
Host, vectors and, 116
HPV. *See* Human papillomavirus
H7N9. *See* Avian influenza H7N9 virus
      strain
HSV. *See* Herpes simplex virus
HSV-1. *See* Herpes simplex virus type 1
HSV-2. *See* Herpes simplex virus type 2
Human immunodeficiency virus (HIV),
      67, 69, 70, 190, 226
  antiretrovirals in treatment of, 226, 226*t*
  antivirals in treatment of, 194
  RNA viruses and, 189

symptoms of, 226
treating, 176
tuberculosis and, 253
Human metapneumovirus, pneumonia
      and, 246*t*
Human papillomavirus, 65*f*
Humoral immune response, 20, 21, 22*t*, 23*f*
Hydration, sulfonamide antibiotics and, 185
Hydrogen peroxide, 102*f*
  effect, mode of action, and uses for, 105*t*
  infection prevention and control and, 102
Hypertet, 169*t*

I

Ibuprofen, otitis media and use of, 207
Imidazole, 82
Imipenem, 176, 213*t*
Imipenem-cilastatin, 179
Imipenem/cilastatin +vancomycin,
      necrotizing skin and soft tissue
      infections treated with, 216
Immune response
  integrated, 23*f*
  role of, 168–169
Immune system, 17–22
  circulatory and bloodstream response, 19
  innate and adaptive immune responses,
      20–22
  protective barriers and, 18–19
Immunity
  active, 66, 169
  artificial, 66
  artificial passive, 67
  defined, 168
  natural active, 66
  passive, 66, 169
Immunization(s), 66, 168–170
  defined, 66
  passive, agents for, 169*t*
Immunoglobulins, 22, 169, 169*t*
Imogam, 169*t*
Incineration, 99
Incivek, 193*t*
Incubation, 51, 51*f*
Incubator, 52
Independent variables, 38
Indinavir, 195*t*, 226*t*
Indirect contact
  defined, 115
  disease transmission and, 25
Infection prevention and control, 40,
      93–107. *See also* Hand hygiene/
      hand washing
  basic definitions for, 95–97
  Clostridium difficile colitis patients
      and, 220

cough etiquette and respiratory hygiene,
      124, 126–127
  defined, 94
  disinfect and sterilize methods, 98–104,
      104*t*–105*t*
  droplet precautions, 126*f*
  expanding outside of hospital, 94
  issues related to killing organisms, 98
  safe handling of potentially
      contaminated surfaces or
      equipment, 127–128
  safe injection practices, 127
  standard precautions, 121, 122–123, 125*f*
  transmission-based precautions, 121,
      128–131
Infections, 24–27
  bacterial, 56
  bone and joint, 228–229
  cardiovascular, 210–212
  defined, 24, 95
  direct and indirect disease transmission,
      25–26
  of eye, 209–210
  fever and inflammatory response, 27
  genitourinary tract, 223–226
  gram-positive and gram-negative, 57
  health care-associated, 39, 40, 95–96
  intra-abdominal, 216–222
  nosocomial, 40, 95, 96
  opportunistic, 40
  upper respiratory system, 235–238
  urinary tract, 227
Infectious diarrhea, 221–222
  defined, 221
  microorganisms as cause of, 222*t*
  risky foods and, 221*t*
Infectious diseases, of head and neck,
      202–208
  encephalitis, 204
  meningitis, 203–204
  otitis media, 205–208
  parotitis, 208
Infectious diseases, of lower respiratory
      system, 238–253
  acute bronchitis and bronchiolitis,
      239–241
  pneumonia, 241–251
  tuberculosis, 252–253
Infectious diseases, of skin and soft tissues,
      213–216
  cellulitis and erysipelas, 213–215
  necrotizing skin and soft tissue
      infections, 215–216
Infectious Diseases Society of America, 251
  CAP treatment guidelines, 242, 243
  cellulitis guidelines, 215
  empiric therapy guidelines, 250

Infectious mononucleosis, 65
Infectious proteins, 8
Infectious waste
  containers for, 141f
  defined, 140
  disposal of, 91, 140–141, 142t
  types of, 141t
Inflammation, defined, 95
Inflammatory response, 20, 27
Influenza A, 191
Influenza B, 191
Influenza C, 191
Influenza vaccine, 170, 189
Influenza virus, 65, 67, 190, 236
  antivirals used in treatment of, 69,
    190–192, 193t
  bronchitis and, 240
  detecting, 157
  droplet precautions and, 131
  pneumonia and, 246t
  reporting on and tracking, 38, 38f
  RNA viruses and, 189
  spikes on type of, 189f
  treatment of, 191
  types of, 191
Inhaled drug hazards, 191
Injections
  safe practices for, 127
  swabbing before, 101f
Innate immune response, 20
Inoculum, 26
Institutional Review Board, 36
Integrase inhibitors, 71t
Integrase strand transfer inhibitor, 194, 226
Intelence, 195t
Interleukins, 20
Intermediate-level disinfectants, 96
Intra-abdominal infections
  acute cholecystitis, 217
  appendicitis, 216–217
  Clostridium difficile colitis, 219–221
  diverticulitis, 218–219
  infectious diarrhea, 221–222
Intubation, health care-associated bacterial
    pneumonia and, 247, 248, 249
Invanz, 179
IRB. *See* Institutional Review Board
Isolation procedures, 94
Isoniazid, 187, 252, 253
Isopropyl, defined, 100
Itraconazole, 83

J

Jenner, Edward, 36, 37
Jock itch, 80, 83t, 195
Joint infections. *See* Bone and joint infections

K

Kaposi sarcoma, 194
Keflex, 178t
Keratinase, 82
Keratitis, defined and treatment of, 210
Ketek, 183
Ketoconazole, 82, 197t
Kidney infections, treatment of, 227
Killer T lymphocytes, 23f
Kingdoms, 8
Klebsiella, acute cholecystitis and, 217
Klebsiella pneumoniae
  parotitis and, 208
  urinary tract infections and, 227
Koch, Robert, 36
Kuru, 86

L

Lamivudine, 195t, 226t
Lancets, safe disposal of, 127
Larvae, of parasites, 73
Larynx, 235
Latency, 67, 190
Leeuwenhoek, Antonie van, 32, 35
Legionella pneumophila, 242, 243
Legionella spp., 183, 242
Legionnaires' disease, airborne
    transmission of, 26
Leprosy, 49
Levaquin, 181
Levofloxacin, 181
  cystitis treated with, 227
  kidney infections treated with, 227
  osteomyelitis treated with, 228
  pneumonia treated with, 244, 250
Linezolid, 175t, 184, 185, 214t, 215, 250
Liposomal amphotericin B, 197t
Lister, Joseph, 37
Listeria, 56
Loracarbef, 176
Louse (lice), as vectors of disease, 116f
Lower respiratory system, primary
    function of, 235, 238–239.
    See also Infectious diseases,
    of lower respiratory system
Low-level disinfectants, 96
Lyme disease, 46, 183
Lymphedema, cellulitis and, 214
Lysosomes, 14, 15t, 19
Lysozyme, 18

M

Macrolides, 175t, 182–183
  pneumonia treated with, 243
  resistance to, 172

Macrophages, 19, 21
Malaria, 26, 73
  diagnosis and treatment of, 74
  mosquitoes and transmission of, 78, 116
Malarial parasite, in red blood cell, 75f
Mallon, Mary ("Typhoid Mary"), 113
Mantoux tuberculin skin test, 252, 252f
Masks, 124f
  Bloodborne Pathogen Standard and, 133
  HEPA-filtered, 131, 131f
Mastoiditis, untreated pharyngitis and, 236
Maxipime, 178t
MBC. *See* Minimum bacterial concentration
Measles vaccine, 66, 189
Mebendazole, 76
Mechanical vector, 26
Mechanical ventilation, health care-
    associated bacterial pneumonia
    and, 247, 248, 249
Medical asepsis, defined, 147
Medical hand hygiene, surgical hand
    hygiene *versus*, 148t
Medical microbiology
  defined, 39
  evolution of, 38
Medical training records, Bloodborne
    Pathogen Standard and, 134
Medical Waste Tracking Act, 141
Medicare, 96
Mefloquine, 74
Mefoxin, 178t
Memory cells, 21
Memory T lymphocytes, 23f
Meningitis, 82, 203–204
  community-acquired, common causes
    of, 203t
  defined, 203
  hospital care-associated, common causes
    of, 204t
  treatment of, 204
  viral causes of, 204t
Meropenem, 176, 179, 208
  kidney infections treated with, 227
  pneumonia treated with, 250
Merrem, 179
MERS. *See* Middle East Respiratory
    Syndrome
Methicillin-resistant *Staphylococcus
    aureus*, 171
  cellulitis and, 215
  cutaneous abscess of knee caused
    by, 182f
  epiglottitis and, 237
  pneumonia therapy and, 249, 250
  quinupristin-dalfopristin in treatment
    of, 185
  scanning electron micrograph of, 182f

treatment of, 178, 208
vancomycin for, 182
Metronidazole, 74, 175*t*, 186
   Clostridium difficile colitis and, 220, 221
   diverticulitis and, 219
MIC. *See* Minimal inhibitory concentration
Micafungin, 196, 197*t*
Miconazole, 196, 197*t*
Microbes, infections and, 24, 25
Microbial resistance mechanisms, 171–172
Microbiology
   defined, 6, 32
   evolution of "science" of, 35–38
   history of, 32–33, 33*t*–35*t*
   other fields and applications of,
      40–41, 41*t*
Microorganisms
   classification of, 8, 9*t*
   germicidal susceptibility of, 97*t*
   killing, issues related to, 98
   portals of entry and, 114*t*
Microscope(s)
   invention of, 32–33
   types of, 7*f*
Middle East Respiratory Syndrome, 72, 246*t*
Minimal inhibitory concentration, 53,
      54, 54*f*
Minimum bacterial concentration, 53, 54*f*
Minocin, 183
Minocycline, 183
Mites, 118*f*
Mitochondria, 10*f*, 13, 15*t*
Mitosis, 13
Mixed culture, 51
Moist heat, effect, mode of action, and
      uses for, 104*t*
Mold(s), 64, 79, 84–85
   on bread, 80*f*
   defined, 84
   disease-producing, examples of, 85*f*
Mold therapy, 35
Monistat, 196, 197*t*
Monobactams, 176, 179
Monocytes, 19
Mononuclear phagocyte system, 19
Moraxella catarrhalis, 183
   bronchitis and, 240
   conjunctivitis and, 209
   otitis media and, 207
   sinusitis and, 235
Morbidity, defined, 168
Morphology, 32
Mortality, defined, 168
Mosquitoes, 78, 79*f*, 116, 116*f*, 118*f*
Mouth, 235
Moxifloxacin, 181, 244
MPS. *See* Mononuclear phagocyte system

MRSA. *See* Methycillin-resistant
      Staphylococcus aureus
Mucology, defined, 79
Mucor, 85
Mucor fungus, 85*f*
Mucormycosis, 85, 85*f*
Mucous membranes, 17
Mucus, mucous *versus,* 18
Multidrug-resistant (MDR) bacteria, 121
Multidrug-resistant (MDR) TB, 186, 187
Multipathogen viral detection systems,
      68–69, 69*t*
Mumps vaccine, 189
Mushrooms, 79, 80*f*
Mycamine, 196, 197*t*
Mycobacterium tuberculosis, 252
   x-ray of tuberculosis of lungs caused
      by, 187*f*
Mycology, 39, 79–85
Mycoplasma, 183, 237
Mycoplasma pneumoniae
   atypical pneumonia and, 242, 243
   community-acquired pneumonia
      and, 242
Mycostatin, 195, 197*t*
Myringotomy, 207

N

NAATs. *See* Nucleic acid amplification
      tests
Nafcillin, 177*t*, 212*t*, 213*t*
   osteomyelitis treated with, 228
   spectrum of activity for, 175*t*
Nail infections
   dermatophytes and, 83*t*
   fungal, 81*f*, 82
Naproxen, 207
Narrow-spectrum antibiotics, 175, 175*t*
Narrow-spectrum drugs, 57, 172
Nasal specimens, 157
   defined, 157
   obtaining and processing, 157
Nasal steroids, 235
National Healthcare Safety Network, 96
National Immunization Program, 170
National Nosocomial Infection
      Surveillance System, 96
Natural active immunity, 66
Natural penicillins, 176, 177*t*
Nebcin, 181
Nebulizer equipment, bronchiolitis
      treatment and, 240–241
Necrotizing fasciitis, defined, 216
Necrotizing skin and soft tissue infections,
      214, 215–216, 216*f*
Needleless intravenous systems, 133

Needles
   multidraw, with rubber sheath, 133
   safe disposal of, 127
   self-sheathing, 133
Negative pressure rooms, airborne
      precautions and, 131
Neisseria gonorrhoeae, conjunctivitis
      and, 209
Neisseria meningitidis
   droplet precautions and, 131
   meningitis and, 203–204
Neuraminidase inhibitors, 191
Neutrophils, 19
Nevirapine, 195*t*, 226*t*
Niclosamide, 76
Nizoral, 197*t*
N-95 filtered masks, 131, 131*f*
NNISS. *See* National Nosocomial
      Infection Surveillance System
NNRTIs. *See* Non-nucleoside reverse
      transcriptase inhibitors
Noninfectious waste, 141
Non-nucleoside reverse transcriptase
      inhibitors, 71*t*, 194, 195*t*, 226, 226*t*
Nonsharp infectious waste, 140, 141*t*
Nonsterile gloves, 140
   applying and removing, 141–142,
      143, 143*f*
Nonsteroidal anti-inflammatory agents,
      otitis media and, 207
Normal flora, 6, 24, 32
   intestinal, 18
   pathogens *versus,* 15–16
   representative, body sites and, 16*t*
Norovirus, 129, 222*t*
Norvir, 195*t*, 226*t*
Nose, 235
Nosocomial infections, 40, 95, 96
NRTIs. *See* Nucleoside reverse
      transcriptase inhibitors
Nucleic acid amplification tests, 224
Nucleolus, 13, 15*t*
Nucleoside polymerase inhibitors, 193
Nucleoside reverse transcriptase inhibitors,
      71*t*, 194, 195*t*, 226, 226*t*
Nucleus, 10, 10*f*
   in eukaryotic cells, 13
   function of, 15*t*
Nystatin, 195, 197*t*

O

Occupational Safety and Health
      Administration
   Bloodborne Pathogen Standard, 132–134
   defined, 112
   regulations, 132–134

Olysio, 193*t*
Omnicef, 208
Omnipen, 177*t*
Open method, for applying and removing
    sterile gloves, 142, 144*t*, 145*f*
Opportunistic infections, 40
Oral candidiasis, 195
Oral thrush, 81, 82*t*, 196*f*
Organelles, 10, 10*f*
Oseltamivir, 70, 191, 193*t*, 255
OSHA. *See* Occupational Safety and
    Health Administration
Osteomyelitis, defined and treatment
    for, 228
Otitis media, 205–208, 240
    antibiotics and management of, 207
    in children, factors increasing risk of, 206*t*
    common bacterial pathogens in, 207–208
    defined, 205
    microbial causes of, 206*t*
    schematic drawing of, 205*f*
    untreated pharyngitis and, 236
Ova, of parasites, 73
Oxazolidinones, 184–185

P

Pandemic, defined, 168
Papillomavirus, 189*f*
Papilloma warts, DNA viruses and, 189
Parainfluenza virus, 236
    detecting, 157
    pneumonia and, 246*t*
Parainfluenza virus types 1 and 2, croup
    and, 237
Parasites, 25, 39, 64
    common, route of transmission, and
        disease condition, 117*t*
    ectoparasites, 78
    helminths, 72, 75–76, 75*t*
    major groups of, 118*f*
    protozoa, 72, 73–75
Parasitology, 39, 72–78
Parotid glands, 208
Parotitis, defined and treatment for, 208
Passive immunity, 66, 169
Passive immunization, agents for, 169*t*
Pasteur, Louis, 36
Pasteurization
    disinfecting and sterilizing with, 99
    effect, mode of action, and uses for, 104*t*
Pathogenic, 6, 32
Pathogenic flora, body sites and, 16*t*
Pathogenic organisms, 39
Pathogens
    defenses against, 17–18
    identifying, 52

normal flora *versus,* 15–16
    virulence of, 24
Pathological waste, 141*t*
Patient care items, infectious waste and, 141*t*
Patient care rooms, safe handling of,
    127–128
PBPs. *See* Penicillin-binding proteins
Pegasys, 193*t*
Peginterferon, 71, 193
Peginterferon alfa-1a, 193*t*
Pelvic inflammatory disease, 224
Penicillinase-resistant semisynthetic
    penicillins, 176, 177*t*
Penicillin-binding proteins, 176
Penicillin G, 175*t*, 177*t*, 212*t*
Penicillin-resistant *pneumococcus,*
    epiglottitis and, 237
Penicillin-resistant pneumonia strains, 243
Penicillin(s), 80*f,* 216
    aspiration pneumonia treated with,
        250, 251
    commonly used, 177*t*
    discovery of, 56
    inactivation of, 172
    pharyngitis treated with, 236
    prophylaxis and, 177
    side effects of, 176
    subdivisions of, 176
Penicillin V, 177*t*
Pentamidine, IV, *Pneumocystis jiroveci*
    pneumonia treated with, 251
Peptic ulcer disease, 183, 186
Peripheral intravenous catheters, 212
Peritonitis, appendicitis and, 216
Personal protective equipment, 91
    airborne precautions and, 131, 131*f*
    Bloodborne Pathogen Standard and, 133
    contact precautions and, 128–129
    droplet precautions and, 131
    examples of, 124*f*
    standard precautions and, 122, 123
Petechiae, endocarditis and, 211, 211*f*
Petri dish, 51
    with sheep's blood agar culture
        inoculated with *Yersinia pestis*
        bacteria, 46*f*
Phagocytes, 19, 23*f*
Phagocytosis, 19, 20*f*
Pharyngitis (sore throat), 157, 235–236, 236*f*
    defined, 235
    diagnosis of, 236
    untreated, complications of, 236
Phenolics, effect, mode of action, and uses
    for, 105*t*
Phenols
    effect, mode of action, and uses for, 105*t*
    infection prevention and, 101

Phenylphenol, 101, 102*f*
Phisohex, 101
Phlebotomy, safe injection practices
    and, 127
PID. *See* Pelvic inflammatory disease
Pink eye. *See* Conjunctivitis (pink eye)
Pinocytic vesicles, 14
Pinworms, 76*f*
    root of transmission, testing, and disease
        related to, 75*t*, 117*t*
    treatment of, 76
Piperacillin, 177*t*
Piperacillin-tazobactam, 177*t*, 208,
    213*t*, 214*t*
    acute cholecystitis and, 217
    appendicitis and, 217
    diverticulitis and, 219
    kidney infections treated with, 227
    necrotizing skin and soft tissue
        infections and, 216
    pneumonia treated with, 250
Piperacillin-tazobactam + penicillin,
    aspiration pneumonia treated
    with, 251
Pipracil, 177*t*
PIs. *See* Protease inhibitors
Pityrosporum, 119
PJP. *See Pneumocystis jiroveci* pneumonia
Plague, as bioweapon, 253
Plasma cells, 23*f*
Plasma or cell membrane, function of, 15*t*
Plasmodium falciparum, 74
Plasmodium spp., 74, 74*t*, 75*f*, 117*t*
Plasmodium vivax, 74
Pleural effusions, pneumonia and, 241
Pneumococci, croup and, 237
Pneumocystis carinii, 251
Pneumocystis jiroveci pneumonia, 194
    in AIDS patients, 184
    clindamycin in treatment of, 186
    HIV infection and, 251
Pneumonia, 241–251
    adult, empiric antibiotic choices for, 244*t*
    antibiotic therapy for health care-
        associated pneumonia, 249–250
    aspiration, 250–251
    atypical, 242–244
    chest x-ray of, 241*f*
    community-acquired, 241–242
    defined, 241
    health care-associated, 246, 248
    hospital-acquired, 248
    normal chest x-ray and x-ray
        showing, 171*f*
    Pneumocystis jiroveci, 184, 186, 194, 251
    preventing, precautions for, 247*f*
    signs and symptoms of, 170

therapy guidelines for, keeping up to date with, 251
ventilator-associated, 248
viral, 245, 246*t*
Polio, 65
morbidity rate for, 168
RNA viruses and, 189
Polio vaccine, 189
Polymerase chain reaction, 68, 204, 220, 225, 245
Polymerase inhibitors, 71
Polymyxin/trimethoprim eyedrops, 210
Polyvinyl chloride, 104
Portals of entry, 112–114
defined, 94, 112
with examples of related microorganisms and diseases, 114*t*
major types of, in body, 113*f*
respiratory tract as, 116
Postexposure evaluation, Bloodborne Pathogen Standard and, 134
Potassium hydroxide, 82
PPE. *See* Personal protective equipment
Praziquantel, 76
Prednisone, 251
Pressure, altitude and, 99
Primaquine, 251
Primary culture, 51
Primaxin, 179
Prions, 8, 64, 86
Probiotics, 17
Prognosis, defined, 168
Prokaryotes, 8, 9, 11–12
Prokaryotic bacterial cell, 11*f*
Prophylaxis, penicillins and, 177
Protease inhibitors, 71, 71*t*, 194, 195*t*, 226, 226*t*
first-generation, 193
second-generation, 193
Proteins, infectious, 8
Proteus mirabilis, urinary tract infections and, 227
Protista kingdom, 8
Protists, 8
Protozoa, 9*t*, 72, 73–75, 118*f*
Pseudomembranes, *Clostridium difficile* colitis and, 220
Pseudomonas aeruginosa, 178, 250
germicides and, 102*f*
tracheobronchitis and, 246
Public health data, communicating, 38
Puerperal (childbed) fever, 37
Pure culture, 51
Purified protein derivative (PPD) test, 252
PVC. *See* Polyvinyl chloride
Pyelonephritis, 227
Pyrantel pamoate, 76

Pyrazinamide, tuberculosis treatment and, 253
Pyridoxine (vitamin B$_6$), 187
Pyuria, 227

Q

Quaternary ammonium compounds
effectiveness of, on various pathogens, 102*f*
infection prevention and control and, 102
Quaternary ammonium salts, effect, mode of action, and uses for, 105*t*
"Quick strep test," 236
Quinine, 74
Quinolones, 180–181
Quinupristin-dalfopristin, 185

R

Rabies, 65, 189
Rabies immune globulin (human), 169*t*
Radiation
disinfecting and sterilizing with, 104
effect, mode of action, and uses for, 105*t*
Rapid antigen detection test, 236
Rebetol, 193*t*
Red blood cells
with plasmodium parasite, 75*f*
scanning electron microscope image of, 7*f*
Red man syndrome, 171, 182
Reduviid bugs, as vectors of disease, 116*f*
Relapse, defined, 168
Relenza, 70, 191, 193*t*, 255
Remission, defined, 168
RES. *See* Reticuloendothelial system
Reservoirs of infection
defined, 113
types of, 114
Resident flora, 118, 119, 152
Resistance. *See also* Antibiotic resistance
to antimicrobials, mechanisms of, 172
defined, 57
Resistant pneumococcus, 243
Respiratory hygiene, cough etiquette and, 124
Respiratory illnesses, prescreening patients for, 127
Respiratory syncytial virus, 70
antivirals in treatment of, 191–192, 193*t*
bronchiolitis and, 240
bronchitis and, 240
croup and, 237
detecting, 157
pneumonia and, 246*t*

Respiratory system
lower, infectious diseases of, 238–253
upper, infections of, 235–238
Respiratory tract
as main portal of entry, 116
protective barriers in, 18
Reticuloendothelial system, 19
Retropharyngeal abscess, 236
Retrovir, 195*t*, 226*t*
Reyataz, 195*t*, 226*t*
Reye syndrome, 207
Rheumatic fever, acute, untreated pharyngitis and, 236
Rhinovirus, 236
Rhinoviruses
bronchitis and, 240
detecting, 157
Rhizomucor, 85
Rhizopus, 85
Rhonchi
acute bronchitis and, 239
pneumonia and, 241
Ribavirin, 71, 192, 193, 193*t*, 240, 241
Rickettsiae, defined, 9*t*
Rifampin, 187, 204, 253
Rifaximin, 221
Rimantadine, 70, 191, 193*t*
Ringworm (tinea corporis), 83*t*, 195, 196*f*
Ritonavir, 195*t*, 226*t*
RNA viruses, 65, 189
Rocephin, 178*t*
Rocky Mountain spotted fever, 78, 183
Rotavirus, infectious diarrhea and, 222*t*
Roundworms, 118*f*
Routes of transmission, 115–118
airborne route of, 116
common vehicle route of, 115
contact routes of, 115
vector route of, 116–117
RSV. *See* Respiratory syncytial virus
Rubella, 189

S

Saliva, 18
Salmonella
infectious diarrhea and, 222*t*
stool specimens evaluated for, 155
Salpingitis, chlamydia and, 224
Sanitization, 94, 96
San Joaquin Valley fever, 83
Saprophytic molds, 85
SARS. *See* Severe acute respiratory syndrome
Scanning electron microscope, 7*f*
Science, defined, 35
Scientific hypotheses, 37

Scientific inquiry, 36
Scientific theories, 37
Second-generation cephalosporins, 178
Second-generation protease inhibitors, 193
Self-sheathing needles, 133
Semmelweiss, Ignaz, 37
Septic arthritis
    defined, 228
    diagnosis and treatment of, 229
    of finger, 229f
Septra, 184
Serodiagnosis, 69
Serology, 41
Severe acute respiratory syndrome,
    71–72, 246t
Sexually transmitted diseases, 223–226
    chlamydia, 224
    defined, 223
    gonorrhea, 224–225
    herpes simplex virus, 225
    human immunodeficiency virus, 226
Sharps
    containers for, 127, 127f, 133, 141f
    as infectious waste, 140, 141t
Shigella
    infectious diarrhea and, 222t
    stool specimens evaluated for, 155
Shingles, 64, 190
Side effects
    antimicrobial therapy, 170
    carbapenems, 179
    daptomycin, 185
    erythromycin, 183
    folate inhibitors, 184
    glycopeptides, 182
    influenza agents, 191
    metronidazole, 186
    peginterferon and ribavirin, 193
    penicillins, 176
    quinolones, 180
    quinupristin-dalfopristin, 185
Signs, defined, 167
Simeprevir, 193, 193t
Simple stains, 47
Sinusitis, untreated pharyngitis and, 236
Skin
    fungal infections of, 82
    infectious diseases of, 213–216
    as protective barrier, 18
Smallpox, 36
Sneezes, aerosol produced by, 26f, 116f
Soap detergent, effect, mode of action, and
    uses for, 105t
Social ethics, 36
Sofosbuvir, 71, 193, 193t
Soft tissues, infectious diseases of, 213–216
Sore throat (pharyngitis), 157, 235–236

Sovaldi, 193t
Species, 43
Specimen collection, 46–55, 150–158
    bacterial staining, 47, 49
    blood cultures, 152–153
    cerebrospinal fluid (CSF) cultures, 153
    clinical application, 47
    culturing, 51–52
    general principles of, 151
    growing and testing bacteria, 50–55
    guidelines for, 46–47
    identification, 52
    information for, 151t
    nasal specimens, 157
    safety in handling specimens, 47
    sites of specimen samples and potential
        pathogens, 48t
    sputum cultures, 153, 154t
    stool specimens, 155–157, 157t
    susceptibility testing, 52–55
    throat cultures, 157, 158f, 158t
    wound cultures, 154, 155t, 155f
Specimen containers, labeled examples
    of, 152f
Spiders, 118f
Spirilla, structure and morphology
    of, 44, 46
Spirochetes, 46, 183
Spontaneous generation theory, 36
Spores, 12, 12f, 44, 44f, 80, 95
Sporozoan, 118f
Sputum cultures
    defined, 153
    obtaining, 153
Sputum specimen collection, 154t
Standard precautions
    Bloodborne Pathogen Standard and, 133
    chart, 125f
    defined, 96, 121
    hand hygiene, 122–123
    personal protective equipment, 122, 123
Staphylococcus aureus, 43, 45, 119
    binary fission of, 42f
    bronchitis and, 240
    conjunctivitis and, 209
    croup and, 237
    germicides and, 102f
    osteomyelitis and, 228
    parotitis and, 208
    septic arthritis and, 229
    tracheobronchitis and, 246
Staphylococcus bacteria, gram positive, 50f
Staphylococcus epidermidis, 43, 45, 119, 182
Staphylococcus hominis, 119
STDs. *See* Sexually transmitted diseases
Steam and pressure, disinfecting and
    sterilizing with, 99–100

Steam heat, 98
Sterile field
    defined, 149
    establishing and maintaining, 148
    guidelines for, 149t
Sterile gloves, 140
    applying and removing, 142, 144
    applying and removing with closed
        method, 146f–147f, 146t
    applying and removing with open
        method, 144t, 145f
Sterile principles, defined, 149
Sterilization, defined, 97
Sterilization and disinfection of medical
    equipment and facilities, 98–104,
    104t–105t
    boiling water and, 98, 99
    gas sterilization and, 98, 103
    heat and, 98–99
    pasteurization and, 98, 99
    radiation and, 98, 104
    steam and pressure and, 98, 99–100
    surgical instruments and, 148
    various liquids and compounds for, 98,
        100–102
Steroids
    fungal infections and, 79
    nasal, 235
    Pneumocystis jiroveci pneumonia and, 251
    topical, otitis media and, 207
Stethoscopes, safe handling of, 127
Stool specimens, 155–157, 157t
Streptococci, 44
Streptococcus pneumoniae, 183
    bronchitis and, 240
    community-acquired pneumonia
        and, 242
    conjunctivitis and, 209
    otitis media and, 207
    sinusitis and, 235
Streptococcus pyogenes, 157, 236
Streptogramins, 185
Streptomycin, 253
Sulfacetamide eyedrops, 210
Sulfonamide antibiotics, hydration
    and, 185
Sulfonamides, 184
Sunusitis, defined and treatment for, 235
Super bacteria, 57, 171
Superinfections, 180, 181
Superpathogens, 172
Suprax, 178t
Surfactants, effect, mode of action, and
    uses for, 105t
Surgical asepsis, 147
    defined and goal of, 148
    hand hygiene for, 148

Surgical attire, 148
Surgical hand hygiene, medical hand hygiene *versus,* 148*t*
Surgical hand scrub, 148
Surgical masks, droplet precautions and, 131
Susceptibility testing, 52–55
Sustiva, 195*t,* 226*t*
Swab cultures, 151
Symmetrel, 70, 191, 193*t*
Symptoms, defined, 167
Syndrome, defined, 167
Synercid, 185
Syphilis, 46, 225
Syringes, safe disposal of, 127

T

Tamiflu, 70, 191, 193*t,* 255
Tapeworms, 76*f,* 118*f*
   beef or pork, 75, 75*t*
   segmented portion of, 73*f*
TB. *See* Tuberculosis
T cells, 21, 22, 22*t*
Teflaro, 178*t*
Telaprevir, 71, 192, 193, 193*t*
Telavancin, 182
Telithromycin, 183
Tendon injury, quinolones and, 181
Tenofovir, 195*t*
Tequin, 181
Tetanus, 45
Tetanus immune globulin, 169*t*
Tetracyclines, 175*t,* 183, 243
Theophylline, quinolones and, 180
Third-generation cephalosporins, 178
3TC, 195*t,* 226*t*
Throat culture, 157, 158
   defined, 157
   obtaining, 158*f*
   procedure for, 158*t*
Thrush, 81, 82*t,* 195, 196*f*
Ticks, 78, 79*f,* 116*f,* 118*f*
Tigecycline, 183
Tinea capitis, 83*t*
Tinea corporis, 83*t*
Tinea cruris, 83*t*
Tinea imbricata (Tokelau), 81*f*
Tinea pedis, 83*t*
Tinea ungulum, 83*t*
Tinidazole, 74
T lymphocytes, 23*f*
TMP-SMX. *See* Trimethoprim-sulfamethoxazole
Toadstools, 80*f*
Tobramycin, 181, 250, 251
Toenail fungus, 81*f*
Tonsil infections, 236

Toxins, 24, 55–56
Tracheobronchitis
   defined, 245
   treatment for, 246
Training for workers, Bloodborne Pathogen Standard and, 134
Transient flora, defined, 148
Transmission-based precautions, 128–131
   airborne precautions, 130–131, 130*f*
   contact precautions, 128–129, 129*f*
   defined, 121
   droplet precautions, 131
   types of, 122
Travelers' diarrhea, 222
Trimethoprim-sulfamethoxazole, 175*t,* 184, 214*t,* 215
   cystitis treated with, 227
   diverticulitis and, 219
   Pneumocystis jiroveci pneumonia treated with, 251
   sinusitis treated with, 235
Trophozites, 73
True allergies, adverse reactions *versus,* 188
Truvada, 195*t*
Tuberculosis, 45, 49, 186, 187*f,* 252–253
   airborne transmission of, 26
   defined, 252
   multidrug-resistant, 186, 187, 253
   preventive therapy for, 252–253
   risk factors for, 253
   skin test for, 252*f*
   treatment of, 187–188, 253
Tubes in the ears, 207
Tumor necrosis factor, 20
Tygacil, 183
Tympanostomy tubes, in ears, 207
Typhoid fever, 45

U

Ultraviolet light, effect, mode of action, and uses for, 105*t*
Ultraviolet rays, disinfection with, 104
Unasyn, 177*t*
Unipen, 177*t*
Upper airway, diseases related to, 234*f*
Upper respiratory airway infections, 235–238
   croup, 237–238
   epiglottitis, 237
   pharyngitis, 235–236
   sinusitis, 235
Urinalysis, 227
Urinary tract infections, 45, 227
Urine cultures, 227
Urine sample, in biohazard bag, 155*f*
Urine specimens, 155

clean-catch midstream collection technique, 156*t*
containers for, 46*f*
Urethritis, chlamydia and, 224
UTIs. *See* Urinary tract infections

V

Vaccination(s)
   active immunity and, 169
   prevention of viral infections by, 189
   research, 36–37
   for young child, 170*f*
Vaccines, 66
   defined, 66
   HIV, 71, 226
   influenza, 170
   keeping up-to-date on, 170
Vaginal yeast infections, 196
Valacyclovir, 190, 193*t,* 225
Valacyclovir (Valtrex), 70
Valtrex, 190, 193*t*
Vancocin, 182
Vancomycin, 171, 175*t,* 182, 208, 212*t,* 213*t,* 214*t,* 215
   Clostridium difficile colitis and, 220–221
   osteomyelitis treated with, 228
   pneumonia treated with, 250
   septic arthritis treated with, 229
Vancomycin-resistant *Enterococcus faecium* infections, 185
Vantin, 208
VAP. *See* Ventilator-associated pneumonia
Variant Creutzfeldt-Jakob disease, 86
Varicella-zoster immune globulin, 169*t*
Varicella zoster virus, pneumonia and, 246*t*
Variconazole, 197*t*
vCJD. *See* Variant Creutzfeldt-Jakob disease
Vector route of transmission
   biological form of, 116
   mechanical form of, 116–117
Vectors, 25
   arthropod, 116, 116*f*
   biological, 25–26
   defined, 116
   mechanical, 26
Veetids, 177*t*
Vegetative growth, endocarditis and, 211*f*
Vegetative organisms, defined, 95
Venous insufficiency, cellulitis and, 214
Ventilator-associated pneumonia
   antibiotics for, 249–250
   defined, 248
   empiric antibiotic choices for, 244*t*
Ventilators, tracheobronchitis and, 245
Ventriculostomy, 203

VFEND, 196, 197*t*
Vibativ, 182
Vibramycin, 183
Victrelis, 193*t*
Videx, 195*t*, 226*t*
Vinegar, 100, 101, 101*f*
Viral identification, 67–69
    cell culture, 67
    direct detection, 68
    multipathogen detection systems, 68–69
    serodiagnosis, 69
Viral infections
    classification of, 67, 189
    signs and symptoms of, 65–66
Viral load, 69
Viral pneumonias, 245, 246*t*
Viramune, 195*t*, 226*t*
Virazole, 192, 193*t*
Virology, 39, 64–72
Virulence, 6, 24, 32
Viruses, 8, 39, 188–189
    as causes of meningitis or encephalitis, 204, 204*t*
    defined, 9*t*, 64–65
    hidden, 67
    latency and, 67, 190

pharyngitis and, 235–236
resulting disease, artificial immunization status, and, 66*t*
schematic representation of, 65*f*
various types of, 189*f*
Vital signs, defined, 167
Vopegus, 193*t*
Voriconazole, 85, 196
Vulvovaginitis, 82*t*

W

Warning labels, Bloodborne Pathogen Standard and, 134
Warts, 65
Wart virus, 189*f*
WBCs. *See* White blood cells
West Nile virus, mosquitoes as vectors for, 116
White blood cells, 19, 27
White distilled vinegar, 101, 101*f*
Whooping cough, droplet precautions and, 131
Work practice controls, Bloodborne Pathogen Standard and, 133
World Health Organization, on SARS outbreak, 71

Wound cultures
    common techniques with, 154
    defined, 154
    obtaining specimens of, 155*t*, 155*f*

X

X-rays, effect, mode of action, and uses for, 105*t*

Y

Yeast infection, in armpit, 81*f*
Yeasts, 64, 79, 81–83, 119

Z

Zanamivir, 70, 191, 193*t*, 255
Ziagen, 195*t*, 226*t*
Zidovudine, 195*t*, 226*t*
Zinacef, 178*t*
Zithromax, 183
Zone of inhibition, 53
Zosyn, 177*t*
Zovirax, 70, 190, 193*t*
Zyvox, 184